TRAUMATIC BRAIN INJURY

Volume I
Pathophysiology
and Neuropsychological
Evaluation

TRAUMATIC BRAIN INJURY

Volume I
Pathophysiology and Neuropsychological Evaluation

RALPH M. REITAN

Neuropsychology Laboratory
Tucson, Arizona

Professor of Psychology
University of Arizona
Tucson, Arizona

DEBORAH WOLFSON

Neuropsychology Laboratory
Tucson, Arizona

Anthony M. Pazos

Medical Illustrator

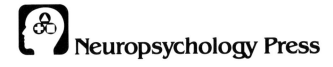Neuropsychology Press

Neuropsychology Press
1338 East Edison Street
Tucson, Arizona 85719

Made in the United States of America.

ISBN 0-934515-06-9
Library of Congress Card Number: 86-60951
Great care has been taken to maintain the accuracy of the information contained in the volume. However, Neuropsychology Press cannot be held responsible for errors or for any consequences arising from the use of the information contained herein.

PREFACE

Head injury affects a tremendous number of people and produces difficult and complex medical, psychological and social problems for its victims. The diverse and complicated nature of the condition has required the efforts of many specialists, ranging from neurosurgeons to experts in rehabilitation. The problems facing the head-injured person change as time progresses after the injury. In many cases, the effects of head injury evolve into residual long-term or permanent deficits, and the neuropsychologist is asked to evaluate the patient and develop a cognitive rehabilitational program.

The two volumes of this book are principally concerned with these long-term problems and are based on the conviction that the specialists who deal with the problems facing the head-injured person must be informed about the full range of conditions that may accompany a head injury. Volume I of *Traumatic Brain Injury* reviews the epidimiology of head injury and addresses the immediate biological and pathophysiological consequences (primary and secondary damage to the brain). The next section of the book is concerned with the neurological methods of evaluation of the primary and secondary effects of head injury. A review of diagnostic procedures (such as computed tomography and cerebral angiography) provides important information for the specialist who will be concerned with long-term effects, particularly

post-traumatic epilepsy and neuropsychological deficits.

The principal purpose of this book is to communicate information, training, and the development of skill in neuropsychological assessment using the Halstead-Reitan Neuropsychological Test Battery. Volume I features a detailed presentation of a neuropsychological model of brain-behavior relationships and considers the ways in which various neuropsychological tests relate to this model as either general or specific indicators of brain dysfunction.

Next, the neuropsychological literature is reviewed (to the extent possible) within the general framework of this neuropsychological model. We then present a series of test results and interpretations for 31 head-injured persons. We disagree with the contention of some writers that the only way to develop skills in neuropsychological interpretation is through personal clinical contact with the patient and that one cannot develop proficiency in interpretation by studying case material. We believe that case studies can provide invaluable information for both the novice as well as the experienced practitioner and should be utilized to increase one's knowledge of the range of diverse effects that head injury can have on cognitive functions.

Careful attention was given to the selection of the 31 head-injured case examples so that they would represent the wide range of primary and secondary lesions resulting from head injury. From our total of 639 subjects who had received a complete Halstead-Reitan Battery (as well as a neurological examination documenting their medical condition) we were able to select cases illustrating a diverse range of conditions. For example, we have included young as well as older adults, persons representing a range of intelligence levels, and subjects who have conditions (such as alcoholism, drug abuse, cerebral vascular disesase and peripheral nerve damage) complicating their head injury.

The reader will notice that we have not reported individual Glasgow Coma Scale scores or estimated the durations of post-traumatic amnesia; we believe that while these measures may be useful guides in some specific instances, they are distinctly limited in their informational base compared with a comprehensive neuropsychological evaluation and provide minimal information about the way in which a head injury has affected an individual's brain-behavior relationships.

The neuropsychological evaluation of individual cases may be viewed as a series of single-case experiments rather than the usual case-history presentations. The cases can provide meaningful information because we have developed a framework that eliminates the permissiveness usually found in evaluation of individual subjects. The interpretations presented here are based on generalizations developed from earlier scientific studies which have been used to structure a framework for individual clinical evaluation. The case interpretations may be used to test the applicability of the scientific generalizations to the individual subject. In this sense, clinical evaluation of individual subjects, as validated against independent criterion information, represents a critical level of scientific validation.

Great interest exists in the biological mechanisms of recovery from head injury, clinical studies of outcome and recovery, development of accurate prognostic indicators, spontaneous recovery, facilitated recovery or methods of brain re-training, and rehabilitation. These are important issues that deserve extensive consideration and are addressed in Volume II of this book.

The reader may also be interested in related publications that complement and augment some of the features of this book. *Aphasia and Sensory-perceptual Deficits in Adults* (Reitan, 1984) provides a review of the area of aphasia and research results based on the Reitan-Indiana Aphasia Screening Test as well as instruction in interpretation of the results obtained on examination of individual subjects. *The Halstead-Reitan Neuropsychological Test Battery: Theory and Clinical Interpretation* (Reitan & Wolfson, 1985a) provides detailed instruction in interpretation of the entire Halstead-Reitan Battery across a broad range of neurological conditions. Clinicians who wish to develop expertise of this type in the area of head injury must necessarily acquire knowledge of other conditions of brain disease and damage for comparative purposes. In addition, this volume presents a description of the various tests used in the Halstead-Reitan Battery and the manual for administration and scoring. Finally, *Neuroanatomy and Neuropathology: A Clinical Guide for Neuropsychologists* (Reitan & Wolfson, 1985b) was written to provide basic information of human neuroanatomy, neurology and neuropathology, and provide an introductory review of neuropsychological correlates of a wide range of neurological and other conditions (e.g., aging) that may compromise brain functioning.

Several persons have made invaluable contributions to the production of this book. Jacquelyn Tarpy endured many long days and nights of organizing and editing, and offered many helpful comments and suggestions. Kathleen Whitwer typed the entire manuscript, often under the pressure of a deadline. We are pleased to include the original medical illustrations drawn by Anthony M. Pazos. We are grateful to Frank Wallis and Sharon

Flesher for sharing their technical expertise with us.

We also wish to acknowledge the continued support of Steve Mackie, James LeRoy, Kerry Wilcoxon, and Michele Redmond of the Neuropsychology Laboratory in Tucson.

Ralph M. Reitan
Deborah Wolfson

CONTENTS

Head injuries of long duration

Examples of spontaneous recovery

Head injuries in persons with prior conditions of alcoholism, drug abuse, hypertension, stroke, peripheral nerve injury and suspected conversion hysteria

INDEX OF PLATES

I

EPIDEMIOLOGY OF
HEAD INJURY

Head injury is a major public health problem, both in terms of mortality and morbidity. Many severely head-injured patients die before reaching the hospital. Survivors often have serious long-term after-effects (including post-traumatic epilepsy and neuropsychological deficits).

Trauma is the leading cause of death in youth and early middle age and is the third most common cause of death in the United States; it is exceeded only by vascular disease and cancer (U.S. Department of Health Education & Welfare, 1974). When death is caused by trauma, head injury is a significant contributing factor in more than half of the cases. In patients who have multiple injuries, the head is the part of the body most commonly injured and in fatal accidents injury to the brain occurs in nearly 75% of the cases (Gissaine, 1963). Although the incidence of head injury is highest among persons aged 15 to 25 years, it still exceeds stroke as a cause of death in males aged 45 to 64 years. Obviously, many of the victims of head injury would have had many years of life remaining; instead their lives were cut short or they live with significant neurological and neuropsychological deficits.

Epidemiological data and the characteristics of head-injured persons have been reviewed recently by Jennett and Teasdale (1981) and Levin, Benton, and Grossman (1982). The reader should be aware that epidemiological data must be evaluated carefully because of the many problems in the initial recording of information. In the individual case, information is usually incomplete and limited in detail. Part of the problem is the lack of uniform terminology for describing head injury. The number of deaths due to head injury is difficult to determine because many patients die at the scene of the accident and there is no hospital record. There is a tremendous degree of variability regarding severity of cerebral damage; many patients who have mild injuries are not admitted to the hospital or are discharged within a relatively short period of time. All of these factors lead to unreliable statistical data regarding incidence and prevalence of head injury and undoubtedly contribute to variability among individual studies.

The incidence of head injuries has had variable estimates. Some investigators reported about 200 persons with head injury per 100,000 population (Kalsbeek, McLaurin, Harris, & Miller, 1980) and others have estimated as many as 600 head-injured persons per 100,000 population (Caveness, 1977).

These differences are probably due to the researcher's definition of "head injury"; using a criterion such as "a head blow that leads to restricted activity for at least one day" will naturally produce higher figures than a criterion such as "loss of consciousness or presence of post-traumatic amnesia." When the injury is sufficiently severe to require hospitalization, estimates have been in the vicinity of 300–350 cases of head injury per 100,000 members of the population, although approximately half of these patients were discharged within 24 hours of admission (Hawthorne, 1978). The National Head and Spinal Cord Injury Survey of head injuries in the United States in 1974 estimated about 404 head injuries per 100,000 members of the population, with a distribution of 272 males and 132 females (Anderson, Kalsbeek & Hartwell, 1980).

Similar figures were reported by other investigators (Annegers, Grabow, Kurland & Laws, 1980), who estimated 274 cases per 100,000 among males and 116 cases per 100,000 among females. Caveness (1976) estimated that in 1974 approximately 8.1 million Americans had head injuries and of this number about 1.9 million persons had injuries sufficiently severe to suggest the possibility of brain damage. Although these figures vary rather widely, it is apparent that injury to the head constitutes a major public health problem.

There have been some studies of the conditions under which head injuries occur, although there are also difficulties in obtaining accurate data in this area. Road and traffic accidents almost certainly represent the major cause of head injuries in the civilian population and probably account for nearly 50%. Among persons injured in traffic accidents, approximately 70% have been estimated to have sustained a head injury. Domestic accidents or falls account for about 20%; about 10%

result from industrial injuries; 10% represent cases of assault; and sport injuries represent approximately 5% of the cases. The remaining 5%–10% are caused by other factors.

In terms of the age distribution, head injuries are known to occur more frequently among younger persons, particularly males. In the 15 to 25 year age range there appears to be a peak incidence among males that far exceeds the female distribution (Annegers, Grabow, Kurland & Laws, 1980). Caveness (1976) found that head injury was the leading cause of death in males under the age of 35 and the leading cause of death among females under the age of 25. Kraus (1980) reported that hospital admissions for head injury were about four times as frequent among males as females.

Additional reports have indicated that head injuries are more common among persons in lower socioeconomic levels (Klonoff, 1971) and alcohol abuse has been noted as an especially significant factor. Levin, Benton, and Grossman (1982) report that about 20% of their head injury hospital admissions have significant problems with alcohol or drug abuse, psychiatric disorders, or intellectual retardation. While these figures suggest that victims of head injury have many pre-existing problems and do not appear to represent a cross-section of the population, a large number of otherwise healthy persons, particularly in the younger parts of the age distribution, suffer significant and permanent cognitive losses due to head trauma. When the number of years of potentially productive living are considered, head injury takes a very high toll. While various estimates have been made regarding the economic costs of head injuries (in terms of days lost from work, hospitalization expenses, etc.), the principal loss to society is probably represented by the long-term neuropsychological deficits among survivors.

II

MECHANISMS AND TYPES
OF HEAD INJURY

Reitan and Wolfson (1985b) have reviewed the principles, mechanisms and pathophysiology of head injury, including compression, penetration, tension, and shearing of tissues; acceleration and deceleration injuries; focal and diffuse tissue damage (including cerebral atrophy, damage to blood vessels and contre-coup effects); cerebral concussion; evaluation of coma; clinical manifestations; neurological diagnostic procedures; and post-traumatic epilepsy, electrical injuries, birth injuries, and whiplash injuries. The present review will also focus on these issues in greater detail and emphasize the information pertinent to the needs of neuropsychologists.

There is a close association between the various types of head injuries and the mechanisms that caused them; therefore, we will consider these variables conjointly. Closed head injuries and penetrating wounds (as well as focal and diffuse damage) have a number of common mechanisms. We shall identify some of the mechanisms responsible for brain damage in instances of head injury and the various kinds of brain injury that occur.

Head injuries may be classified in a number of ways. It is common to refer to acceleration injuries and deceleration injuries. *Acceleration injuries* occur when the head is relatively motionless and is struck by a more rapidly moving object. *Deceleration injuries* occur when the head itself is moving rapidly and strikes a fixed or solid object. In either case there may be linear or rotational gradients of force that cause damage to the brain and, in each case, movement of the brain within the skull may result in sudden contact with bony prominences (ridges) or the edges of dural membranes.

Much of the early work that led to a realization of the type and location of damage to the brain sustained by movement within the skull was done by an English physicist, Holbourne (1943; 1945). Holbourne, using gelatin models of the brain encased in a skull, delivered blows of measured intensity to various points of the skull. He reported that the irregular internal contour, ridges, and dural partitions of the skull play a role in determining the distribution of forces on the brain resulting from blows to the head.

Shear strain also occurs in addition to compression injuries and damage to the brain tissue as it moves over the irregular surfaces of the internal table of the skull. As noted by Jennett and Teasdale (1981), Holbourne drew attention to this tearing effect on brain tissue and likened it to the way a pack of cards might differentially distribute themselves in response to a swinging force. This shearing effect, represented by sliding of brain tissue over bone and other structures, is responsible for much of the diffuse damage that occurs with both closed and open head injuries. If the blow causes a pressure gradient in a straight line, relatively little shearing effect is to be expected. However, when the external force causes rotational movement of the brain, wide-spread damage may result (depending to a considerable extent upon the overall force of the blow).

Therefore, in addition to acceleration and deceleration injuries, head blows which cause rotation and shearing can be considered another classification, even though these latter effects may occur in either acceleration or deceleration injuries. Rotation and shearing effects may cause not only widespread damage to the cerebral cortex and to axons in the white matter but may also injure the diencephalon and mesencephalon. Damage to blood vessels may occur in any of these areas.

To summarize, the major forces by which head trauma causes brain injury include: (1) direct compression of brain tissue, in which the tissues are penetrated by a propelled object or pushed together in some other manner; (2) tension or tearing tissues apart; and (3) shearing or sliding of tissues over other tissues either as a result of differential pressure gradients (acting on tissues of approximately the same density) or movement of brain tissues across tissues of greater density (such as bony ridges).

In acceleration injuries the force of the moving object against the relatively stationary skull induces a pressure wave that spreads through the brain from the point of impact. The highest pressure occurs at the point of impact on the skull and the lowest pressure (which may be negative) is directly opposite the point of impact. In fact, cavitation may occur opposite the point of impact and result in tearing of tissues and contrecoup injuries.

As noted above, movement of the brain within the skull may cause bruising or contusion at any point, including areas of the brain stem. The superior surface of the cerebellum may be damaged as it moves against the edge of the tentorium. The upper surface of the corpus callosum is sometimes damaged as it makes contact with the edge of the falx. The inferior surface of the occipital lobes may be damaged by direct contact with underlying bony ridges. The tips of the frontal and temporal lobes and the orbital surface of the frontal lobes are particularly vulnerable; when they move in either an anterior-posterior or superior-inferior direction they strike various bony ridges on the interior surfaces of the skull.

Widespread damage to brain tissue may also occur with deceleration injuries of the head. When the moving head strikes a fixed object (as in a fall), generally the result is differential areas of damage, depending upon whether the back or front of the head is struck. When a person falls on the back of his head contusions frequently occur in the frontal and temporal lobes, due to inertia of the cranial contents. This consequence also reflects negative pressure in the area of the injury and rotational effects may result in shearing of frontal and temporal lobe brain tissue against bony ridges. A fall impacting on the frontal region of the skull usually does not cause damage in the occipital areas, probably because of the relatively smooth contour of the interior surface of the skull (Ommaya, Grubb, & Naumann, 1970). It is not uncommon to find contusions in the opposite temporal lobe when the lateral aspect of the head strikes a fixed object. Damage to the midbrain and brain stem may also occur when softer tissues collide with more dense tissues.

As commonly found in the pursuit of scientific knowledge, a great deal of experimental research has been done to elucidate relationships between variables. Many factors are significant in determining the nature of the brain injury, including brain bulk, compartmentalization and density of cerebral tissue, the anatomy of the internal surface of the skull, the force of the blow, the transmission of forces, and the acuteness of the striking object.

Investigators have attempted to produce experimental injuries under variable conditions, particularly manipulating the force of blow, the acuteness of the object which strikes the head, and the point of impact. Of course, when injuries of this kind are experimentally induced, the subject is an animal rather than a human and the variables which relate to anatomy (shape of the head, thickness of the skull, characteristics of brain structure) are different. The rhesus monkey, which has been used extensively for this type of experiment, has a rather thin skull which damages easily. The chimpanzee, which has been used less frequently because of the expenses involved, has a thick skull that is more similar to man's.

Both acceleration injuries (in which the relatively immobile head is struck by an object) and deceleration injuries (in which the head is propelled into a fixed object) have been investigated. Although large sums of money have been spent injuring animals in order to simulate "real life" head injuries in human beings, Jennett and Teasdale (1981) indicate that it has been very difficult to produce pathological lesions in animals that closely resemble the lesions that occur in man. They also point out that producing prolonged unconsciousness in animals has "largely defeated all attempts at solution." Finally, the neuropsychological consequences of traumatic brain damage in primates — especially in terms of higher-level cognitive functions and their potential for recovery — are of almost no relevance to man because of the tremendous gap that exists between the higher-level brain functions of primates and human beings.

There may be some value in learning about relationships between independent and dependent variables (conditions of damage and the actual damage sustained by the brain); however, when a monkey is strapped into fixed position and hurled at a pre-determined speed into a specifically designed, immovable object in order to strike a preselected part of its head, a question must be raised regarding the value of this information in relation to the price that is paid to achieve it.

Statistics have documented the fact that there is no shortage of human beings who have damaged their brains by striking their heads against a fixed object. Neurosurgeons who specialize in the evaluation and treatment of craniocerebral trauma have gained extensive information about the types of damage and clinical consequences of brain trauma from the thousands of patients who survive such injuries as well as from the thousands of victims in whom autopsies are performed. There is therefore no lack of human material from whom the biological consequences, pathological changes, or clinical manifestations of head injuries can be learned.

Admittedly, in instances of human head injury, it is often difficult to learn the exact point of impact, the velocity of impact, and other factors that may be of significance. However, it is valid to ask whether specific knowledge concerning these independent variables and their effects upon production of the lesion are, in fact, significant questions compared to the need for more information regarding the end result of the damage in human beings and the repair, remediation, and rehabilitation of injured brains. These comments in no way reduce the importance of preventive measures that may limit the likelihood of head injury, minimize the injuries that are sustained when impact occurs, and reduce secondary damage that may be sustained after the injury.

Head injuries may also be classified as closed or open. In *closed head injuries* the blow to the head has not caused a direct pathway from the outside through the soft tissue to the brain. Linear skull fractures may or may not be present in a closed head injury. In an *open* or *penetrating brain wound* an external object penetrates through the scalp and skull directly into the brain.

Intermediate injuries also occur, particularly in the case of depressed skull fractures. In such instances there may actually be a direct route through soft tissue into the brain substance, although in some cases the skull is so minimally deformed that surgical elevation is unnecessary. Closed head injuries may be of the acceleration or deceleration type, frequently involve rotational forces, and may result in extensive diffuse damage or focal lesions. The injury may be so minor that no brain damage is sustained or so severe that the result is irreversible brain damage with gross clinical consequences.

Damage resulting from closed head injuries may have variable but extensive effects, including primary brain stem damage; diffuse damage throughout the cerebral cortex, white matter, and lower structures; injuries to blood vessels of the brain; secondary adverse effects on brain stem function; damage to cranial nerves; and injuries which result in leakage of cerebrospinal fluid.

Gilroy and Myer (1979) point out that the brain is able to tolerate deceleration forces only to a limited extent and for a limited time period. When deceleration stresses go beyond this limit, the pressure wave passes to the level of the brain stem and toward the spinal canal. The foramen magnum requires that the pressure wave be dissipated in the spinal canal and the result is a sudden downward movement of the brain stem through the foramen magnum. These factors may result in very serious damage to the brain stem and long-term coma.

Closed head injuries may cause diffuse brain damage, resulting from injury and severance of axons (caused by shearing forces resulting from the impact to the head). As discussed in more detail below, neuropathological studies have indicated the presence of diffuse lesions throughout the brain in *every* instance of significant brain stem damage.

Damage to blood vessels is not uncommon in instances of closed head injury. In fact, the development of traumatic aneurysms involving all of the major intracranial arteries and their branches have been reported, and such lesions increase the risk of subarachnoid hemorrhage in the post-traumatic period (Cockrill, Jiminez, & Gorse, 1977).

Following a closed head blow the most common form of injury to an intracranial artery is damage to the internal carotid artery as it enters the base of the skull. Such injuries may result in a traumatic aneurysm with eventual rupture into the cavernous sinus. The basilar artery may also be injured in a similar manner, or a thrombus may occur with infarction of the pons. Subarachnoid hemorrhages or intracerebral hematomas may occur at any site in the brain as a result of tearing of intracerebral arteries or veins. The cortical veins have relatively little capacity for movement at the point of entry into a venous sinus and bleeding from torn veins may produce a subdural hematoma.

As explained below, damage to capillaries is extremely common in closed head injuries. The orbital surfaces of the frontal lobes and the anterior temporal lobes may be bruised and torn as they move across bony prominences and result in capillary rupture. Injury to blood vessels may represent a significant source of brain damage and dysfunction in both closed and open head injuries.

Secondary damage to the brain is common in instances of closed head injury and include consequences such as intracranial bleeding, brain swelling, subarachnoid hemorrhage, hydrocephalus, and cerebral ischemia. These pathological changes will be considered below.

Secondary brain stem damage may also occur as a result of increased intracranial pressure and intracranial hemorrhage. When the intracranial pressure is sufficiently increased and results in increased volume in only one cerebral hemisphere, herniation of the cingulate gyrus beneath the falx cerebri may occur. When the supratentorial contents of the brain expand, there may be transtentorial herniation with displacement of the diencephalon and upper midbrain through the tentorial notch. In turn, this displacement of the brain stem may stretch the penetrating arteries that arise from the basilar artery and the circle of Willis. In this manner, cerebral edema may have a secondary adverse effect on brain stem arteries and cause ischemia, arterial necrosis, and brain stem hemorrhage.

Increased pressure above the tentorium may also cause the midline structures to move away from the site of the lesion and place the uncus of the temporal lobe over the free edge of the cerebellar tentorium. This may cause herniation of the uncus, displacement of the midbrain, and compression of the third nerve and posterior cerebral artery on the side of the herniation. In fact, any of the cranial nerves are susceptible to injury by shearing forces resulting from injury to the head.

Cerebrospinal fluid rhinorrhea may also accompany closed head injury, even without skull fracture. This complication is often due to the combination of a sudden increase of intracranial pressure and shearing forces.

Relatively focal lesions may involve the tissue underlying or close to the point of impact (coup lesions) or on the opposite side of the brain (contrecoup lesions). Gurdjian (1975) has discussed the mechanics of these types of lesions, noting that coup contusions are caused by inbending of bone as a direct result of impact and damage to underlying brain tissue.

Contrecoup contusions are usually the result of movement of brain tissue against irregular and rough bony surfaces. In acceleration injuries, when the head is in a relatively fixed position, a blunt impact causes a coup lesion and there is no contrecoup damage. However, when the head is free to move, a blunt impact may cause a contrecoup lesion with little or no coup effect (Gurdjian, 1975).

Lindgren (1966) has studied the relative frequency of coup and contrecoup lesions in relation to injury sustained at various sites of the head. When the blow is delivered to the occipital region, coup lesions are rare and the resulting damage is almost always contrecoup. Both coup and contrecoup lesions are relatively frequent when the blow is delivered to the frontal area. Contrecoup lesions occur more frequently than coup lesions with blows to the side of the head, particularly when they involve the temporal areas. With blows to the vertex, contrecoup lesions are often located in the orbital region. Injury to the corpus callosum may also occur in such instances.

Ommaya, Grubb, and Naumann (1970) produced experimental head injuries in monkeys, delivering the blows to various points of the head. Their results indicated that contusions were most common in the frontal-temporal areas regardless of whether the skull was struck from the front or behind. Many investigators (Bakay & Glasauer, 1980) have noted that contusions were more common on the side of the skull fracture, particularly if the fracture was depressed.

The skull has some degree of elasticity and may be flattened or indented when struck with a blunt object; however, if the blow is sufficiently severe, the skull may be fractured, depressed, or penetrated. A factor even more important than the force of impact (velocity) is the size and surface of the object striking the skull. If a pointed object of high density is delivered with high velocity, it may perforate the skull and penetrate the brain; a large, blunt object striking the head with the same velocity may cause a depressed fracture of the skull.

In some instances there may be depressed fractures or even penetration of the skull and dura without significant damage to the underlying cerebral cortex. Frequently, though, there is focal tissue destruction and secondary consequences at the point of penetration. For example, penetration of the brain by metallic pieces and bone fragments is often followed by a rapid rise in intracranial pressure. The pressure wave set up by the force of impact may cause impairment of brain stem functions (in accordance with the mechanisms described above) and a fall in systemic blood pressure. These factors (including intracranial pressure and reduced systemic blood pressure) result in a marked reduction of cerebral perfusion pressure.

There may also be a loss of autoregulation of blood flow with a reduction in cerebrovascular resistance. This combination of factors may increase cerebral blood volume, which adds to and sustains the increased intracranial pressure. This results in cerebral edema and, in severe injuries, death may result from the continued increases in intracranial pressure. In less severe injuries the brain stem begins to function again, systemic blood pressure rises, autoregulation is restored, and the patient gradually improves, even though cerebral edema continues to be present and intracranial pressure is increased.

It should be clear from the above comments that head injuries may cause focal cerebral damage, diffuse damage, or both focal and diffuse damage, depending upon the nature and characteristics of the injury. In terms of neuropsychological findings it is important to recognize that diffuse tissue damage is usually present when there is a head injury, even with focal lesions (coup or contrecoup).

In the earlier neuropsychological studies of penetrating head injuries it was presumed that the limits of the lesion were restricted to the area of tissue damage observed at surgery. It is now known that small diffuse lesions, quite characteristic in their appearance, can be identified by the neuropathologist and occur throughout the white matter. Jennett and Teasdale (1981) have described the pathological features of these lesions in some detail. The brain may look almost normal to the naked eye when there is this type of damage, but

these authors indicate that on coronal slicing there is always a small lesion observable in the corpus callosum and another in or adjacent to the superior cerebellar peduncle, with about half the patients having the latter lesion bilaterally. In some instances patients have been described as having primary brain stem injury, particularly on the basis of cranial nerve dysfunction that was apparent on clinical examination. Adams and his co-workers (1977) have studied the brains of such patients at autopsy and did not find a single patient in whom lesions were confined to the brain stem.

It is clear from these results that diffuse axonal injury occurs in most (if not all) cases of significant head injury and appears to be due to a shearing mechanism produced by differential movement of various components of the brain. This type of movement would be caused particularly by rotational acceleration injuries. In addition, certain investigators (Ommaya & Gennareli, 1974; Greenberg, Becker, Miller, & Mayer, 1977; Adams, Graham, Murray, & Scott, 1982) suggest that such damage is more severe in the cerebrum than in the brain stem.

Considering the fact that higher-level neuropsychological deficits are most pronounced with lesions of the cerebral cortex, secondarily impaired with lesions of the white matter, generally less severely impaired with anterior brain stem lesions, and probably not significantly impaired at all with lesions below the central aqueduct, it is apparent that the mechanics of craniocerebral trauma emphasize the importance and significance of neuropsychological evaluation.

Differences in Type of Head Injury Depending Upon Type of Accident

Neurosurgeons have observed that the type of head injury that occurs is related to the circumstances that produce it. Most civilian head injuries are associated with moving vehicle accidents, either to vehicle drivers or passengers or pedestrians.

When a pedestrian is involved in an accident involving a moving vehicle, the victim is usually struck below the level of the head and toward the center of his/her gravity. The force from the moving vehicle frequently causes the victim's head to move toward the vehicle and strike the hood, windshield, or side of the car. The pedestrian's body is often propelled against the vehicle, causing a combination of both deceleration and acceleration injury to the brain, usually with a substantial degree of rotation. Pedestrian injuries frequently involve widespread brain damage and may result in both diffuse and focal lesions. The victim may suffer further deceleration damage upon hitting the pavement or other surface.

Motorcycle and bicycle accidents usually cause deceleration injuries and often involve rotational factors. In these cases the point of impact may be of definite significance, depending upon whether the front or back of the head strikes an immobile object or surface. In any case, there are likely to be injuries to the anterior frontal, orbital frontal, and anterior temporal areas. Frontal injuries may result in less contusion of cerebral tissues than posterior injuries.

The most common type of head injury in moving vehicle accidents occurs to car occupants. Injury to the head occurs in 70% of persons who sustain injuries; an estimated 26% of those who sustain a head injury have at least moderately severe damage (Ryan, 1967). If a person who is not wearing a seat belt is involved in a head-on collision, he/she usually strikes the instrument panel of the vehicle with his/her knees. This forces the body upward and causes the head to strike the upper part of the windshield. If the impact is delivered to the side of the vehicle, the victim's head may strike the inside of the door.

Head injuries caused by moving vehicle accidents are usually due to impact of the moving head against the interior of the car frame or windows (including the rear-view mirror). These injuries are principally of an acceleration type. When injuries of this type are fatal there is frequently damage to both the head and neck at the level of the craniocervical junction or the upper two cervical vertebrae.

Head injuries also occur in contact sports and range from relatively mild damage to severe concussion or contusion. Injuries are not uncommon in boxing and appear to have a cumulative effect (Corsellis, Burton, & Freeman-Browne, 1973).

Football has a preponderance of head injuries; however, severe brain injuries are relatively uncommon and occur most frequently in high school players and relatively inexperienced college athletes rather than among more experienced or professional players.

The incidence of serious head injuries in football have been surveyed and the most common injuries are extradural and subdural hematomas, cortical contusions, and intracerebral clots (Schneider, Reifel, Crisler, & Oosterbaan, 1961). As with other head injuries, cerebral ischemia may result from direct trauma to blood vessels (including the major arteries and venous tributaries). It should also be noted that severe injury to the brain can be caused by violent motion of the neck, even if no direct blow to the head has occurred (Ryan, 1967).

III

PRIMARY STRUCTURAL DAMAGE

Scalp and Skull Damage

Because injuries to the scalp constitute a potential route for intracranial infection and meningitis, they must be carefully evaluated by medical personnel. Because the scalp is so highly vascularized, injury to the scalp can lead to extensive blood loss.

As neuropsychologists, our principal concern is with brain-behavior relationships, and scalp injuries are obviously not directly involved in this consideration. Nevertheless, observation of the effects of superficial involvement may be significant in discerning the associated damage to the skull or brain. For example, bruising around the eyes (raccoon eyes) or behind the ears (Battle's sign) is an indication of basilar skull fracture in the anterior fossa (suborbital bruising), or in the middle fossa (postauricular bruising).

Scalp wounds should be evaluated carefully in the initial medical examination because even a small scalp wound may provide a clue to penetration of the brain, a fractured skull, or torn dura, any of which could lead to meningitis or brain abscess.

Although the skull is principally composed of dense bone and is remarkably strong, it may fracture or break when an object strikes it with sufficient velocity. It should be noted, however, that in most cases the presence of a skull fracture *per se* probably does not have great significance concerning underlying damage of the brain. In other words, significant brain damage may occur even if the skull has not been fractured and there is frequently no evidence of a skull fracture in cases of severe diffuse damage (Adams, Mitchell, Graham, et al., 1977).

Although skull fractures may be associated with other lesions, some investigators have concluded that the presence of a skull fracture, without evidence of other neurological abnormalities, is of limited clinical significance (Harwood-Nash, Hendrick, & Hudson, 1971). However, Miller and Becker (1982) emphasized that the neurosurgeon should be careful not to underestimate the importance of skull fractures, because they may give some indication of the site and type of impact and, more importantly, may reveal information about the underlying brain injury and possible complications, such as hemorrhage and infection.

There are three broad categories of skull fracture: linear, depressed, and penetrating or perforating. About 20%–25% of all skull fractures are of the linear type. These fractures result from an inbending of the skull at the site of impact and an outbending of the bone around the point of impact. Stresses on bone tissue initiate linear fractures in the outbending area and the fracture extends toward the point of impact and in the opposite direction toward the base of the skull.

The deformation of the skull caused by a linear fracture may also cause remote effects. For example, a blow to the occipital or temporal bone may produce a fracture in the anterior cranial fossa, usually involving the orbital roof (Hirsch & Kaufman, 1975). Deformation of the skull caused by linear fractures may result in tearing of the dura and laceration of the scalp, either of which can lead to serious infection. In many cases epidural hematomas are also associated with linear fractures.

Linear fractures of the cranial vault may extend to the basal area of the skull and result in complications, particularly if the dura mater is torn. Complications include meningitis or cerebrospinal fluid rhinorrhea. Depending upon the location of the injury, cerebrospinal fluid may drain through the nose (rhinorrhea) or the ear (otorrhea).

Depressed or comminuted fractures constitute about 25%–30% of all skull fractures. Depressed fractures are usually the result of impact to a relatively small area of the skull. In these cases the force breaks the skull bone and drives a part of the bone below the level of the remaining skull. As would be expected, depressed skull fractures are quite variable and may range from only a small indentation to instances of bone fragments driven into the brain tissue. Obviously, the effects range from minimal damage to focal injury with dural tearing and, in some instances, widespread brain damage. Miller and Jennett (1968) reviewed 400 civilian cases of depressed skull fracture and found that 25% of the victims had never been unconscious, even though the dura had been penetrated in 60%.

Factors that may lead to complications and require surgical intervention in cases of depressed skull fracture include scalp laceration, penetration of the dura, in-driven bone fragments or other potentially contaminating material, hemorrhage and contusion in the damaged area underlying the fracture, and possible involvement of major dural venous sinuses. About 9%–10% of patients with depressed skull fractures have complications that involve infections, 7% have intracranial hematomas, and 11%–12% have complications involving the venous sinuses (Miller & Jennett, 1968). In total, complications were present in about 25% of the sample and were in turn associated with significant increases in mortality and morbidity.

Damage to the Dura Mater, Surface Blood Vessels, Pituitary Body, and Hypothalamus and Systemic Injuries

Tearing of the dura mater in the vicinity of the dural venous sinuses may lead to the formation of an acute subdural hematoma, especially in cases of closed head injuries. In older persons who have evidence of cerebral arteriosclerosis, small arteries on the cortical surface may actually break and bleed, leading to a subdural accumulation of blood. In most cases, however, subdural hematomas result from laceration of the brain and blood vessels due to pulling and shearing effects.

Damage may also occur to the hypothalamic-pituitary axis and probably occurs frequently in cases of severe head injury. Injury to the hypothalamus is represented by petechial hemorrhages in the supraoptic and paraventricular nuclei and mammillary bodies, infarction in the infundibulum, and subependymal hemorrhage in the wall of the third ventricle. Petechial hemorrhages as well as acute infarctions may occur in the pituitary.

Autopsy studies of head-injured patients have demonstrated that the effects of direct trauma and ischemic damage may involve the pituitary gland and hypothalamus (McLaurin & King, 1975). Levin, Benton, and Grossman (1982) presume that such injuries may have distinctly adverse effects on functional aspects of the hypothalamic-pituitary system, resulting in diabetes insipidus, signs of hypopituitism, and abnormal secretion of antidiuretic hormone, and cite references to support these conclusions. However, diabetes insipidus appears to occur in less than 1% of persons with head injury (Porter & Miller, 1948) and panhypopituitarism following head injury is rare. Therefore, although there is considerable evidence of pathological lesions in this area, the clinical manifestations are not well known. The presumption by Levin, Benton, and Grossman (1982) that damage to the hypothalamic-pituitary axis is a factor complicating recovery from head injury and is a cause of persistent depression, psychomotor retardation, and diminished sexual function are consequences that have not yet been clearly demonstrated.

Frequently there are significant injuries associated with craniocerebral trauma that involve other systems of the body. Obviously it is important that these problems associated with multiple trauma be handled competently so that secondary insult to the already damaged brain can be avoided.

A detailed review of these systemic factors which may adversely affect brain function has been presented by Watts and Pulliam (1982). These authors stress the importance of maintaining respiratory function, attending to chest and lung injuries as well as later respiratory complications (such as pulmonary embolism and thrombophlebitis, aspiration pneumonia, pulmonary infection, atelectasis, and adult respiratory distress syndrome). Cardiovascular injuries may be of great significance and the trauma patient must be carefully evaluated for peripheral vascular injuries. Management of fluid abnormalities and acid-base balance may also be a significant factor in the management of the head-injured person.

Illingworth and Jennett (1965) found a low incidence of shock in patients with head injuries seen within six hours of the injury. When shock did occur, it was possible to identify substantial blood loss, usually in the chest, abdomen, or pelvis. Blood loss from a scalp wound contributed to arterial hypotension in only three of the 470 patients in the study. Nevertheless, patients with head injury must be monitored closely to detect any signs of hypovolemic shock (decreased volume of fluid in the intravascular system), vasogenic shock, cardiogenic shock, neurogenic shock, and septic shock. A number of conditions can also give rise to acute renal failure, particularly when interacting with results of body trauma. Fat emboli, seen most frequently in patients with multiple fractures of long bones, may also constitute a significant problem.

In terms of additional insult to the injured brain, the various systemic factors that may have adverse effects usually contribute to cerebral ischemia and may be due to arterial hypotension, cerebral anoxia due to systemic anoxia, cerebral fat emboli, and mediastinal block impeding venous return and resulting in increased cerebral venous pressure.

Concussion and the Post-Concussion Syndrome

Concussion

It has been difficult to obtain evidence of brain concussion following closed head injuries. The head injury is usually not severe in cases of concussion and clinical neurological examination shows no objective evidence of deficit. The bases for presuming biological impairment of brain functions usually centers on the subjective complaints of the patient. This set of circumstances is sometimes complicated by litigation and an attempt to recover damages; it is often presumed that the patient sustained no significant biological damage of the brain and the complaints and subjective symptoms are a reflection of a traumatic neurosis with a psychogenic basis. Nevertheless, the complaints of patients who have suffered even relatively minor closed head injuries tend to have a common thread; these victims often report symptoms of headache, dizziness, fatigue, memory deficit, impaired concentration, irritability, anxiety, insomnia, concern about bodily functions, and hypersensitivity to both light and noise.

Research over the past 25 years by Ommaya (1982) and other investigators has supported the validity of concussion as a clinical entity. There have been reports of diffusely distributed petechial lesions in the brains of victims of closed head injuries, including persons who sustained relatively minor head blows and whose brains were studied only after the victims died from other causes (Oppenheimer, 1968). The increasing volume of neuropsychological evidence points rather definitely to impairment of higher-level brain functions even in patients who sustained rather minor head injuries and showed no neurological findings (Levin, Benton, & Grossman, 1982; and evidence presented in this volume).

Ommaya (1982) identifies concussion as the basic phenomenon in head injury along with other primary factors such as skull fracture, contusions, and hemorrhages of the brain. He refers to secondary factors of head injury (discussed in more detail below) as *epiphenomena*. The diffuse effects of cerebral concussion represent a fundamental characteristic of brain damage and the eventual outcome of the individual patient relates to an interaction of these effects with various factors.

Ommaya (1982) differentiates between the linear forces and the rotational effects of concussion. He believes that focal lesions may be caused by potent linear forces but the diffuse injuries characteristic of concussion are caused by rotational effects. In practical terms, both linear and rotational effects are usually present in the individual case of head injury and combine to produce the resulting pathology by shear, tensile, and compressive strains. Cerebral concussion, however, is represented by diffuse effects resulting from rotational forces.

Ommaya notes that such effects, based on theoretical physics, would be (1) maximal on the surface of the of the brain and diminished toward the center; (2) most prominent where there are boundaries or sudden transitions between the density of tissues (the damaging effects of bone or dura as the brain moves against them); and (3) less severe in areas where the interior of the skull is smooth and there are no venous attachments. Obviously, these principles correlate with the early studies of gelatin models of the brain by Holbourn (1943) as well as observations of principal areas of cerebral damage at autopsy.

Ommaya (1982) has proposed six grades of cerebral concussion based upon the degree and type of symptoms and theoretically related to levels of brain involvement (superficial to deeper structures). *Grade I* is characterized by a degree of confusion but no loss of consciousness or amnesia for the head injury. *Grade II* is manifested by confusion of higher-level functions following the injury as well as a degree of anterograde (post-traumatic) amnesia. As in Grade I, there is no loss of consciousness but the return to normal cognitive functioning is somewhat more prolonged.

Related to Ommaya's postulate that the effects of concussion are greatest at the surface of the brain and decrease toward the core, Grades I and II of cerebral concussion would represent a temporary disconnection of the functional relationships between the cortex and the white matter of the cerebral hemispheres. Ommaya proposes that the resultant shear strains progressively affect deeper parts of the brain as the strength of the blow to the head increases.

Grade III concussion is represented by the confusion and post-traumatic amnesia which characterizes Grade II and, in addition, includes retrograde amnesia (inability to remember events which occurred before the accident). Grades II and III imply not only a degree of disconnection between cortical and subcortical tissues but also a diencephalic disconnection.

Grades IV, V, and VI of cerebral concussion are characterized by coma (including sensorimotor paralysis). *Grade IV* is manifested by coma, confusion followed by a gradual recovery of consciousness, post-traumatic and retrograde amnesia, and a gradual recovery of brain functions with persistent retrograde amnesia.

A *Grade V* concussion results from a more forceful blow to the head and includes a persistent vegetative state in addition to the coma and the other symptoms described above. In this condition there is presumably some degree of recovery of brain stem functions but there is a severe disconnection of outer brain layers and brain stem function.

In *Grade VI* concussion the force of the blow extends through the external structures of the brain and irreversibly damages the vital functions of the brain stem. Even in such cases there have been reports of post-mortem examination revealing no visible brain lesions. This had led to a characterization of concussion as coma and paralysis resulting from a head blow but without concomitant structural tissue damage. Ommaya contends that such a description does not accurately represent the facts and that in these cases the patient died before the primary lesions had an opportunity to develop.

In summary, Ommaya's conceptual view of cerebral concussion describes the clinical phenomena as a continuous representation from very mild injury to death, orders the clinical phenomena in a sequence from reversible to progressively less reversible consequences, and attempts to relate the clinical manifestations in an orderly fashion from involvement of surface areas (cerebral cortex) in a sequential manner to lower areas within the brain.

While noting that the post-traumatic (post-concussion) syndrome is puzzling because of the lack of objective clinical deficits, Ommaya postulates that patients with this syndrome represent the functional effects of the diffuse strains of brain tissue in cerebral concussion and proposes that the same mechanisms of injury may also be present in whiplash injuries. He notes that the effects of "microtrauma" must always be supplemented by neuropsychological studies; in significant head injuries (where brain stem function is temporarily lost at the time of cerebral concussion), there is probably always persisting diffuse impairment at higher levels of the brain, possibly due to disorganization of neural cell assemblies (as contrasted with damage only at the cellular level).

The Post-Concussion Syndrome

Investigators have varied conclusions about the neurological and emotional bases of the post-concussion syndrome. Levin, Benton, and Grossman (1982) emphasize that although there is no consensus on the question, the most widely held opinion is that post-concussion symptoms persisting more than two or three months after an injury are most likely reflecting an exacerbation of a previous neurotic condition (Guttmann, 1946; Lishman, 1973). They also point out, however, that the concept of concussion as a fully reversible injury with no corresponding structural alteration of the brain has legitimately been challenged and the current available evidence favors the view of concussion as a severity continuum of diffuse injury.

Jennett and Teasdale (1981) believe that the symptoms of the post-concussion syndrome have an organic basis, but that they subside quite rapidly in most cases. They believe that only a few victims have persistent symptoms and go on to develop depression or anxiety. Jennett and Teasdale conclude that, "It is now accepted that even brief concussion usually entails some structural damage to the brain."

McLaurin and Titchener (1982) observed the "traditional disputes" regarding whether the syndrome arises "principally from mental and emotional reactions to head trauma or from disordered neurophysiological mechanisms and brain damage" and go on to point out that such conflicts can be avoided by recognizing that complex causal chains are involved in concussion, including neurophysiological, psychophysiological, psychiatric, and probably unknown factors. This conceptual framework in turn leads McLaurin and Titchener to discuss the syndrome in terms of "organic" and "psychic" causes.

Headache constitutes a very common symptom of the concussion syndrome, although among individual patients there is considerable variation in its nature and severity. Jacobsen (1963) reported that 78% of the 297 subjects in his sample had headaches in the post-traumatic period. When the headaches were localized, the part of the head that had been struck was frequently cited as being the most painful area; frequently, though, the headaches were of a generalized nature. The headaches were continuous or intermittent and often were aggravated by emotional and physical stress.

In a study of the relationship between headaches and post-traumatic amnesia Jacobsen found no difference in the incidence of headaches in patients with or without post-traumatic amnesia. In his study the duration of post-traumatic amnesia did not relate to variables describing the headaches, a finding which confirmed the earlier results of Brenner, Friedman, Merritt, and Denny-Brown (1944). Although there are many possible organic causes for persisting headache after head injury — including pain in the areas of scalp injury, neuralgia of occipital or supraorbital nerves, precipitation of migraine in subjects who have previously had such headaches, and occasionally more serious intracranial complications (such as hydrocephalus or chronic subdural hematoma) — many of the studies on headache in the post-concussion syndrome conclude that etiological factors relate more to

emotional and psychiatric types of problems than to a neurological disorder (Jennett & Teasdale, 1981).

Dizziness or a disorder of equilibrium is the second most common symptom of the post-concussion syndrome and is estimated to occur in approximately 50% of patients (McLaurin & Titchener, 1982). These authors note that when this symptom occurs in patients with post-concussion syndrome it differs from "true spontaneous vertigo," which is invariably associated with brain stem or vestibular-cochlear damage. In the post-concussion syndrome these symptoms are reported as sensations of giddiness, faintness, or unsteadiness, and occur after sudden movements of the head or movements of the environment with relation to the patient. Jacobsen (1963) found that the incidence of vertigo was correlated with the severity of the head injury. Cartlidge (1978) reported that subjective complaints of dizziness were of labyrinthine origin (as demonstrated by electronystagmographic recordings).

From this point on the factors included in the post-concussion syndrome become much more difficult to identify in specific terms on the basis of routine clinical examination. As noted above, they include fatigue, impaired ability in concentration and memory, irritability, anxiety, insomnia, hypochondriasis, and sensitivity to noise and light. Although head-injured patients frequently report problems of this kind, such symptoms are difficult to evaluate in objective and quantitative terms and to consistently relate to more objective variables.

These factors have lead many investigators and clinicians to conclude that the post-concussion syndrome principally represents a psychiatric rather than neurological problem. McLaurin and Titchener (1982) offer a summarical description of at least some patients with post-traumatic syndrome: "The patient's physical symptoms become the center of his life; he notices and is interested in very little else about himself, most poignantly, about his personal interactions or loss of meaningful relations with others. He literally becomes a headache and a dizziness, assuming the role of the sick, head-injured person, though he once may have been an active, interesting, participating individual with flexibility in social roles, enthusiasms in vocation, enjoyment of marriage and sexuality, and a pleasure in social relations. More specific and narrowed changes in personality include paranoid and counterphobic acting-out traits that replace previous ways of adapting."

These authors go on to present a model of the post-traumatic (post-concussion) syndrome, starting with the "massively threatening situation" represented by injury to the head, a specific type of severe anxiety noted many years earlier by Schilder (1934). This model begins with the trauma, resulting coma, gradual recovery during a period of stupor and confusion, possible amnesia for the injury, and a feeling of acute distress. At this time the patient's intellectual functions (including judgment, thinking, memory, and orientation) may be disorganized. From a biological point of view he is essentially helpless.

McLaurin and Titchener postulate that the problem moves from this biological stage of helplessness to its psychological counterpart as a result of "actual flooding of the psychic apparatus with the terror of the moment." They note that injuries to other parts of the body are regularly accompanied by some form of traumatic neurosis which consists of "a flooding of the psychic apparatus with levels of excitation beyond its capacity to respond."

McLaurin and Titchener state that the individual attempts to recover from this condition by "mastering the traumatic event"; the victim relives the accident in dreams as well as in the waking state and maintains an intense vigilance to protect himself against any further stimuli which might overwhelm his adaptive apparatus. The next step in this process is found in those persons in which

the disorder becomes severe and chronic and results in somatisization of the traumatic neurosis. The focus of neurotic reactions to the trauma then become more generalized and integrated with any pre-existing neurotic tendencies that the individual may have had. For example, any pre-injury tendencies toward depression will blend with elements of the traumatic neurosis and become intensified. Pre-existing paranoid tendencies may not only center around somatic complaints but become more generally expressed as well.

All of these factors lead to increased feelings of defensiveness, limitation of interest, and change of relations with the outside world. McLaurin and Titchener identify these changes as representing a personality constriction in which the individual is principally interested in protecting himself against every sort of change, resisting novel experiences, and narrowing his range of experience.

At this stage the head-injured person begins to view all aspects of his life in terms of his injury. For example, he may relate every personal inadequacy to the head injury. Any personal or professional difficulty may automatically be attributed to the cerebral trauma. Obviously, these kinds of problems have a seriously disabling effect on the individual in terms of efficiency of independent functioning, family interactions, and the general character of his lifestyle.

Although there may be some individuals who experience this sequence of events and circumstances during the post-injury period, there is little known about frequency with which individuals are so affected. Aita and Reitan (1948) studied a series of approximately 500 consecutive head injury cases, most of them soldiers who had sustained relatively severe injuries. These researchers identified only four patients with psychotic reactions during the first year following the head injury. However, a review of the pre-injury personality adjustments, personal interactions, and behavior patterns of each of these men indicated that their post-traumatic psychosis (which developed after the immediate confusional state and over a period of months after the injury was sustained) represented an elaboration of pre-existing personality and behavioral deviations.

For example, one patient was extremely paranoid and had severely unrealistic ideational processes (paranoid schizophrenia). He had a pre-injury history of distinct paranoid tendencies and distrusted others to the extent that he stayed in his own bedroom most of the time, would not eat unless his mother brought food to his bedroom, and so forth. It must be noted, though, that such severe behavioral disturbances are seen rarely in patients who have sustained head injuries and are not characteristically a part of the post-concussion syndrome. Nevertheless, there appears to be a distinct interaction between the customary "neurological" and "psychiatric" effects of head injury and this situation almost certainly would represent a basis for expecting discrepancies among individual experts with respect to assessment of etiology, especially among patients with the post-concussion syndrome.

A number of factors can be identified that would contribute to such discrepancies. First, investigators compare their samples of patients from various populations. Some samples, for example, may include disproportionate numbers of persons who were neurotic or emotionally disturbed before the injury. If head injuries exacerbate previous emotional disturbances (as it appears to do in some cases), the "psychiatric" aspect of the patient's difficulties would become the most prominent symptom. Other subgroups of head-injured persons include those who are interested in recovering losses through litigation. Much has been written in the literature to the effect that these subjects may tend to exaggerate their symptoms, complaints, and disabilities; in fact, patients who have unresolved claims for compensation appear to lose much more time from normal work than those who have no such claims (Jennett & Teasdale, 1981). Therefore,

both pre-injury and post-injury emotional and situational factors may be significant in determining the outcome for any individual patient.

Second, as with recovery from any injury, a considerable degree of variability would be expected among patients, either in terms of residual deficits or the time-scale for recovery. In effect, it is probably impossible to achieve a complete understanding of the patient's residual symptomatology.

The pre-morbid emotional status of the patient should be explicitly mentioned as a third factor. Head injury victims have a great range of personalities and often include persons with deviant or unstable characteristics. Thus, pre-injury personality adjustment, which is very difficult to assess retroactively, appears to be an important factor in the recovery process and residual symptomatology of every individual.

Finally, the customary clinical methods for evaluating residual effects of head injury are rather gross and insensitive. Many persons do not demonstrate any abnormalities on the neurological examination or electroencephalogram. In these cases there may be a natural tendency to conclude that no neurological deficits were sustained as a result of the injury and the patient's complaints are often thought to have a psychiatric origin. As more sensitive methods of neurological evaluation of brain functions are developed (e.g., Ommaya, 1982) researchers and clinicians are realizing that their previous methods of evaluating the symptoms of head-injured persons were generally inadequate for differentiating between neurological and psychiatric etiologies.

As noted above, investigators such as Jennett and Teasdale (1981) have concluded that even mild concussion usually results in some structural damage of the brain. This conclusion is based on diversified findings. Oppenheimer (1968) demonstrated the presence of diffusely distributed pathological lesions in the brains of persons who had sustained even relatively mild head injuries and later had died of non-related (non-neurological) causes. An increasing number of neuropsychological studies show evidence of impairment of higher-level functions which, in some instances, even correlate with the recovery process (Gronwall & Wrightson, 1974; Rutherford, Merritt & McDonald, 1977). Careful and systematic reviews of head-injured patients, including those with post-concussion syndrome, reveal clinical neurological deficits (Kay, Kerr, & Lassman, 1971; Rutherford, Merritt, & McDonald, 1977). Neuro-otological studies, based upon nystagmography, showed definite impairment of the vestibular-cochlear apparatus, often in even mild head injuries. Therefore, evidence from a number of different sources supports the hypothesis that organic damage to the brain may result from even relatively mild head injuries.

Additional evidence supporting this hypothesis is found in the sequence of complaints of head-injured persons. In the early post-injury period complaints are essentially similar among persons who will show a complete recovery and persons who will develop post-concussion syndrome. It would appear that some initial basis of brain impairment has been sustained in both groups. Of course, in the latter group, pre-existing emotional factors or post-injury circumstances may lead to a perpetuation of symptoms that were initially produced by organic impairment.

Merskey and Woodford (1972) studied two groups of patients with similar post-concussion symptoms. The group without pending litigation had either no claims or claims that had already been settled; nevertheless, their symptoms were quite similar to the symptoms reported by the subjects who had litigation pending. Although many earlier research reports proposed that the post-concussion syndrome was heavily dependent upon (if not the result of) existing litigation and claims for compensation, the Merskey and Woodford study suggests that this is generally not the case

(although there is undoubtedly a strong relationship in some instances). Obviously, resolution of these kinds of problems depends upon the availability and validity of objective methods of examination which can identify organic impairment without being influenced by the subjective complaints of the victim.

The mechanisms or etiology of the various symptoms included in the post-concussion syndrome are not subject to specific (one-to-one) explanation. Dizziness may be related to labyrinthine dysfunction (Toglia, 1969; Toglia & Katinsky, 1976). Evidence of intellectual impairment, even in persons with relatively mild head injuries, has been amply documented in the literature. However, the results of the initial examination are not necessarily conclusive of cognitive impairment, even when using sensitive and complete neuropsychological test batteries. The degree of impairment in persons with even mild head injuries can be definitively determined by serial examinations which document the initial deficit (Reitan & Wolfson, in press). Pre-existing emotional problems undoubtedly contribute to the victim's post-injury complaints and the injury may, in fact, precipitate pre-existing neurotic or psychotic tendencies. In addition, impairment of the intellectual functions resulting from the head trauma may create problems of adjustment in the individual's personal and occupational setting and result in emotional maladjustments.

Obviously, the presence of emotional difficulties may have important clinical ramifications. In most cases a complete neuropsychological evaluation can differentiate between emotional problems and the neuropsychological deficits due to brain damage.

Although headache is the most frequent complaint of patients with post-concussion syndrome, they are caused by various etiologies and frequently are never adequately explained. It is not likely that the cause of headaches of most patients with post-concussion syndrome can be determined.

Contusions of the Brain

Gross examination of the injured brain frequently shows obvious signs of primary brain damage, generally represented by contusions. The severity of cerebral contusions ranges from a minor bruise involving the crest of a single gyrus to widespread damage of much of the surface of the cerebral hemisphere. Contusions may also be accompanied by lesions that penetrate the white matter and midbrain. These lesions are usually hemorrhagic (although sometimes necrotic) and when they are present the patient's cerebral spinal fluid is frequently bloody.

The distribution of cerebral contusions seen at autopsy has been studied in detail (Adams, Scott, Parker, Graham, & Doyle, 1980). Regardless of the site of impact, cerebral contusions occur most frequently in the frontal lobes, particularly involving the orbital surfaces. The lateral surfaces of the temporal lobes are also frequently damaged, and bruises may occur over the convexity of the cerebral hemispheres as well. Contusions sometimes involve the medial surfaces of the hemispheres and the corpus callosum may be contused by contact with the falx or tentorium.

Significant contusion of the cerebral cortex is always associated with edema of the underlying white matter. Of course, diffuse primary structural damage to the white matter may also occur (Adams, Mitchell, Graham, & Doyle, 1977) and damage to the corpus callosum and brain stem has been reported.

Damage to the white matter may occur independently of cerebral contusions and is caused by stretching and tearing of nerve fibers in the white matter of the cerebral hemispheres or brain stem. This results in diffuse axonal injury, as described below (Oppenheimer, 1968; Strich, 1961).

Except when caused by a depressed skull fracture with in-driven bone fragments, contusions are not commonly found directly under the site of the blow. Although contusion hemorrhages are sometimes solitary, they usually occur in several places. Electron-microscopic studies have shown necrotic endothelial changes in the walls of small blood vessels (Testa, Bollini & Columella, 1970) and though the hemorrhages are initially perivascular, they become more widespread and sometimes coalesce, usually in the depths of the sulci. Areas of necrosis resulting from contusions are usually wedge-shaped, with the point of the wedge extending toward or into the white matter (Lindenberg & Freytag, 1957).

When contusions occur following head trauma, they develop almost immediately on impact and may increase in size during the first several hours following the injury. Necroses are usually not visible until about 12 hours post-injury (Bakay & Glasauer, 1980) and gradually reach their greatest size in about one week. They subside over a period of a few months and eventually become small cavities in the cortex and white matter.

Although larger hemorrhages may become cystic, smaller lesions induce phagocytotic microglial reactions within the first two days post-injury and are later followed by astrocytosis. Small lesions are eventually absorbed completely or leave a small scar.

Systematic serial neuropsychological examinations of patients who have sustained cerebral contusions show that a significant recovery effect occurs during the first 12 months post-injury; however, a considerable number of these patients demonstrate deterioration of cognitive abilities in the 12 to 18 months following the head injury (Reitan & Wolfson, in press). The exact mechanism of this deterioration of neuropsychological functions is undoubtedly related to the long-term biological changes described above, but the sequence of events is presently unknown. In some cases it has been documented that computed tomography demonstrates severe late atrophy associated with reabsorption of damaged brain tissue.

When a patient sustains a head injury that results in cerebral contusion, his/her state of consciousness is usually impaired, although complete loss of consciousness does not often occur. The patient may be comatose or semi-comatose for a variable period of time and may be confused, restless, or delirious. As in other cases of head injury, emergence from a comatose state in instances of contusion is a relatively gradual process and includes variable periods of initial confusion and retrograde amnesia.

As might be expected with cerebral contusion (because of tissue damage of the cerebral cortex), focal neurological signs are demonstrated frequently and depend on the location of contusion. Frontal contusions occur often but focal neurological deficits are less commonly associated with these lesions than damage involving the somatosensory or visual areas of the cerebral cortex.

Contusions are rarely seen in the occipital lobes. Homonymous defects of the visual field may occur in patients with contusions in the middle parts of the cerebral hemispheres extending into the white matter and involving the geniculostriate tract.

Finally, it should be noted that it is not uncommon to encounter patients who have experienced circumscribed local contusions (or even lacerations of the brain) and have suffered no loss of consciousness, even temporarily, as an immediate effect of the injury.

Damage to the Poles of the Brain

We have previously noted that the frontal and temporal poles are often damaged in rotational injuries, resulting from shearing forces, movement of the brain within the skull, and tearing of the cerebral cortex as it passes over the rough surfaces in the interior of the skull. Because such injuries occur frequently in closed head injuries, we will describe them more specifically.

When the brain moves within the head, the poles (as contrasted with more central regions) experience the greatest forces and changes in position. As noted, Holbourn (1943), based on his studies of gelatin models of the brain, believed that the frontal and temporal poles were particularly vulnerable to damage, especially as a result of the shearing forces which occur during sudden and severe rotation of the head. Movement of the frontal poles against the anterior fossa and the temporal poles against the sphenoid bones can also cause contusion or laceration of the brain tissue. Although there is usually more damage on one side of the brain than the other, bilateral damage is common (Miller & Becker, 1982). Observing a shift of midline structures on radiological examination does not rule out the possibility of bilateral damage; it may only indicate which hemisphere is more severely involved.

In terms of their nature, cerebral lesions involving the frontal or temporal poles do not differ from other surface contusions and lacerations. In a contusion there is a rupture of small vessels below the pia mater accompanied by swelling of the involved area. At surgery the area appears necrotic, soft, and hemorrhagic. It is sometimes difficult to differentiate between contusions and lacerations; lacerations are customarily associated with tearing of the pia mater.

In the early post-injury period polar lesions frequently show a tendency to swell and/or bleed and act as an intracranial expanding lesion which may in turn cause secondary brain dysfunction. The clinical neurological manifestations of polar lesions are often rather minimal unless the lesion extends to the motor or sensory areas or has a direct effect on the functional status of these regions.

Historically, these lesions have been referred to as "silent." However, neuropsychological evaluation with the Halstead-Reitan Battery demonstrates impairment on the general tests of the integrity of the cerebral cortex with any of these lesions: at least mild dysphasia will be demonstrated in most cases of left hemisphere lesions; in instances of right anterior temporal lesions impairment of finger tapping speed and complex psychomotor skill performances (Tactual Performance Test) will be impaired; and in cases of anterior frontal damage, a relative absence of focal signs is often observed (even though the general indicators are significantly impaired). Clinical neuropsychological examination frequently is able to make unique contributions in the assessment of focal polar brain lesions.

Cerebral Damage at the Cellular Level

Miller and Becker (1982) have proposed a cellular-level model of primary damage of the traumatically injured brain. Their conceptualization explains many of the mechanisms of cerebral injury and has significance for both short-term and long-term recovery processes. This model is also consistent with the clinical neuropsychological findings of diffuse effects (and focal deficits when they are present) in nearly every case of significant head injury and correlates with the post-injury recovery gradient.

We should note, however, that the Miller and Becker model is not relevant to the neuropsychological deterioration which often occurs 12 to 18 months after the injury. This finding of long-term deterioration has only recently been discovered and documented (Reitan & Wolfson, in press).

The model proposed by Miller and Becker begins with recognition of axonal damage of neurons. This leads to the process of chromatolysis, which starts to occur shortly after injury. Chromatolysis is a series of changes in the cell body that includes swelling, dissolution of Nissl bodies, and displacement of the nucleus to the periphery of the cell.

If the damage to the neuron is sufficiently severe, these changes may cause complete dissolution of the cell. With less severe damage the process may be arrested and eventually reversed, with recovery occurring over a period of months.

The process of chromatolysis is undoubtedly important concerning the documentation of statistically significant recovery of neuropsychological functions (compared with the retesting results obtained from control subjects within the first 12 months following injury) (Reitan & Wolfson, in press).

Recent studies indicate quite clearly that trauma to a neuron may result in death of the cell or cause the cell to remain in a marginally functional state for some time before it eventually recovers. It appears that the concept of chromatolysis represents circumstances that work toward repair of injured cells through increased cellular metabolism (Ducker, Kempe, & Hayes, 1969).

As pointed out by Miller and Becker (1982), this concept of damage with the potential of recovery over an extensive period of time should not be confused with the consequences of complete disruption or severance of the axon. In this latter instance, wallerian degeneration (degeneration of the part of the axon from the point of injury that is distal to the cell body) occurs, resulting in breakdown of the myelin sheath, absorption of the axon cylinder, and phagocytosis of fatty droplets.

A series of changes occur in this type of injury, with early indications of axonal damage represented by the appearance of retraction balls (formed from the axoplasm of torn and damaged axons). Using special histological methods, it is also possible to demonstrate discontinuity of axons. Within a few days a number of changes occur, including histological changes that result in microglial stars around small tissue tears (Oppenheimer, 1968). Eventually these changes result in demyelination and gliosis.

The role of damage to glial cells is relatively unknown. There is no doubt that glial swelling occurs when the brain is damaged (Grossman, 1972; Grossman & Seregin, 1976) and it has been hypothesized that this process reflects uptake of potassium (or possibly even neurotransmitters released from damaged neurons) into the extracellular space. In addition to injury of neurons and glial cells, trauma of the brain may also disrupt cerebral blood vessels and cause gross and microscopic hemorrhages.

Experimental evidence has suggested that local injuries to the cortical surface may result in arterial hypertension; this in turn may produce brain swelling and extracellular edema. Other complications may also result from breakdown in specific areas of the blood-brain barrier. Therefore, in addition to damage to the walls of blood vessels and hemorrhage, the integrity of the vascular system and its relationship to the blood-brain barrier is often compromised in instances of cerebral damage.

It has been proposed that the cause of cerebral edema following blunt head injury is the breakdown of the blood-brain barrier; however, experimental studies have indicated that there may be such an alteration of the blood-brain barrier without significant concurrent evidence of brain edema. In addition, some reports have suggested that biochemical disorders of neuronal function, possibly represented by the neurotransmitter system, may be a significant factor related to coma and other aspects of neurological dysfunction.

Although evidence has accrued to explain some of the injurious effects of head trauma at the cellular level and clarify certain basic biological deficits associated with head injury, many additional questions and problems remain for future investigation.

Diffuse Injury of the Brain

Earlier in this chapter we reviewed the evidence indicating that diffuse tissue damage of the brain may occur in severe head injuries even if there is no evidence of ischemic or hypoxic brain damage or increased intracranial pressure.

In animal studies, using gelatin models of the brain and a lucite model of the calvarium (Pudenz

& Sheldon, 1946), researchers have directly observed the movement of the brain during an impact. Widespread movement of the brain is associated with shearing and tearing of axons and myelin sheaths in the white matter of the cerebral hemispheres. On autopsy the brains of such patients look normal grossly, with few (if any) surface contusions.

During the first two weeks following the injury (based upon autopsies done at that time) microglial stars representing small clusters of hypertrophied microglia are often seen along with numerous retraction balls. Such lesions are very prominent and are found diffusely scattered throughout the white matter of the cerebral hemispheres, the cerebellum, and the brain stem.

After approximately two weeks retraction balls are no longer observable. The brains of persons who expire six to eight weeks post-injury show wallerian degeneration of the white matter involving both ascending and descending tracts in the brain stem. These lesions are so characteristic in appearance that they can be identified by the neuropathologist quite easily (Adams, Mitchell, Graham, & Doyle, 1977).

As noted by Miller and Becker (1982), these pathological changes form a sequential series of events in patients with severe closed head injuries. The retraction balls and microglial stars appear first and are followed by axonal degeneration and demyelination approximately six to eight weeks post-injury.

As noted above, Ommaya and Gennarelli (1974; 1976) postulated that neuronal damage would involve the cerebral cortex and extend inward toward the brain stem in cases of closed head injury involving increased impact. This finding corresponds with the observations of Adams, Mitchell, Graham, and Doyle (1977), who reported that every patient who had a lesion of the brain stem also had a lesion involving the cerebral hemispheres. This diffuse brain damage is considered to be responsible for prolonged periods of unconsciousness in patients who have sustained severe closed injury without complications of focal or mass lesions of the brain.

Penetrating Brain Injuries

Penetrating injuries of the head can be classified as low velocity or high velocity and are extremely variable in the brain damage they produce. *Low velocity* injuries are characterized by stab wounds. The brain damage they cause is primarily limited to the track of entry and may involve only the outer aspects of the brain tissue or may penetrate deeply into the cerebrum. Patients with wounds of this kind do not ordinarily lose consciousness.

It is important that the wounding instrument (e.g., a knife) is not removed from the victim's head until careful surgical preparations have been made for the consequences. Skull x-rays should be obtained and cerebral angiography may be necessary if it appears that the instrument has damaged a major blood vessel. After the penetrating instrument has been removed massive hemorrhage is always a possible complication; surgical preparations to expose the track of the wound should be made.

High velocity injuries are usually represented by bullet wounds. More extensive brain damage occurs with higher-velocity wounds because bone fragments, skin, hair, and other foreign objects may have been pushed into the brain tissue by the penetrating object. The penetrating missile may spin irregularly through the brain and cause widespread damage, even ricocheting from the opposite side of the skull and causing additional laceration and contusion.

Missiles of very high velocity produce extreme shock waves that extend in every direction from the missile track and cause a great amount of damage. A number of factors (besides the penetrating wound) are significant regarding of the outcome of these injuries. These factors include hypoxemia, hemorrhage, intracranial hypertension, and brain shift. Bullet wounds are more frequently fatal than injuries caused by lower-velocity instruments, such as fragments of grenades or mines. Guns with muzzle velocity of 2,000 or more feet per second kill almost instantly (Hammon, 1971).

Although the entry wound may be rather small in high-velocity missile injuries, the skull may shatter from within, beginning along suture lines. Because of the force involved in penetrating the cranial cavity, there may be transient cavity formation of the brain. The transmission of energy per unit of time depends upon the velocity of the entering agent (usually a bullet); higher velocities will cause larger transient cavitation with damage along the path of the missile as well as in much more widespread areas. Cavity formation causes compression and stretching of tissues both adjacent to and remote from the missile path and generates greatly increased intracranial pressure that may result in respiratory and cardiac failure and death.

There have been extensive studies of missile velocity in military casualties and the importance of velocity has been clearly demonstrated (Hammon, 1971). Civilian penetrating wounds are generally from lower-velocity missiles and are associated with less tissue damage. Nevertheless, penetrating brain wounds among civilians have a high mortality rate, ranging from 40% to 55% in various studies.

Raimondi and Samuelson (1970) have shown that a delay in definitive treatment leads to significant deterioration of the patient's neurological status and increases the likelihood of a fatal outcome. Delay in treatment is associated with progressive respiratory depression.

Early definitive treatment also leads to control of intracerebral bleeding and the edema which may compress adjacent brain tissue. Most hematomas will be located along the missile track but may also occur at distant locations and computed tomography is helpful in identifying these various areas of damage. In most civilian injuries the patient arrives at the hospital promptly and can be in surgery within two hours of the injury, before deep infection can occur. The basic principles of neurosurgical treatment — including debridement of the scalp wound, removal of hematoma and control of bleeding, removal of any pulped brain and any in-driven bone fragments or other foreign substances, watertight closure of the dura mater and scalp closure without tension on the skin — contribute to the eventual outcome.

Complications associated with penetrating injuries are essentially similar to those seen with depressed skull fracture and include infection, intracranial hemorrhage, bleeding from dural venous sinuses, problems related to distant distribution of bone or missile fragments and distant hemorrhages due to the penetrating agents. In terms of immediate care, the principal danger from such injuries probably relates to infection, particularly in instances of discrete perforating penetration of the skull.

Brain Stem Injury

Brain stem injury, particularly when caused by compressive forces resulting from the transmission of energy from a blow to the head, may be quite severe and result in disruption of vital functions and eventual death. There has been a tendency in the literature to describe the effects of closed head injuries only in terms of brain stem damage. This particular characterization has gained a considerable amount of acceptance and is still currently used in published articles as well as clinical practice. However, as we noted above, more recent scientific evidence has suggested that when brain stem injury occurs, there is always corresponding widespread damage throughout the cerebral hemispheres.

First we will suggest briefly why emphasis on brain stem injury gained such a widespread acceptance; the great importance placed on the ascending reticular activating system (ARAS) and its relationship to alertness and maintenance of consciousness was probably an important factor.

Following the report of Moruzzi and Magoun (1949) describing the significance of the brain stem reticular system and its influence on activation of the electroencephalogram, there was a surge in interest in the ARAS and its role in alertness and presumably in its function in the more complex aspects of psychological functioning. It was presumed that loss of consciousness corresponded with temporary impairment of the ARAS. In addition, reports of animal studies had proposed that the effects of blunt head blows were largely restricted to the brain stem.

Finally, in terms of clinical examination, evidence of impaired cranial nerve function (particularly with respect to extraocular eye movements) were frequently apparent. Therefore, when the clinician recognized that these nerves and their nuclei were located in the brain stem and then observed objective evidence of cranial nerve impairment, the indication of brain stem damage (even though probably reversible) was inescapable.

Damage involving the brain more generally, particularly with diffuse involvement of the cerebral hemispheres, was much less apparent in terms of specific deficits that would have localization value. Cerebral involvement tended to become identified only in instances of penetrating lesions or contusions which involved the cerebral cortex and caused the patient to demonstrate focal neurological signs.

Thus, in terms of clinical evaluation, there was a tendency to base diagnostic conclusions on the immediately available and observable evidence. Closed head injuries were generally described as causing brain stem damage; open head wounds were related to cerebral damage more generally.

These results have long been inconsistent with findings based on the neuropsychological examination. First, neuropsychologists who have examined patients with focal lesions at various levels of the brain (including the cerebral cortex, cerebral white matter, anterior brain stem, midbrain, and the lower parts of the brain) have observed that lesions at the midbrain level (approximately at the level of the aqueduct of Sylvius) or lower have produced relatively few manifestations of neuropsychological deficit. Lesions involving the anterior brain stem frequently cause mild, generalized neuropsychological impairment in the early stages of lesion development, and lead to gross functional impairment (including akinetic mutism) as they mature.

The lesions that appear to involve the white matter exclusively cause somewhat more specific deficits (depending on their location) and may produce relatively serious cognitive impairment. Lesions directly involving the cerebral cortex, reported by the surgeon to show pathological changes at the time the cerebral cortex is exposed, cause the greatest focal deficits and the most severe neuropsychological impairment.

Considering the fact that patients with closed head injuries show specific and focal losses in association with areas of focal tissue damage as well as widespread diffuse cerebral dysfunction involving the cerebral hemispheres, it was not consistent to propose a concept implying that closed head injury damage was related rather exclusively to brain stem injury without evidence of focal cerebral tissue damage. Neuropsychological studies strongly indicated that patients who were diagnosed clinically as having only brain stem injury actually had generalized involvement of the cerebral hemispheres.

More recent pathological studies have indicated that structural lesions located exclusively in the brain stem, without evidence of primary damage elsewhere in the brain, occur rarely (if ever). Mitchell and Adams (1973) studied the brains (including the brain stem) of a group of patients who had died after blunt head injury and in whom increased intracranial pressure and brain shift did not appear to have been significant factors. These researchers concluded that localized brain stem damage, without more extensive involvement of the brain, does not exist as a pathological entity. They noted that the clinician's reference to primary brain stem damage should be defined as manifestations of brain stem dysfunction occurring soon after the injury.

Adams, Mitchell, Graham, and Doyle (1977) studied a series of 152 fatal head injuries and confirmed the findings of widespread damage in the brain whenever the brain stem has been injured. In addition, the widely-cited study of Oppenheimer (1968) showed that there were microscopic lesions diffusely distributed in the white matter of the cerebral hemispheres in patients who had died of other causes after recovering from even relatively mild closed head injuries.

There is no doubt that brain stem injuries occur, but it seems that their appearance is in conjunction with more widespread damage throughout the brain. From a neuropsychological point of view, brain stem injuries do not generally appear to have major significance concerning impairment of higher-level cognitive brain functions.

IV

SECONDARY STRUCTURAL DAMAGE

As noted previously, primary damage to the brain results from the direct forces of a blow to the head. In contrast, secondary damage is caused by a space-occupying lesion that occurs in response to the primary damage. Secondary damage is frequently caused by hematomas (epidural, subdural or intracerebral), brain swelling (either focal or diffuse), or brain abscess (localized necrosis) due to bone, skin, hair or foreign material driven into the brain tissue in a penetrating head injury. Secondary damage to the brain should be suspected if a patient's condition deteriorates suddenly after the initial response to the head injury.

Mechanisms of Secondary Damage

Expanding brain lesions caused by a head injury may be either relatively focal or diffuse and are generally represented by bleeding (hematoma), infection (abscess), or swelling (edema). Such lesions vary in location; they may be intracerebral or occur in the epidural or subdural space, and can be supratentorial or infratentorial. In addition to producing increased intracranial pressure, these lesions usually cause some shift and distortion of brain structures. If the secondary factors (including intracranial pressure) are not relieved, herniation of the brain may result.

Displacement of Brain Structures

The more rapidly a mass lesion expands, the higher the degree of intracranial pressure with relation to brain displacement or distortion. For example, an acute subdural hematoma may lead to a very rapid increase in intracranial pressure; a chronic subdural hematoma, which has developed over a longer time interval, is often associated with normal intracranial pressure.

The corresponding neuropsychological effects of acute and chronic lesions have also been studied in detail (Fitzhugh, Fitzhugh, & Reitan, 1962a; 1962b; 1963). Research has demonstrated that acute lesions are customarily associated with focal, more pronounced neuropsychological deficits and poorer levels of performances. The majority of expanding lesions caused by head injury are supratentorial and frequently occur bilaterally. Of course, supratentorial lesions are much more likely to show corresponding evidence of neuropsychological deficits than lesions below the tentorium.

Although the neurological deficits that occur with secondary mass lesions are often attributed to a rapid increase in intracranial pressure, some researchers have suggested that they are more closely related to brain displacement (Miller &

Becker, 1982) and neuropsychological testing tends to confirm this hypothesis: Many patients, particularly those having lesions at the level of the aqueduct of Sylvius or below, show little evidence of neuropsychological impairment despite having severely increased intracranial pressure.

A mass lesion in the epidural or subdural space will exert pressure on the underlying cerebral cortex, flatten gyri against the dura mater and compress surface vessels. When this occurs, the subarachnoid space is compressed and subarachnoid cisterns decrease in size. The lateral ventricle on the side of the lesion may also become narrowed.

Essentially these same effects occur when the lesion is intracerebral in location. The free-flowing nature of cerebrospinal fluid permits some degree of compensation for increased intracranial pressure caused by an expanding lesion. However, occlusion of fluid spaces may occur at the level of the midbrain and interfere with both flow and absorption of cerebrospinal fluid. This mechanism results in an uneven distribution of pressure above and below the tentorium, with the infratentorial pressure, which may be close to normal, serving as an invalid basis for inferring supratentorial pressure. A build-up of supratentorial intracranial pressure, as a result of this mechanism, may lead to the death of the patient.

Midline Shift

Midline shift occurs when an expanding mass lesion, located predominantly on one side of the brain, expands in size and pushes brain structures to the side of the tentorium opposite the lesion. The degree of midline shift can be determined by various techniques which demonstrate tilting of the third ventricle, the intraventricular septum, and the pineal gland (when calcified) away from the mass lesion.

Herniation of cerebral tissues may occur if increased intracranial pressure (which causes shifting of the brain) becomes severe. The cingulate gyrus is particularly susceptible to herniation under the edge of the falx cerebri. The medial portion of the temporal lobe, especially the uncus and hippocampal gyrus, may become pressed against the side of the midbrain, causing damage to these structures, and the entire process may lead to tentorial herniation.

Tentorial Herniation

Tentorial herniation results from compression and expansion of the brain. The most commonly recognized form of tentorial herniation (referred to as lateral or uncal tentorial herniation) occurs when the uncus and medial portion of the hippocampal gyrus bulge and herniate over the free edge of the tentorium, compressing the midbrain and possibly the opposite cerebral peduncle against the tentorial edge on the other side of the brain. Damage to the opposite cerebral peduncle may, in fact, cause ipsilateral hemiparesis, a condition sometimes seen in cases of chronic subdural hematoma. Herniation of the brain may also impair the function of the oculomotor nerve and cause infarction of the posterior cerebral artery. Involvement of the posterior cerebral artery may in turn cause damage to the ipsilateral medial occipital cortex.

Clinically, when lateral tentorial herniation occurs, the patient may show an additional impairment of consciousness, contralateral (or sometimes ipsilateral) hemiparesis that may progress to a state of decerebrate rigidity, and ipsilateral pupillary dilatation accompanied by loss of the pupillary response to light and loss of extraocular movements other than abduction. Expanding lesions of the temporal lobe are most likely to produce this clinical picture.

Posterior tentorial herniation may occur in patients with bilateral cerebral lesions or lesions restricted to the frontal or occipital areas. In these cases, herniation of medial temporal areas is more posterior in location or on both sides so that the herniated tissue affects the quadrigeminal plate at the level of the superior colliculi rather than involving the oculomotor nerve and the posterior cerebral artery. Clinically, these patients appear drowsy; their eyes are closed or partly closed as a result of bilateral ptosis, and when the eyelids are raised it is apparent that upward gaze is defective. The pupil's responsiveness to light is usually preserved.

When lateral or posterior tentorial herniation occurs the entire brain stem is shifted downward toward the foramen magnum, a condition referred to as *central or axial herniation of the brain stem.* This downward shift of the brain stem results in stretching and elongation of branches of the basilar artery which in turn may produce ischemia and hemorrhage. The patient may demonstrate arterial hypertension, bradycardia, and irregular respiration. Mechanical distortion of the lower brain stem and brain compression may also contribute to this clinical response. In addition, stretching of the oculomotor nerves may also occur, producing the type of response that is frequently seen with lateral tentorial herniation.

Tonsillar herniation may occur following tentorial herniation if supratentorial compression continues to increase or if the expanding mass lesion is located below the tentorium. In this condition the cerebellar tonsils are forced through the foramen magnum, obliterating the cisterna magna and compressing the medulla oblangata. Clinically this is manifested by apnea. When the tentorial opening is small it is likely that indications of tentorial herniation may be prominent and the patient may show little evidence of tonsillar herniation. However, when the tentorial opening is large and the tentorium can be displaced downward, tonsillar herniation may occur with little prior indication of a tentorial herniation. In such instances temporal lobe swelling, as a secondary response to head injury, may result in rather sudden symptoms of apnea.

Increased Intracranial Pressure

Increased intracranial pressure is a frequent complication of head injury, resulting from space-occupying lesions such as epidural hematoma, subdural hematoma, contusion, or swelling. In a series of fatal head injuries that included a large proportion of patients with intracranial hematoma, Adams (1975) found that 83% of the victims had increased intracranial pressure. Miller, Becker, Ward, et al. (1977) reported that as many as 30% of patients with diffuse brain damage also have unequivocal intracranial hypertension. Many factors and their interactions lead to increased intracranial pressure.

The basic cause of increased intracranial pressure in cases of head injury is a pathological increase in volume occurring within the relatively fixed confinement of the skull. These volume increases interact with the brain's potential for accommodation, which is represented by displacement of cerebrospinal fluid and venous blood and the capacity of brain tissue to stretch in response to volume increases.

Pathological volume increases are influenced by (1) the amount of blood in a hematoma or contusion; (2) the volume of blood contained in distended veins in the congested, swollen brain (engorgement of cerebral vessels); (3) the amount of extracellular fluid around a contusion in brain edema; and (4) the volume of swollen cells in areas of ischemic or necrotic brain tissue.

In the early stages these pathological increases in volume cause relatively little increase in intracranial hypertension because of the effectiveness of the displacement mechanisms. In other words, the cerebrospinal fluid and venous blood may be displaced by the bleeding or swelling with relative maintenance of normal pressure. However, as the accommodation mechanism is exhausted, pressure begins to increase in an accelerating fashion. At this point the elastic properties of the brain (the capacity of brain tissue to stretch) represents an additional factor and the inflexibility of the brain contributes to even greater increased hypertension. The elastic properties of the brain may be influenced by a number of factors, including a rise in blood pressure.

These various mechanisms causing intracranial hypertension are superimposed on the production, absorption, total volume and flow characteristics of the cerebrospinal fluid (Reitan & Wolfson, 1985b), arterial pressure, local cerebral metabolism, and intrathoracic pressure, as well as the tissue alterations caused by the injury itself. Obviously, many variables are significant in the production of intracranial hypertension following head injury. These variables may interact in a number of ways and lead to the interindividual variability that is observed.

Adams and Graham (1976) have studied the relationship of premorbid increased intracranial pressure and autopsy findings. These researchers consistently found an area of tissue necrosis along the line of the edge of the tentorium in one or both parahippocampal gyri. Some patients also have evidence of necrosis in the cingulate gyrus and infarction of the medial occipital cortex. One question that has arisen is, What are the effects of intracranial hypertension alone compared to the effects of brain herniation or shift or distortion of the brain stem? Many patients with sharply elevated intracranial pressure show relatively few focal neurological signs despite symptoms of headache, vomiting, drowsiness, bradycardia, arterial hypertension, and irregular respiration.

The interaction of brain herniation, brain stem shift, and intracranial pressure is complex, intertwined, and difficult to dissociate. Brain herniation may cause a loss or reduction of transmission of pressure gradients between the cranial and spinal compartments. In addition, supratentorial lesions (the most common) may also alter pressure gradients in the supratentorial (as compared with infratentorial) and spinal compartments.

Although it has generally been thought that brain shift or distortion results from pressure gradients from the mass lesion — and this almost certainly is a significant factor — research studies have failed to demonstrate that pressure gradients (supratentorial, infratentorial, and spinal compartments) have a very striking influence on brain shift. However, large pressure variations occur in the supratentorial, infratentorial, and spinal compartments (across the divisions of the tentorium and the foramen magnum), with the supratentorial compartment being principally affected by pressure increase. The results of these various investigations suggest that intracranial pressure by itself has less effect on neurological status than intracranial pressure combined with brain shift and distortion.

Intracranial hypertension may also impair neurological status by reducing cerebral blood flow. In some patients with head injury, intracranial pressure may increase to the point that it is equivalent to arterial pressure and this situation may reduce cerebral perfusion pressure to zero. The result is a sharp reduction of cerebral blood flow and eventual impairment of neuronal function. These circumstances are sometimes responsible for a patient's sudden deterioration of neurological status.

Factors which contribute to reduced cerebral flow as a result of intracranial hypertension include disrupted local and general levels of oxygen metabolism of the brain, changes in arterial pressure, impaired autoregulatory mechanisms of cerebral blood flow occurring on either a general or focal basis (Reitan & Wolfson, 1985b) and brain edema. Thus, a number of factors may influence maintenance of cerebral perfusion levels in patients with head injury. The interaction of these variables is quite complex, and clinical studies have shown a wide range of cerebral blood flow levels in individual patients. However, when intracranial pressure is strikingly increased, cerebral blood flow falls below normal levels in almost all cases. A very important clinical problem in the management of patients with severe head injury concerns reduction of intracranial hypertension when cerebral blood flow is compromised.

Brain Ischemia Following Head Injury

Ischemia refers to a deficiency or impairment of blood supply; ischemic necrosis is the death of tissue caused by a deficiency of blood supply. Ischemic lesions occur very frequently in the brains of persons with severe head injury and are due to a number of causes. Brain shift may produce lesions of the anterior or posterior cerebral arteries (especially with lateral tentorial herniation, described above) as well as vascular damage of the brain stem. Severe intracranial hypertension may also be a factor, interacting with arterial pressure and failure to maintain adequate cerebral blood perfusion. Ischemia may also be produced by brain edema. Arterial spasm has also been implicated in the production of focal brain ischemia and anemia due to blood loss and hypoxemia resulting from inadequate oxygenation.

It is apparent that many of these factors may co-exist and have complementary effects in producing neurological deficit or death. For example, secondary pathology within the brain may make brain structures quite vulnerable. Damage to the brain tissue can result from even relatively minor reductions of arterial pressure which otherwise would not have a very profound effect. In addition, the brain's excellent autoregulatory functions of maintaining cerebral blood flow may also be compromised by minor changes of arterial pressure (Reitan & Wolfson, 1985b).

While ischemic brain damage due to infarction, occlusion, hemorrhage and fat embolism has long been recognized, more recent evidence has indicated that generalized neuronal necrosis and other types of infarctions also occur commonly. In detailed pathological studies of 100 consecutive head injuries, Graham and Adams (1971) found ischemic foci in the cerebral cortex of 46% and

ischemic foci in the basal ganglia and hippocampus in 80% of head-injured cases.

Graham, Adams, and Doyle (1978) performed a similar investigation in 151 consecutive cases and found evidence of ischemic damage in 91%. They found focal cerebral lesions in the cortex (46%), basal ganglia (79%), hippocampus (81%), and cerebellum (44%). Obviously, many individual brains had multiple lesions and the ischemic lesions were usually widespread. Ischemic lesions of the medial occipital cortex were found in 33% of the patients and each of these patients also had hypoxic lesions elsewhere in the brain. The boundary zone between the major cerebral arteries were affected in 54% of the cases and infarcts in the distribution of the anterior or middle cerebral arteries were found in 27% of the subjects and were bilateral in nearly half of the cases. Instances of neocortical necrosis that appeared to be associated with episodes of cardiac arrest occurred in 11% of the patients.

Post-Traumatic Hydrocephalus

Hydrocephalus is a condition characterized by an abnormal increase in the amount of cerebrospinal fluid. There are three types of hydrocephalus that may occur following head injury. The first type, *ex vacuo,* results from atrophy of the white matter of the brain after severe injury. The second type, *obstructive,* results when the normal flow of cerebrospinal fluid is obstructed. *Normal pressure hydrocephalus,* the third type, is less well understood in terms of etiology; it usually develops weeks or months after a head injury.

Hydrocephalus ex vacuo appears to occur when shearing damage of the white matter results in wasting of cerebral tissue. Although rare, obstructive hydrocephalus may be a reaction of fibrosis and scarring between the pia and the arachnoid, resulting from blood in the subarachnoid space, much in the same way that fibrosis results from purulent meningitis and occludes the subarachnoid and cisternal cerebrospinal fluid pathways

(Reitan & Wolfson, 1985b). In some instances obstructive hydrocephalus will resolve spontaneously following head injury; in other cases it is necessary to treat the condition surgically, using a shunting procedure to bypass the obstruction.

Injuries that penetrate the ventricles occasionally result in intraventricular scars which may also cause hydrocephalus. Displacement of brain structures may also limit the flow of cerebrospinal fluid, particularly when transtentorial herniation has occurred.

The mechanism of normal pressure hydrocephalus is unknown, although it has been postulated that the first stage of the process is an initial period of increased intraventricular pressure resulting in dilatation of the ventricles. When the pressure returns to normal, the cerebral ventricles are enlarged and the patient shows clinical signs of hydrocephalus even though the intracranial pressure is within normal limits.

Types of Secondary Damage

Intracranial Hemorrhage

Bleeding within the brain sometimes occurs as a complication of blunt head injury in the patient who has recovered consciousness after a severe injury or, in some instances, has sustained only a minor impact or damage. Intracranial hemorrhage may become a life-threatening situation within a matter of hours and may require rapid surgical intervention.

Intracranial hematoma may be classified according to the location in which the bleeding occurs (epidural, subdural, subarachnoid, intracerebral, or intraventricular) or, in some instances, by the amount of time elapsed since the injury (acute, subacute, or chronic). There is no close agreement concerning the time frame used by various authors. In general, acute lesions develop within one to three days after the injury; chronic lesions have been present for more than two to three weeks;

subacute lesions are those that occur in the intervening period.

Approximately 70% of hematomas (particularly subdural) are diagnosed and surgically evacuated within three days of the injury: 50% within the first 24 hours and 20% within the next two days. Within the first two weeks most hematomas can be removed through burr holes. After two weeks most clots have solidified and a craniotomy must be performed to remove them.

The frequency with which different types of hematomas occur is distinctly related to chronological age. Extradural hematomas occur frequently (about 40%) in persons under 20 years of age; bleeding below the dura mater occurs more commonly in people aged 30 to 50 years. Although hematomas are classified according to the level of the brain involved, it must be emphasized that there is a considerable degree of overlap. For example, while pure subdural hematomas may occur (i.e., without underlying cortical laceration), they are frequently a combination of subdural bleeding and an intracerebral clot with cortical lacerations. Lesions classified principally as epidural in location also often have intradural components. Hematomas occur bilaterally in approximately one-third of cases.

Teasdale and Galbraith (1981) have reviewed reports from a number of investigators regarding the differential frequency of various types of traumatic hematomas and have found that (1) epidural hematomas are slightly more common than epidural plus intradural hematomas, with the total of these locations representing approximately 20% of all cases; (2) subdural and subdural plus intracerebral lesions are approximately equivalent in frequency in about 70% of the total; and (3) instances of bleeding limited to intracerebral locations constitute the remaining 10% of hematomas. Only 2%–3% of hematomas following head injury are in the posterior fossa.

It has been estimated that nearly 50% of patients who develop intracranial hemorrhage following a head injury were not unconscious immediately after the injury; however, most patients who have a subdural hematoma in combination with intracerebral bleeding did experience a period of unconsciousness. In cases of pure extradural, subdural, or intracerebral hematoma, over 80% of the patients reportedly showed some degree of decreased alertness and awareness, as manifested by impaired verbal communication following the injury (Jamieson & Yelland, 1968).

Although patterns of consciousness vary among individual patients, the possibility of intracranial bleeding should always be considered whenever a patient demonstrates a progressively deteriorating level of consciousness. Sometimes a progressive weakening of the contralateral lens also occurs and headache, vomiting and nuchal rigidity are frequently reported symptoms. A clinical diagnosis of developing hematoma is difficult to make accurately.

Epidural Hematoma

An epidural hematoma is a collection of blood between the skull and the dura mater. In the majority of cases epidural hematomas are caused by traumatic injury of the middle meningeal artery. Bleeding from this artery (and sometimes two or three of its accompanying veins) is almost always unilateral and causes a separation of the dura from the internal table of the skull as the hematoma enlarges. Depressed skull fractures and penetrating injuries of the skull can also sever arteries or veins and result in epidural bleeding.

Depending upon the fracture (deformation) of the skull and the branch of the middle meningeal artery that is torn, epidural hematomas may be frontal, temporal, or occipital-parietal in location. The most common site is the temporal area (50%–60% of all cases). As noted previously, epidural hematomas occur most frequently in males with a median age of 24 years. These lesions occur

in approximately 1%–3% of head-injured patients and in a substantially greater number when the injury is fatal.

The size and weight of the hematoma may vary considerably and is related to the ultimate damage that results. For example, as the size and weight of the hematoma increases there is a greater likelihood of herniation of the uncus and hippocampus under the edge of the tentorium. Rapidly developing hematomas, even if small, may cause sudden compression of the brain and result in death; slowly developing lesions are associated with less pronounced signs of brain dysfunction. The majority of patients who develop an epidural hematoma have a skull fracture, but there is no evidence of fracture in approximately 10% of the cases. Fractures that cross the middle meningeal groove or a dural sinus or show evidence of depression in the parietal-temporal area are frequently associated with an epidural hematoma.

Although a considerable degree of interindividual variability exists, Bakay and Glasauer (1980) have described the typical course of events in patients who develop an epidural hematoma. Initially the patient is unconscious; he regains consciousness for 1 to 24 hours, and then relapses into a comatose state. During the episode of regained consciousness the patient shows a progression of signs and symptoms, the most significant of which is a gradual impairment of consciousness. Other frequent symptoms include headache, restlessness, nausea, vomiting, dizziness, and confusion. Epileptic seizures sometimes occur before the patient progresses into a comatose state. Additional focal neurological signs, stemming particularly from the location of the lesion, may also develop during this so-called lucid interval.

Cerebral angiography was frequently used in the past because of its accuracy in diagnosing epidural hematomas. Computed tomography is now being used more commonly and demonstrates an epidural hematoma as a hyperdense shadow, usually having a crescent shape. In addition, the CT scan may also identify other types of intracranial pathology.

The mortality rate in cases of epidural hematoma is reported to be about 27% (McKissock, Taylor, Bloom, & Till, 1960).

Subdural Hematoma

A subdural hematoma is an area of bleeding into the subdural space. Such bleeding is usually caused by linear and rotational acceleration which results in a tear in a venous channel. Most instances of severe head injury have some subdural bleeding as well as some accumulation of blood in the subarachnoid space. Bleeding in the subdural space is associated with many types of brain injury; however, when the bleeding in the subdural space is sufficiently extensive to act as a compressive lesion on the brain, subdural hematomas are usually associated with closed head injuries. Subdural hematomas occur in approximately 1% of all head injuries, although in severe brain injuries the incidence has been reported to be much higher.

Subdural hematomas are almost always associated with trauma to the head, although the injury may be relatively slight (particularly among older people). Bleeding in the subdural space appears to occur more frequently with frontal or occipital blows rather than with impact to the side of the head. Subdural hematomas are mainly venous in origin and therefore often develop more slowly than epidural hematomas.

It has been estimated that subdural hematomas are present in about 25% of all penetrating head wounds, although small subdural clots are probably present in nearly all such injuries. Although open fractures of the skull involving the dural sinuses may result in extensive subdural bleeding, there are many instances in which subdural hematomas form without a skull fracture. These lesions have been frequently reported in whiplash injuries, resulting from tearing of cortical veins where they enter the more stable tissues of the dural sinuses (Ommaya & Yarnell, 1969).

In some instances, small cortical veins are torn as a result of tensile and shearing stresses caused by rotation of the head and movement of the brain within the skull. The brain damage associated with these injuries may be mild and following surgical evacuation of the subdural hematoma the patient may show only minimal evidence of neuropsychological deficit.

The most common cause of subdural hematomas is hemorrhagic contusion of the cerebral cortex, which is usually associated with lacerations of the arachnoid and dura as well as cortical tissue. These patients generally have severe, diffuse brain injury. The subdural hematoma forms adjacent to the damaged and necrotic brain tissue and is often continuous with an intracerebral hematoma. Therefore, many subdural hematomas are associated with severe focal damage of the cerebral cortex and diffuse involvement of the white matter, cerebral edema, and an interaction of cerebral edema with pressure and midline shifts resulting from the space-occupying hemorrhage. These patients may demonstrate significant neuropsychological deficits.

Contusions of the brain, seen in conjunction with subdural hematomas, frequently involve the frontal-temporal junction, the orbital surfaces of the frontal lobes, and the frontal and/or temporal poles. The most common site of subdural hematomas is in the center of the convex surface of the hemisphere in the frontal-temporal-parietal region. The hemorrhage most commonly occurs over the upper part of the hemisphere, but the bleeding may spread diffusely over the entire hemisphere. These lesions are usually unilateral, but various investigators have reported them to be bilateral in 15%–35% of the cases.

Clinical signs and symptoms of subdural hematomas are quite variable, undoubtedly because of the differing degree of intracranial damage which is associated with these lesions. Petechial hemorrhages, large cerebral clots, epidural hematomas, and subarachnoid hemorrhages have been reported in 24% of patients with subdural hematomas (Jamieson & Yelland, 1972). Thus, these additional lesions, plus any cerebral displacement and herniation that may have occurred, produce most of the clinical manifestations.

Chronic subdural hematomas are often not recognized in older persons and are frequently misdiagnosed as a primary neuronal degenerative disease, such as Alzheimer's disease. It appears that even a minor blow may cause a subdural hematoma, especially among older people. The decreased brain bulk in these persons may allow the hematoma to become quite large before any significant increase in intracranial pressure occurs. In addition, a slowly progressive hematoma tends to give the brain time to adjust to the increased volume without producing clinical symptoms until the hematoma has reached a large size. Thus, even though the patient may show considerable higher-level deterioration, the lesion can cause severe distortion and displacement of brain structures before any significant increase in intracranial pressure can be detected.

The overall mortality rate in subdural hematomas has been quite variably reported, ranging from 22% to 69% (Johnson & Sinkler, 1961).

Subarachnoid Hemorrhage

Bleeding into the subarachnoid space generally arises from damage to the superficial cortical vessels and contusions over the orbital surface of the frontal lobes and the tips of the temporal lobes. As with other instances of intracranial bleeding resulting from trauma, subarachnoid hemorrhage is frequently associated with subdural bleeding or brain laceration.

Subarachnoid hemorrhage (and resulting blood in the cerebrospinal fluid) is a very common form of intracranial bleeding. Traumatic subarachnoid hemorrhage is usually diffuse and thin and does not generally form a specific, space-occupying lesion. Even relatively minor head injuries showing no apparent damage to the skull or cerebral tissue may lead to subarachnoid hemorrhage and ultimately result in death. Such instances have frequently been associated with minor head injuries sustained by persons who are acutely intoxicated (Simonsen, 1963).

Even though autopsy examinations of these patients indicated that an abnormal vessel had bled in 20%, the source of bleeding was not demonstrable in most of the remaining subjects and raises the question of whether an increase of blood pressure and dilatation of cerebral arteries in alcoholic intoxication was a precipitating factor. In subarachnoid hemorrhages the blood is usually diluted by the cerebrospinal fluid and removed by phagocytic action. Patients with subarachnoid bleeding clinically show symptoms of severe headache, restlessness, nuchal rigidity, elevated temperature and Kernig's sign (inability to extend the leg completely when lying down with the thigh flexed upon the abdomen; a sign of meningeal irritation).

Subarachnoid hemorrhage usually does not require any specific treatment; however, it may lead to at least temporary hydrocephalus, which occurs as a result of impaired cerebrospinal fluid flow due to fibrosis of the meninges.

Intracerebral Hematoma

Intracerebral hematomas represent bleeding within the substance of the brain tissue. On the basis of autopsy studies, Courville (1962) classified intracerebral hematomas according to the type of injury.

The first category includes hematomas caused by a depressed skull fracture and laceration of the brain. In such injuries tissue damage and in-driven bone fragments may cause extensive damage, tear vessels, and result in an accumulation of blood that forms a separate clot.

Courville's second category is represented by hematomas caused by a penetrating wound in which the blood clot lies in the path of penetration (usually toward the end of the path).

The third classification encompasses hematomas resulting from acceleration or deceleration closed head injuries. In these cases the bleeding may be associated with contusions either toward the surface of the cerebral tissue or deep in the white matter.

Intracerebral hematomas had previously been considered to be a severe complication of head injury; however, computed tomography scans of the brain have shown that these lesions occur quite often, even though estimates are variable. Intracerebral hematomas may be single or multiple. They can be located subcortically or deep in the white matter, and may act as expanding lesions or, in some cases, be remarkably silent in their demonstration of symptoms.

The mechanisms by which subdural hematomas are produced relate principally to penetration, movement of brain tissue following a head injury, and pressure forces (including rotational acceleration). These lesions are more commonly seen in instances in which a discrete blow applies force over a relatively small area of the head, including missile injuries, perforating wounds, and depressed skull fractures.

Although blunt head injuries more commonly cause subdural or epidural hematomas, in some instances they may also lead to intracerebral bleeding. Damage to a major vessel (such as a branch of the middle cerebral artery) is the cause of intracerebral bleeding only in a minority of instances. In most cases the bleeding occurs as a result of rupture of small vessels within the brain tissue in a manner similar to the bleeding associated with cerebral contusions.

Intracerebral hematomas are most frequently located in the frontal or temporal areas, but may also occur in the cerebellum and brain stem. Intracerebral hematomas resulting from frontal or temporal lacerations often include some element of subdural hematoma as well. When in the frontal lobes, these lesions are most often caused by blows to the occipital area and much less frequently by direct frontal impact. Blows to the side of the head are more frequently associated with intracerebral hematomas in the temporal and parietal areas. In many cases, intracerebral bleeding is at the point or in the path of penetration; however, in closed head injuries, approximately two-thirds of intracerebral lesions are caused by contrecoup mechanisms (Adams, 1975). Surgical evacuation is the treatment of choice but, as with other vascular lesions, intracerebral hematomas may resolve spontaneously, leaving a scar formed by glia and connective tissues. Large intracerebral hematomas may eventually result in intracerebral cysts.

The general sequence of events in patients who have traumatic intracerebral hematoma is (1) loss of consciousness for at least a short period of time following the injury; (2) a lucid interval later followed by stupor, disorientation, irritability, agitated restlessness, and even aggressiveness. Careful clinical monitoring of the patient is necessary because intracerebral hematomas may be rapidly expansive and cause additional secondary damage associated with increased intracranial pressure and brain herniation and may lead to death. Depending upon the location of the lesion, focal neurological signs may be elicited in persons whose state of consciousness permits clinical examination.

Intraventricular Hemorrhage

Traumatic intraventricular hemorrhage, which usually resulted in death, had previously been recognized only in instances of massive rupture of large intracerebral hematomas into the ventricular system. It has also been recognized that penetrating wounds of the brain, with a missile track crossing aspects of the ventricular system, may also cause bleeding into the ventricles. However, computed tomography scans have shown that intraventricular hematomas are not rare and may occur in patients who have sustained even relatively minor head injuries and only mild impairment. In these instances the bleeding may originate in the ventricular walls and not be associated with any massive injury elsewhere in the brain. In such instances intraventricular hemorrhage does not cause any known specific neurological signs.

Computed tomography scanning clearly shows the fresh blood in the ventricular system in contrast with the low density cerebrospinal fluid. There may be some enlargement of the lateral ventricles in instances in which an intracerebral clot has partially escaped into the ventricle, although such instances may not be associated with any displacement of brain structures. Intraventricular clots usually liquefy and become absorbed in time; therefore, they are rarely evacuated using surgical procedures.

Brain Edema

Brain edema (excess fluid in the brain) is a frequent complication of head injury. If the edema is extensive, intracranial pressure may be sharply increased. This in turn may lead to transtentorial and cerebellar herniations. Increased intracranial pressure may also lead to a decrease in cerebral blood flow as well as impairment in the electrical excitability of neurons and glia. In conjunction with other adverse effects, edema is one of the most common causes of death in head-injured patients.

Brain edema results from circumstances that cause accumulation of excess water in the brain tissue. The water content of normal gray matter is approximately 80%, and in the white matter, where the fat content is higher, approximately 70%.

There are a number of types of cerebral edema, depending upon their cause (Klatzo, 1967). *Vasogenic edema* is the type principally associated with head injury. In this condition the source of excess water is the bloodstream and results from damage to capillaries as well as larger arteries and veins. Cerebral edema is customarily associated with cerebral contusion and the multiple small hemorrhages in the contused area allow the flow of fluid into the extracellular space. The arterial pressure therefore becomes a significant factor in

the degree of cerebral edema; increased arterial pressure leads to an increase in edema.

Although a contusion may be located principally in the gray matter, it is not uncommon to see no widespread cerebral edema in the cerebral cortex. This appears to be due to the compactness of tissue in the gray matter. However, plasma from the wound in the cerebral cortex gradually oozes into the white matter and spreads the myelin sheaths, which are easily separated by mechanical force. The fluid may gradually extend into the white matter and involve an extensive area.

Although edema following head injury is usually found in the area of contusions and hematomas, it may spread more generally and involve an entire lobe or hemisphere or even both hemispheres. Although the principal outflow is to the extracellular space, studies using electron microscopy have shown that the excess fluid is located both within (intracellular) and between (extracellular) cells (Lee & Bakay, 1966).

The areas principally affected by cerebral edema correspond with the areas most frequently involved in cerebral contusions, namely, the poles of the frontal and temporal lobes and the orbital surface of the frontal lobes where the brain may be injured against the internal table or bony prominences of the skull. With lateral blows to the head, edema may be more prominent in the contralateral cerebral hemisphere, just as contusion may result from contrecoup injury. Larger and more generalized contusions, as well as penetrating injuries (particularly from high-velocity missiles) lead to diffuse edema involving the entire brain.

CT scans frequently show areas of decreased density, most prominently represented by the contusion and radiating out from the affected area. Extensive cerebral edema can develop within a few hours post-injury and continue for weeks, but in most instances the process is maximal from about the first to third day post-injury and then gradually subsides.

Brain Infections

Brain infections following head injury may be focal (epidural, subdural, or intracerebral abscess) or generalized (meningitis, tetanus).

Epidural abscesses are usually associated with a penetrating injury of the head and an accumulation of pus or infected granulation tissue between the skull and the dura mater. These infections, which are not usually apparent until the wound has completely healed, are characterized by progressive fever, headache, and increased lethargy. Increased intracranial pressure will eventually develop and, depending upon the location of the lesion, focal neurological signs may become evident.

Epidural abscesses can be identified by computed tomography scans and have an appearance similar to epidural hematomas. The dura serves as an effective barrier against infection of the brain tissue, but in some instances the infection may spread through the dura and into the brain tissue. Treatment consists of surgical evacuation of the lesion and systemic antibiotic treatment.

As with epidural abscesses, subdural abscesses are rare complications of head injury but occur particularly when a compound wound of the brain is not properly debrided soon after the injury. Subdural abscesses are more commonly seen as a complication of severe sinusitis. These infections spread much more widely than epidural abscesses and meningitis is also frequently present. Swelling of the brain may occur concomitantly and lead to additional disadvantages of brain compression. In these cases the mortality rate is over 30%. Computed tomography is effective in making the diagnosis and cerebral angiography may also be helpful. Acute subdural abscesses are considered to be one of the most imperative neurosurgical emergency conditions because of the potential for rapidly developing brain edema, increasing intracranial pressure, and ultimately, death.

Intracerebral abscesses are generally associated with penetrating head wounds having indriven hair, bone fragments, or foreign bodies. Under these conditions, preventing an abscess depends upon early operation, complete removal of in-driven tissue and foreign bodies, debridement of necrotic and contaminated tissue, tight closure of the dura, and skin closure without excessive tension.

As with subdural abscesses, intracerebral abscesses lead to edema and expansion of the surrounding white matter with increased intracranial pressure, possible herniation of the brain, and deficits related to these complications. Once the abscess has developed, surgical evacuation is necessary.

It should be noted that most brain abscesses occur with depressed skull fractures and penetrating injuries in which contaminated material has been driven into the brain. They tend to occur rarely with brain wounds caused by high-velocity missile fragments, apparently because the penetrating materials in these instances are rendered sterile by the heat of explosion (Bakay & Glasauer, 1980).

Meningitis, a rare complication of head trauma, sometimes occurs in cases of compound skull fracture and is frequently associated with leakage of cerebrospinal fluid. When meningitis develops it usually occurs within two weeks of the injury. Clinically it is characterized by headache, vomiting, fever, irritability, and varying degrees of impaired consciousness (the usual signs of meningeal irritation). The complications of traumatic meningitis may be quite serious and the mortality rate is estimated to be 30% or higher.

Tetanus involving the brain is rare but may occur in penetrating injuries of the head. The prognosis is poor and the mortality rate is high.

Osteomyelitis of the skull is another condition that may occur in cases of head injury and lead to brain infection.

V

ADDITIONAL INSULTS
TO THE BRAIN

Birth Injuries

A great number of adverse events may influence brain structure, function, and development of the fetus, including such factors as maternal alcoholism (which may result in the fetal alcohol syndrome). In addition, there may be traumatic insult to the fetus resulting from many unidentified sources. In some instances external impact to the maternal abdomen results in blunt injury or penetration of the fetus' head. However, these prenatal events are rarely documented in detail, and damage to the cranium and brain occurs more commonly during the birth process.

Frequently an extensive molding of the fetal skull results from cephalic rotation and compression forces during labor. If permanent damage to the brain occurs, the pathology is frequently vascular in nature and is represented by intracranial hemorrhage. Recent findings have suggested that trauma as a cause of brain damage at birth has probably been overestimated; nevertheless, such injuries appear to be responsible for about 10% of the deaths that occur at birth.

Factors pre-disposing the fetus to cerebral damage include abnormal presentations, precipitated delivery, prolonged labor, and the use of obstetric forceps. Trauma to the head of the neonate may impair function of the respiratory center in the medulla oblongata and result in respiratory irregularity and periods of apnea. Therefore, anoxia is viewed as the major factor complicating the effects of trauma at the time of birth and subsequent cerebral damage is often due to the effects of anoxia rather than the initial trauma.

The use of forceps and other obstetric maneuvers may cause direct injury to the head and brain as well as excessive compression or molding of the head within the birth canal during labor. Skull fracture is usually due to the use of forceps or excessive pressure to the head during breech extraction. Dural tears may occur and the brain may actually herniate through the fracture site, eventually resulting in the formation of scar tissue and ventricular dilatation (which is more likely to be on the side underlying the damaged brain). Such lesions frequently serve as an epileptogenic focus later in life.

Epidural hemorrhage, a rare condition, may occur in association with a linear fracture of the skull that tears the middle meningeal vessels. Subdural hemorrhage is usually the result of tearing of venous sinuses or of the great vein of Galen. Subarachnoid hemorrhage is common in the newborn but is relatively asymptomatic and the blood is absorbed during the first several weeks of life. Large intracerebral hemorrhages are uncommon and usually result from obvious and severe head trauma.

The majority of infants who suffer traumatic brain injury at birth are reported to develop normally, but careful studies in this regard have been difficult to accomplish. Even small cerebral hemorrhages in the neonate may result in the formation of a porencephalic cyst and depending upon their size and severity, such lesions may be a major factor in limiting normal brain development. Glial scars (particularly involving the temporal lobes) in conditions that have resulted in tentorial herniation may cause impaired intellectual and cognitive development as well as partial complex epilepsy.

Although some studies have reported favorable results with respect to intellectual development after head injury in children (Bruce, Shute, Bruno, Wood, & Sutton, 1978; Fuld & Fisher, 1977), these studies have not been based upon careful and complete neuropsychological evaluation. The reports of eventual unimpaired functioning have used a criterion of whether or not the neonatal injury was sufficient to cause death or whether the child was eventually able to function within the broad limits of normality. Based upon clinical neuropsychological experience, it would appear probable that brain injuries at birth produce more significant and serious intraindividual impairment of potential for normal development than has presently been documented.

Fat Embolism of the Brain

Multiple fat emboli of the cerebrovasculature, a rare complication in patients who suffer fractures of the major long bones of the body, can occasionally develop from extensive soft-tissue injuries even though fractures are not present. Symptoms usually begin one to two days after the injury and are characterized by fever, rapid pulse, a progressive deterioration of consciousness, and signs of respiratory distress, including increased respiration rate, dyspnea, and increased bronchial secretion.

Cerebral edema is commonly due to increased intracranial pressure. Focal neurological signs are unusual and pupillary responses customarily remain normal, even though epileptic seizures sometimes occur. Cerebral fat embolism may be fatal and, in severe cases, carries a high mortality rate.

Air Embolism

Introduction of air into the blood circulation is an uncommon occurrence but has been reported during cardiac surgery, cerebral arteriography, cardiac catheterization, thoracic surgery, and neurosurgical repair of highly vascular tumors. In the conscious patient symptoms include lightheadedness, vertigo, respiratory difficulties, pallor, and sometimes, cyanosis.

When air enters the pulmonary vein or the arterial system, air emboli may be present in many organs. The episode may involve epileptic seizures, focal signs, increasing stupor, coma, and eventually, death. However, the usual course is one of steady improvement even though permanent and irreversible damage to the brain can result.

Electrical Injury

Electrical energy can cause significant damage to the tissues of the body. From the point of contact to the point of exit electrical current always flows via the shortest path of least resistance: spinal fluid, blood vessels and nerves.

Alternating current is considerably more dangerous than direct current and 60-cycle alternating current is particularly dangerous to the heart and respiratory centers. Death may occur if the electrical current passes through the respiratory center of the brain. If the patient survives such an episode, anoxic encephalopathy may be present throughout the central nervous system. In addition, inflammatory changes of blood vessels and meninges, as well as brain tissue, may result. Subarachnoid hemorrhage or thrombosis of vessels may occur within the areas of infarcted tissue. Electrical current resulting in proliferation of microglial cells and replacement by gliosis may cause direct injury to cerebral neurons.

Obviously, the severity of electrical injuries ranges from minimal to severe and may result in death. Neuropsychological evaluation has demonstrated evidence of significant brain impairment in patients who have sustained severe electrical burns; mild injuries of this type may cause no cognitive deficit whatsoever.

Radiation Injury

Irradiation of the head may result in serious damage to the central nervous system and cause long-term impairment. This has been particularly apparent among children who require prophylactic radiation of the head as a treatment for acute lymphocytic leukemia. An increase in the incidence of epilepsy, learning disability, and other kinds of impairment related to brain function has been reported in these children.

Information regarding the effects of irradiation have been derived from studies of patients who have undergone this type of treatment, and the pathological changes to the brain include atrophy with loss of neurons, proliferation of astrocytes, and the presence of macrophages filled with lipid material. White matter may show evidence of demyelination, though axons are relatively well preserved. Blood vessels which have been irradiated tend to have an increase of collagen, causing thickening and endothelial proliferation which may, in extreme cases, actually obliterate the lumen of the vessel.

VI

CLINICAL AND SPECIAL NEUROLOGICAL METHODS OF EVALUATION

Clinical Neurological Evaluation

Neurosurgeons, who customarily perform the initial examination of head-injured patients, agree that clinical neurological examination fails to identify the effects of head injury in many cases. Becker, Miller, Young, et al. (1982) state, "If based solely on the neurological examination, an accurate prognosis in the first hours after injury is limited." Bakay and Glasauer (1980) say, "An accurate diagnosis cannot be made on the basis of the physical examination alone, except on rare occasions."

Initial examination of patients with head injuries requires identification of brain injury and abnormal brain function as quickly as possible in order to determine the appropriate and necessary therapy and to identify mass lesions that require surgical intervention before secondary damage occurs. In the initial examination the neurosurgeon determines which additional special diagnostic procedures should be performed to accurately determine the patient's condition. Many various diagnostic procedures were used in the past, but they have been largely superseded by computed tomography.

To a large degree, the patient's status determines the extent to which a complete neurological examination can be performed. It is usually possible to do a thorough neurological examination if the patient is alert and cooperative. Regardless of the patient's condition, the Glasgow Coma Scale (described below) can be completed because the patient's reactions are rated from "completely normal" to "no response." However, the Glasgow Coma Scale is concerned essentially only with eye opening, motor response, and verbal response, and additional neurological and medical information is obviously needed to completely assess the head-injured individual.

In the initial examination of the head-injured patient the clinician notes the size of the pupils, their equality or inequality, and the presence or absence of reflex response to light. Normally, the pupil constricts sharply when exposed to a bright light and dilates in response to reduced luminous flux. There are two sets of muscles in the iris (the structure that surrounds the pupil, which is only an open space). When the concentric muscles contract they cause diminution (constriction) of the pupillary space; when the radial muscles contract they enlarge (dilate) the pupillary space.

The actions of these two sets of muscles are differentially controlled by sympathetic and parasympathetic pathways within the autonomic nervous system. Therefore, the predominance of one set of pathways (the parasympathetic pupillary constrictor mechanism or the sympathetic dilatation mechanism) in response to injury represents information about intracranial function.

The pupillary light reflex results from stimulation of ganglion cells in the retina with impulses traveling through the optic nerves and to the optic tracts. The reflex pathways bypass the lateral geniculate body and synapse in the nuclei of the pretectum of the posterior diencephalic area, with connections to the Edinger-Westphal nuclei on both sides. Normally, stimulation of one eye with light results in constriction of the pupil of the stimulated eye (which is referred to as the ipsilateral or direct response) as well as the other eye (referred to as the contralateral or consensual response).

Depending upon the location of the damage, various pupillary abnormalities may be observed. Midbrain damage, which frequently occurs in head injuries, produces a dilated and fixed pupil on one or both sides. Lesions involving the third cranial (oculomotor) nerve between the nucleus and the point at which it emerges from the brain stem results in a widely dilated, fixed pupil either on one or both sides. A widely recognized sign of temporal lobe herniation is mild dilation of the pupil and a corresponding sluggish pupillary light response. Pontine lesions interrupt descending sympathetic pathways and result in constricted pupils. Thus, in cases of severe head injury, the size of the pupils and their reaction to light may yield important information regarding underlying brain damage.

Traumatic damage to the third (oculomotor) nerve may be diagnosed by (1) dilated pupils occurring since the time of injury; (2) improving level of consciousness; and (3) weakness of the appropriate extrinsic musculature of the eye. Bilateral dilated and fixed pupils may also be the result of inadequate cerebral vascular perfusion caused by significant elevation of intracranial pressure or hypotension due to blood loss.

Evaluation of abnormal eye movements can also provide considerable information regarding brain injury. If the patient is awake and alert the examination can be performed in response to simple commands and the integrity of the full range of eye movements representing the functional state of the ocular motor system in the brain can be assessed.

In patients who are comatose or in a state of partially depressed consciousness, it may not be possible to depend upon voluntary responses. In these cases, the examination is performed by eliciting oculocephalic or oculovestibular responses. The oculocephalic reflex is elicited by raising the head approximately 30 degrees from the supine position and rapidly rotating the head back and forth. It is sometimes necessary to retract the eyelids manually in order to observe movements of the eyeballs. The normal response of the eyeballs is to maintain their position in space by moving opposite to the rotation of the head. If this reflex response is absent or impaired ("Doll's eyes"), it may be a result of impaired consciousness but usually represents severe midbrain damage.

The oculovestibular reflex is an eye movement response to caloric stimulation of the oculovestibular pathways. This reflex is elicited by injecting cold water into the ear canal while holding the patient's head at about a 30 degree elevation. Normal response to this stimulation is eye movements toward the source of stimulation. A complete absence of eye movements is an indication of severe brain stem dysfunction.

Observation of the position of the eyes of an unconscious patient may also show a lack of conjugation or divergent positioning of the globes. This finding may also signal a brain stem lesion or may be due to damage to nerves that supply the eye muscles. If the eyes deviate toward the side of the brain lesion, contralateral to the side of hemiparesis or hemiplegia, a destructive lesion, possibly in the frontal lobe, may be present. Vertical conjugate gaze is sometimes affected and most often is represented by limitation of upward gaze. This deficit is associated with damage at the junction of the midbrain and diencephalon.

Finally, the initial clinical examination of the head-injured patient should include a brief examination of motor functions. In patients with impaired consciousness, responses to painful stimuli should be observed and recorded. When the patient is sufficiently alert and able to cooperate, motor strength of each extremity should be evaluated and is customarily graded according to normal strength, moderate weakness, severe weakness (insufficient strength to resist gravitational forces), trace movements, and complete paralysis.

When the patient has regained consciousness, alertness, and is able to at least follow simple commands, it is possible to perform the conventional neurological examination. The full details of this examination are described in several sources, including DeMyer (1980) and Talbert (1982) and the content of the examination (including its relationship to neuropsychological evaluation) has been discussed in a recent publication (Reitan & Wolfson 1985b).

In brief, the clinical neurological examination includes evaluation of strength, tone, and fine coordination of the limbs; sensory functions; deep tendon and pathological reflexes; and cerebellar functions. Special attention is given to evaluation of the function of the cranial nerves.

Certain aspects of the clinical neurological examination are emphasized in patients with head injury. Serial examinations are often performed because of changes over time as the patient manifests recovery. Careful examination of the external surface of the head may reveal information concerning skull fracture. The cranial nerves are examined carefully in order to assess olfaction, vision, ocular motility, tactile sensation of the face, equilibrium and hearing, and movement capabilities generally. Tests of visual acuity as well as of the visual fields

are also conducted. Even though it is frequently normal even in cases of severe head injury, careful examination is made of the ocular fundus because sometimes there are indications of intraretinal hemorrhages or papilledema. Various types of traumatic retinopathies have been reported.

The neurological examination also attempts to gain information about aspects of neuropsychological functioning, including memory, speech and language disorders. Attempts are made to determine the presence and duration of *retrograde amnesia* (loss of memory for events prior to the injury) and *anterograde amnesia* (inability to remember events following the injury even after having regained consciousness). In this latter instance it is difficult to separate impairment of consciousness from amnesia following recovery of consciousness. *Post-traumatic amnesia* is a more general term and refers to the interval extending from the time of injury until the complete return of continuous memory functions.

Relationships of Neurological and Neuropsychological Evaluation Following Head Injury

In studies directed toward evaluating the comparative frequency and significance of neurological (physical) and neuropsychological (intellectual, cognitive, and emotional) deficits following head injuries, the results have consistently indicated that neuropsychological losses are of greater significance. Jennett and Teasdale (1981) reported that the physical disability was more prominent than mental losses in only about 25% of the 150 head-injured patients in their study. In more than half of these patients the mental component of disability was judged to be of more limiting significance than physical or neurological deficits (Jennett, Snoek, Bond, & Brooks, 1981).

Other researchers compared physical and mental impairment with regard to social adjustment, including evaluations of work capacity, leisure activities, cohesiveness in the family relationship, and sexual activity (Bond & Brooks, 1976). They found that both types of impairment contribute to handicapped social functions but mental deficits contributed more strikingly to overall social handicap. Considering the fact that these studies were based upon a rather incomplete neuropsychological assessment, the results are all the more striking in their suggestion that higher-level aspects of brain function are of particular importance in determining the eventual recovery and outcome for the individual patient.

The conventional description of neurological deficits among head-injured patients customarily includes hemiplegia, facial weakness, sensory losses (particularly including vision, hearing, and smell), other cranial nerve deficits, dysarthria, and dysphasia. Dysphasia is usually identified only briefly and in rather gross terms, occasionally including notation of specific dysphasic deficits such as dyslexia, dyscalculia, dysgraphia, and dysnomia. More detailed evaluations to identify dysphasia in head-injured patients have usually not been done and have not been related specifically to intellectual and cognitive deficits. There is no doubt, however, that such losses are of definite significance (Reitan, 1984).

The neurological description of neuropsychological deficits is usually given in rather impressionistic terms. Following a head injury sufficiently severe to produce significant coma, initially the patient is generally confused as he begins to recover from the state of impaired consciousness and experiences a period of post-traumatic amnesia (inability to recall events occurring between the time consciousness was lost and the regaining of continuous memory functions).

Some investigators have emphasized that intellectual deficits are not uncommon in patients following the period of post-traumatic amnesia. There have been some generalizations stating that verbal abilities are less severely affected than performance abilities and that verbal abilities also recover more rapidly. In fact, Jennett and Teasdale

(1981) cite Adams (1963) and Jennett (1977) to support their conclusion that verbal intelligence recovers within three to six months (to the extent that recovery is possible) whereas performance intelligence continues to improve for a year or more. Such statements are obviously gross generalizations and have limited meaning for individual patients. For example, verbal intelligence may be much more significantly impaired in patients with left cerebral damage, a finding that has been documented for many years (Reitan, 1955b). The pattern of recovery is also variable for individual subjects, and even demonstrates a biphasic pattern in persons who have sustained cerebral contusion or definite damage of brain tissue (Reitan & Wolfson, in press). Thus, the particular details of relationships between variables that describe the brain lesion and the neuropsychological losses and recovery pattern represent an intricate and complex problem that still needs further elucidation.

Nevertheless, descriptions of intellectual and cognitive impairment, based upon clinical observation rather than detailed neuropsychological testing, is often described as consisting of some degree of intellectual deficit, possible aphasic losses, and various kinds of impairment in the area of memory, attention, and concentration. An additional area of psychological (as contrasted with neurological) loss concerns impaired emotional control and "personality change." Rage responses are not uncommon and have been attributed to temporal lobe damage, particularly involving the amygdaloid nucleus and resulting in a type of epileptic attack. However, this type of epilepsy following head injury is quite rare.

Some patients demonstrate a deterioration in personal hygiene habits, show a loss of insight, impaired ability to persevere and follow through on tasks in everyday living, and general loss of efficiency. It is not uncommon for behavioral changes of this kind to be classified as a psychiatric disorder. Evaluation based upon such relatively gross descriptions of the patient's behavior are not fundamental to the underlying disorder.

Careful neuropsychological assessment shows that many of these deficits are, in fact, related to basic intellectual and cognitive impairment, particularly when one extends the definition of intellectual impairment to go beyond the types of measures included in the Wechsler Scales to include concepts such as those proposed by Halstead (1947) in his description of biological intelligence. More specifically, many of the so-called behavioral or psychiatric disorders are a reflection of impaired insight, understanding, abstraction ability, and ability to understand complex situations in terms of cause-and-effect relationships. In fact, abilities of this type constitute the principal aspect of higher-level brain functions and their impairment results in frank and obvious changes in everyday behavior, even though the underlying deficit is rather subtle and not easily observed.

The neuropsychological deficits demonstrated by persons with a head injury are extremely varied and may involve, differentially or generally, any of the major categories of neuropsychological functioning. It is necessary to perform a complete neuropsychological evaluation of the individual patient in order to understand brain-related strengths and weaknesses. It has been shown repeatedly that the Wechsler Scale — which was devised for assessment of *normal* intelligence — is not adequate (either in terms of range of coverage or methodological approaches) to provide a complete assessment of intellectual and cognitive (neuropsychological) functions for the individual subject.

Reitan and Wolfson (1985a) have presented a conceptualization of brain-behavior relationships that recognizes initially the importance of input (receptor or sensory) variables as well as output (effector or motor) manifestations. (See Chapter 9 for a description of this model.) Obviously, without input to the brain, higher-level brain functions would be meaningless. Correspondingly, unless there is a response element present to represent central processing functions, the higher-level activities of the brain cannot be discerned.

The principal aspects of neuropsychological functioning, however, are represented by central processing that intervenes between input and output. The nature of the these central processing functions has been discerned and classified through study of thousands of individual brain-damaged persons. This is the procedure that has been developed to validate the content and organization of the Halstead-Reitan Battery, testing the results out with individual cases in order to determine whether the test findings accurately reflected the independently obtained neurological information regarding the biological condition of the brain (Reitan & Wolfson, 1985a).

Studies of this kind have indicated that three major areas constitute higher-level brain functions involved in central processing. These include (1) language and verbal abilities (particularly dependent upon the status of the left cerebral hemisphere); (2) visual-spatial, temporal-sequential, and manipulatory abilities (principally dependent upon the right cerebral hemisphere); (3) and abilities in the area of abstraction, reasoning, and logical analysis (which are diffusely distributed throughout the cerebral cortex).

Brain injuries show a tremendous degree of variability, and neuropsychological generalized conclusions about "brain injury" are difficult to support if they involve any degree of specificity. In turn, developing an understanding of the effects of craniocerebral trauma (contrasted with other biologically impairing conditions of the brain) requires comparisons among these various types of damage. Such considerations of neuropsychological deficit with outcome and recovery are sufficiently complex to be considered in detail in a separate volume (Reitan & Wolfson, in press).

Cranial Nerve Deficits

In closed head injuries it is likely that the cerebral hemispheres are principally involved, with lesions represented by contusions, diffuse damage involving the cerebral cortex, and stress and tension effects resulting in shearing lesions of the white matter. Sensory and motor deficits obviously may be affected by cerebral lesions. The nuclei of cranial nerves III through XII, however, lie below the level of the cerebral hemispheres and involvement of these nerves frequently results from secondary damage following head injury.

Impairment of cranial nerve function has received detailed review and evaluation in a number of publications (Fishbone, 1976; Potter & Braakman, 1976; Roberts, 1976; Summer, 1976; Toglia & Katinsky, 1976; Van Vliet, 1976). The reader is referred to these sources in the *Handbook of Clinical Neurology* for more detailed information. In addition, Walpole (1966) has reviewed the effects of injury on the visual pathways and the cranial nerves.

As noted earlier, certain functions of cranial nerves III, IV and VI should be evaluated during the initial examination of the head-injured patient. Even though spontaneous recovery of functions governed by the cranial nerves often occurs, persisting deficits can constitute significant impairment. The damage to cranial nerves may occur at their nuclei (principally in the brain stem) or at their receptor cells. Cranial nerve damage may also result from increased intracranial pressure, by direct injury to the nerves or their blood supply, or as a result of meningeal infection. As noted earlier, the cranial nerve functions of the comatose patient can be examined in certain respects, but a complete neurological examination requires the patient's cooperation and response to the examiner's requests.

Olfactory Function (Cranial Nerve I)

Jennett and Teasdale (1981) report that partial or complete loss of olfactory sensitivity is seen in about 7% of patients admitted to the hospital with a head injury. Damage to the olfactory nerve occurs commonly with relatively mild injuries and the incidence increases with more serious head trauma. Most patients with impaired olfactory sensitivity have sustained a skull fracture (most often frontal) and about 50% of patients having rhinorrhea of cerebrospinal fluid (resulting from fractures involving the frontal sinuses) have anosmia.

Most patients with impaired olfactory sensitivity due to head injuries recovery rather promptly; however, complete recovery is unlikely if the deficit has persisted for two months or more. Patients often report distortion of their olfactory sense during the recovery period.

Appreciation of odors and the taste of food are greatly affected by the functional status of the first cranial nerve. Since subjective appreciation of tastes as well as smell is involved, deficits resulting from damage of the first cranial nerve may have substantial significance.

Optic Nerve (Cranial Nerve II)

Optic nerve damage has been reported to occur in nearly 2% of persons with significant head injuries (Russell, 1960). Damage may involve the optic nerve directly or other parts of the visual system. Impairment ranges from complete blindness to loss of any of the dimensions of functional vision. Recovery frequently occurs within a few days or weeks but failure to show improvement within one month suggests the possibility of permanent impairment. Scotomata of the visual fields are not uncommon and may vary from very small to large areas. The patient with scotomata may notice no significant visual impairment unless injury has occurred to the part of the retina that subserves macular or central vision.

Injuries to the optic nerve are more common in instances of frontal or temporal blows. Bilateral injuries to the optic nerves are rare in instances of closed head injury. Partial impairment of visual function resulting from injury to the optic nerve is more common than complete blindness. Primary optic atrophy often follows blindness that has lasted from three to six weeks and if atrophy occurs vision may be permanently lost.

Homonymous visual field losses imply the presence of a lesion behind the optic chiasm and therefore do not necessarily involve the optic nerves directly.

The Nerves Concerned with Oculomotor Function (Cranial Nerves III, IV, and VI)

Signs of injury to the oculomotor nerve, involving abnormal eye movements, are common in the acute stages of head injury but usually recover rather promptly. The symptoms consist of dilatation of the pupil, loss of reaction to light, and impaired accommodation of the pupil for vision at various distances. However, the symptoms occur without impairment of distant vision, although impairment of extraocular muscular function may limit upward, downward, and inward movement of the eye (which is usually turned laterally).

Third nerve dysfunction often occurs with a fracture of the anterior fossa involving the sphenoid bone and may also indicate an injury to the cavernous sinus or a tentorial herniation. Thus, the damage to the third nerve may be due to direct impact or represent secondary damage. In over 75% of the cases recovery usually occurs within two to three months; however, the impairment is likely to be permanent if the deficit persists for six months or more. Dysfunction of the oculomotor nerve (III) usually occurs without signs of damage to the trochlear (IV) or abducens (VI) nerves, but in individual instances there may be signs of involvement of all three of these nerves.

Diplopia is a frequent complaint following head injury, but there may be many causes for double vision that do not necessarily involve the brain. Damage to the orbit, either directly or as a result of fracture of neighboring bones, may put pressure on the eye and result in diplopia.

Damage to the trochlear nerve is usually associated with fracture of the sphenoid bone. When this nerve alone is involved the patient has double vision with downward gaze.

Damage of the abducens nerve (VI) results in impaired lateral movement and an orbit which is turned inward. With less severe damage the only symptom may be diplopia when the patient attempts to look laterally.

Unilateral involvement of cranial nerve VI is somewhat more common than bilateral impairment. This nerve has a long intracranial course, rendering it more susceptible to irritation from an accumulation of blood in the subarachnoid space, increased intracranial pressure, or meningitis. Damage to the abducens nerve is usually accompanied by fracture of the middle fossa near the petrous area. Recovery of function of the abducens nerve after head injury is good in most cases, even though several months may be required for complete return of function.

Trigeminal Nerve (Cranial Nerve V)

Injury to the trigeminal nerve may be associated with intracranial damage, but deficits involving this nerve more commonly result from crushing injuries to the face and skull. Damage to the supraorbital and infraorbital branches are the most common and often cause numbness over the forehead. The usual course is one of gradual improvement without any specific treatment. The patient may experience severe neuralgia during the course of regeneration of damaged nerve fibers.

Facial Nerve (Cranial Nerve VII)

The facial nerve is injured in about 3% of all significant head injuries (Russell, 1960). The damage may be superficial and occurs in about 20% of patients who demonstrate bleeding from the ear on the same side. More commonly, however, damage to this nerve is associated with fractures of the middle fossa involving the petrous and mastoid areas. Symptoms are represented by weakness or paralysis of the facial muscles. The facial palsy often is delayed in development and does not occur for a number of days following injury, presumably resulting from edema within or around the nerve.

Complete recovery occurs in approximately 75% of patients, partial recovery in 15%, and permanent paralysis in 10%, usually being complete within six to eight weeks after the injury. Recovery is much more common when there is an initial delay of one to two weeks in onset of the facial paralysis after the injury. In cases of facial nerve paresis that occur more promptly, there is a greater likelihood of total transsection of the nerve or more severe damage.

Auditory Nerve (Cranial Nerve VIII)

Hearing impairment is not uncommon among patients who sustain head injuries. The loss is often due to accumulation of blood in the middle ear, resulting principally in a conductive type of deafness. The hemorrhage gradually resolves and hearing improves correspondingly, usually leaving minimal or little disability.

Tinnitus, a constant buzzing or ringing auditory experience, also occurs after head injury and appears to result from damage to the auditory nerve, the labyrinth, or the blood supply to the auditory apparatus. Tinnitus is quite variable in its intensity, nature of the sensation, and duration. At present, no effective treatment is available.

Vertigo and dizziness are also frequent manifestations of closed head injury. They are often associated with significant hearing losses because of the close relationship between the cochlear and vestibular branches of the VIIIth nerve and may be caused by hemorrhage in the labyrinth or direct damage to the vestibular nerve. Vertigo may also result from brain stem injury and in some cases may be sufficiently severe to cause vomiting and horizontal nystagmus. Severe vertigo may be relieved by vestibular suppressant drugs. The symptom usually subsides slowly over a three to four week period.

Glossopharyngeal, Vagus, Spinal Accessory, and Hypoglossal Nerves (Cranial Nerves IX, X, XI, and XII)

Damage to these nerves occasionally occurs in association with fracture of the posterior fossa. However, dysfunction of cranial nerves IX, X, XI, and XII occurs more commonly with extracranial gunshot wounds. Damage to these nerves includes a range of symptoms, including difficulty swallowing, loss of taste on the posterior third of the tongue, partial paralysis of the palate and vocal cord, weakness of the trapezius and sternocleidomastoid muscles, and weakness or paralysis of one side of the tongue.

When the hypoglossal nerve is damaged and causes impairment of tongue movement, enunciation is sometimes impaired. In clinical examination it is important to differentiate between the slurring of speech caused by such peripheral damage and the dysarthria associated with dysphasia (omission of syllables, addition of syllables, or transposition of syllables in enunciation of multisyllabic words) secondary to a cerebral lesion (Reitan, 1984).

Cerebrospinal Fluid Rhinorrhea and Otorrhea

Cerebrospinal fluid rhinorrhea and otorrhea represent drainage of cerebrospinal fluid through the nose and ear, respectively. This occurs because of tears in the dura and is usually associated with fracture of bones of the skull. Cerebrospinal fluid rhinorrhea is usually secondary to a fracture of the frontal bone and adjacent sinuses; cerebrospinal otorrhea customarily occurs in conjunction with a fracture of the petrous ridge of the temporal bone extending into the middle ear. The tympanic membrane is also perforated in these cases, permitting the cerebrospinal fluid to drain from the ear.

In some cases fractures of the middle fossa involve the petrous bone and lead to cerebrospinal fluid drainage via the eustachian tube into the pharynx. Facial fractures are present in approximately 30% of cases of cerebrospinal fluid rhinorrhea. In some cases of cerebrospinal fluid otorrhea the cerebrospinal fluid passes into the middle ear behind an intact tympanic membrane and is referred to as the "closed" variety.

When the tympanic membrane is torn, cerebrospinal fluid otorrhea is obvious as a drainage from the external auditory canal. When the membrane is intact, the fluid is visible through the tympanic membrane.

The onset of these conditions nearly always occurs within two days after traumatic head injury. In some instances, however, there may be a delay of a few weeks before the drainage becomes apparent. Anosmia occurs rather commonly with cerebrospinal fluid rhinorrhea.

Leakage of cerebrospinal fluid through either the nose or ear is a serious complication of head injury because there is a relatively high risk of meningitis occurring concurrently. The probability of infection is increased when the leak persists for more than a week. Meningitis is less likely to occur when the drainage is obvious and continuous; it is more likely to occur when draining is minimal and variable.

Leakage of cerebrospinal fluid after a head injury often stops spontaneously in about one week. However, in about 50% of cases it continues for as long as six months. In some instances it becomes necessary to repair the lesion surgically.

Assessment of Coma and Impaired Consciousness

Impairment of consciousness is a common result of head injury and has been studied for many years as a possible indicator of the degree of cerebral damage (Symonds, 1928). There has been a considerable problem, however, in defining loss of consciousness and in assessing the impaired state with some reasonable degree of consistency. In the individual case the duration of unconsciousness (or impaired consciousness) has varied according to the criteria used.

Although the degree and duration of coma has some significance concerning the severity of brain damage, many patients sustain extensive and severe damage without any loss of consciousness at all. This latter situation occurs most frequently in cases of compound depressed fractures and open head injuries. Therefore, duration of coma may be more closely related to severity of diffuse rather than focal brain damage.

The need for a practical scale using well-defined terms for assessment of coma led to the development of the Glasgow Coma Scale (Jennett & Teasdale, 1977; Teasdale & Jennett, 1974; Teasdale & Jennett, 1976). This scale is based upon simple, observable responses of the patient, factors which allow consistency of ratings between observers. However, the simplified nature of the scale limits its value as any type of comprehensive assessment procedure.

Jennett and Teasdale (1981) point out that the Glasgow Coma Scale is based upon the definition they have offered of coma, and this consists of (1) not obeying verbal commands; (2) not saying any words; and (3) not opening the eyes.

Plum and Posner (1980) have presented a much more extensive consideration of the factors associated with stupor and coma and believe that the cause of impaired consciousness and the site of the responsible lesion are principally reflected by five physiological functions: (1) pupillary reaction; (2) eye movements; (3) ocular reflexes; (4) motor response; and (5) breathing patterns.

Jennett and Teasdale (1981) state that the Glasgow Coma Scale, considered alone, does not adequately describe brain function in the comatose patient but does enable the clinician to define the degree and type of of coma in descriptive terms and allows assessment to be repeated continuously in order to evaluate changes in the degree of impairment of consciousness.

On the Glasgow Coma Scale eye opening is evaluated on 4-point scale ranging from failure to open the eyes under any circumstances (1 point) to spontaneous opening (4 points). Intermediate positions on this scale are eye opening in response to a painful stimulus (2 points) and eye opening by the patient only when spoken to, though not necessarily on command to open the eyes (3 points).

Motor response is graded on a 6-point scale ranging from obeying responses appropriately (6 points) to no motor response whatsoever (1 point). Jennett and Teasdale note that they have avoided descriptive classifications such as "purposeful," "decerebrate," and "decorticate" in describing limb movements and no reference is made to muscle tone.

An emphasis has been made to establish standardized procedures and to observe specific responses, rather than to require interpretation. Thus, if there is some limitation of motor responsiveness, two standardized stimuli are used: pressure on the nail bed using a pencil and supraorbital pressure. If the patient's hand moves above the chin when the supraorbital response is delivered, the movement is scored as a localized response (5 points).

If there is only a flexor withdrawal response without movement toward the source of the pain, a score of 4 points is recorded. If there is preceding extension movement in either arm or leg or if two responses occur among alternatives of stereotype flexion posture, extreme wrist flexion, abduction of the upper arm, or flexion of the fingers over the thumb, an abnormal spastic flexion response is scored (3 points). If only a response of extension at the elbow occurs a score of 2 points is recorded.

Finally, complete absence of motor movement in response to painful stimuli is recorded as a score of 1 point. Sometimes more than one type of response may be observed in a single examination; in this case the score for the *best* motor response

is recorded, since the best response has been found to correlate most closely with eventual outcome.

Evaluation of verbal responsiveness is rated on a 5-point scale. A total absence of verbalization under any circumstances is rated as 1 point and normal verbal responsiveness and conversation rate as 5 points. Confusion in conversation is rated as 4 points; use of inappropriate words which are not related to the existing situation are rated as 3 points; grunts, groans, and incomprehensible sounds, even though in response to verbalization by the examiner, are rated as 2 points; complete absence of vocalization, which might possibly be associated with global aphasia, receives a score of 1 point.

The possible range of scores on the Glasgow Coma Scale is from 3 (no eye opening, motor response, or verbal response) to 15 (normal responsiveness in each of the three areas). A number of investigations regarding outcome have used the Glasgow Coma Scale as an independent variable and these results are summarized in Volume II of *Traumatic Brain Injury* (Reitan & Wolfson, in press).

Special Diagnostic Procedures

Computed Tomography

Computed tomography has been hailed by neurosurgeons as having an unparalleled impact on diagnosis and treatment of the head-injured patient. Bakay and Glasauer (1980) say, "Computed tomography is the single most informative diagnostic modality in the evaluation of the patient with a head injury. The availability of CT scanning has drastically changed the management of patients in institutions where the scanner is available."

Jennett and Teasdale (1981) comment, "Since computer tomography was developed in Britain by Hounsfield and applied in a London neurosurgical unit by Ambrose, the strategy of investigation for suspected intracranial conditions has been revolutionized. The availability of CT scanning alters the clinical approach not only to investigation but to management as a whole. Indeed, it might be said that there are now two kinds of head injury care: with and without CT scanning."

Becker, Miller, Young, et al. (1982) indicate that computed tomography ". . . has revolutionized the diagnostic evaluation of intracranial disorders in general and traumatic intracranial lesions in particular. Computed tomography is a noninvasive technique and requires only 30 minutes to study the entire intracranial cavity with the first-generation scanner manufactured by EMI Medical, Inc. With its unique ability to detect the subtle differences in soft-tissue density, computed tomography proved valuable in detecting various traumatic intracranial lesions: intra- and extracerebral hematomas, infarctions, edema, contusions, and the like."

It is obvious that CT scanning makes a tremendous contribution to the diagnosis of intracranial damage following head trauma, is routinely preferable in initial evaluation to other diagnostic procedures, and is supplemented by other diagnostic studies only when special problems and conditions are present. In fact, Jennett and Teasdale (1981) stress the fact that the clinician must not lose sight of the standard diagnostic evaluation because there are still many hospitals in which CT scanning is not available.

For the neurosurgeon, CT scanning fills a very significant role, particularly because it can provide almost immediate information regarding the presence of space-occupying lesions that may require prompt surgical intervention. Frequently CT scans can also identify other conditions that can be treated in order to minimize further secondary damage of the brain.

However, the situation is quite different for the neuropsychologist. First, space-occupying lesions and structural tissue damage (which is readily identified by CT scanning) have reached a stabilized condition by the time the patient is available for neuropsychological examination. Secondly, CT scanning is within normal limits in a considerable number of persons who have sustained a significant head injury. In many cases the CT scan does not identify extensive small lesions throughout the brain tissue that are commonly present (see section above on diffuse brain damage).

The method of evaluation that is most sensitive to both focal and diffuse damage in the head-injured patient is neuropsychological testing. The domain of evidence produced by neuropsychological evaluation is of additional significance because it relates to the important aspects of behavior concerned with the quality of living, including intellectual and cognitive functions represented by reasoning, abstraction, logical analysis, verbal communication and language functions, adaptability to temporal, sequential, and spatial needs, etc. Neuropsychological evaluation is able to identify the significant cognitive deficits which require remediation in order to help the patient achieve a normal quality of life.

Realistically, brain re-training programs should be based upon neuropsychological findings rather than computed tomography, electroencephalography, or other neurological diagnostic techniques. CT scanning and other neurological diagnostic techniques deal with a different domain of evidence than neuropsychological evaluation, even though the procedures in each area are equally concerned with evaluation of the status of the brain. In neuropsychology, behavior is examined and then inferentially related to the condition of the brain. Neurological diagnostic techniques are farther removed from any behavioral implications, but require less of an inference (i.e., they are more directly representative) of structural aspects of the brain. Physiological monitoring procedures — such as evaluation of cerebral blood flow, cerebral metabolism, and biochemical markers of brain function — represent an intermediate position between structural brain pathology and neuropsychological deficits.

One may postulate that neuropsychological evaluation reflects the consequences of structural cerebral damage and physiological, electrical, and biochemical alterations. In this sense, the many approaches to identification and evaluation of impaired brain structure and function should be viewed as having a complementary role in the integrated understanding of the individual human being.

There are two attributes of computed tomography which contribute to its value in the early examination of patients with head injury. The first of these relates to the ability to differentiate blood from brain tissue and thereby permit diagnosis of intracerebral and extracerebral bleeding.

Second, the CT scan can demonstrate compression of the ventricles and displacement of midline structures which may result from trauma. Thus, on CT scans abnormalities are represented by areas of increased or reduced density, unusually small or large ventricles, or lateral displacement of brain structures. It is beyond the scope of this volume to describe the appearance of individual types of lesions; however, CT scanning has been shown to be very effective in identifying cerebral contusion, intracerebral hematoma, subdural hematoma, epidural hematoma, intraventricular hematoma, the evolution of a hematoma shown by repeated scans, subarachnoid hemorrhage, cerebral edema, hydrocephalus, post-traumatic infarction, abscess, atrophy and cyst formation.

Displacement of brain structures suggests the possibility of a local mass lesion. The lateral ventricles of the brain may be displaced to one side or there may be obliteration of part of one ventricle. With mass lesions the interventricular septum is more often displaced than other midline structures.

The size of the ventricles also provides clues regarding structural brain damage. Following head injury in children, the ventricles are often abnormally small (slit-like) and are sometimes almost invisible. Ventricles that are abnormally large may indicate the presence of a lesion obstructing flow of cerebrospinal fluid, such as a hematoma in the posterior fossa. Of course, the person may have had abnormally large ventricles before the head injury.

The literature has often reported that older people and chronic alcoholics frequently have large ventricles. Enlargement of only one ventricle is often a sign of a contralateral hematoma. In some cases ventricular enlargement is seen some weeks after the injury, particularly in patients with cerebral atrophy resulting from severe diffuse injury. The pineal gland and choroid plexuses in the lateral ventricles are sometimes calcified and are seen on the CT scan as white areas. Their visibility permits evaluation of any displacement associated with the effects of a mass lesion.

As noted above, CT scans are interpreted essentially with respect to indications of abnormally increased or reduced density. Though increased density may be due to calcification or the presence of foreign bodies, it usually indicates an area of hemorrhage. In cerebral contusion, abnormalities are represented by poorly defined areas of mottled density and points or dots of high density mixed with areas of normal brain density, and a surrounding area of edema which has low density. This picture appears to represent minute areas of focal hemorrhage in the brain. With extensive areas of reduced density, representing widespread edema, the ventricles may be extremely depressed in size and possibly not even visible on the scan. Brain infarcts are also less dense than normal tissue and hemorrhagic areas show a reduced density which may gradually improve in time or show permanent residual effects.

Interpretation of the individual scan must consider density abnormalities as well as ventricular shift. When the CT scan demonstrates positive evidence of damage shortly after head injury, it is highly unusual that a corresponding lesion will not be present. Undoubtedly, a small number of false-negative scans occur, possibly due to movement artifacts during the scanning procedure or lesions that are difficult to visualize. CT scans have now made it possible to identify the presence of lesions following head injury and follow their course and resolution. Previously such diagnoses were usually inferred indirectly on the basis of clinical examination or x-rays based on angiography and encephalography. Nevertheless, despite CT scanning's usefulness, it should be remembered that a substantial proportion of persons with significant head injury have normal scans.

A number of studies have been done to determine the frequency of abnormal findings in CT scans in head-injured patients. Becker, Miller, Young, et al. (1982) state that these reports range from 37% (Baker, Campbell, Houser, et al., 1974) to 73% (Paxton & Ambrose, 1974). Obviously the results will depend (at least in part) on the patient's symptoms, the severity of the head injury, and other factors.

French and Dublin (1977) studied 1000 consecutive head-injured subjects and obtained CT scans on 316. Fifty-one percent of these subjects had abnormal CT findings and most of these persons had evidence of more than one lesion. Eighty-five percent of the patients who had impaired consciousness as well as focal neurological signs showed CT abnormalities. Of the patients who were alert and neurologically intact, only 13% had abnormal CT scans. However, it should be noted that in this study nearly 50% of the patients who had abnormal motor activity or were in a deep comatose state also had normal scans.

Other researchers reported that CT scan abnormalities were present in 75% of patients who showed lateralizing findings on neurological examination (Merino, deVillasante & Taveras, 1976). In another study of 140 patients with severe head injury, Sweet, Miller, Lipper et al. (1978) found

abnormal CT scans in 82% of the victims, all of whom had mass lesions, bleeding, or edema.

These findings indicate that completely heterogeneous groups of brain-injured persons do not provide a very meaningful test of the number of false-positives and false-negatives associated with CT scanning. On the other hand, it is clear that many head-injured patients show abnormalities on the CT scan, principally represented by space-occupying lesions and cerebral edema. It appears that approximately 33% of the persons who sustain severe brain injury have no intracranial bleeding and have perfectly normal CT scans. Clinical experience and correlation at autopsy show that severe hypoxic brain damage or severe diffuse damage to the white matter may have occurred in patients who have normal scans. Thus, as pointed out by Jennett and Teasdale (1982), a normal CT scan does not exclude the possibility of either primary or secondary severe brain damage.

Because of the incidence of false-negative CT findings, most authorities recommend that the results of the CT scan be correlated with the clinical findings in order to avoid errors. There are a number of technical and procedural factors that may lead to inadequate CT scanning and errors may occur in the interpretation of the scan. Some injuries, including contusions and hemorrhage within the substance of the midbrain, are rarely recognized on a CT scan.

Finally, it should be emphasized that CT scans reveal areas of specific tissue damage and are far less useful in diagnosing small lesions in the white matter, although there is some evidence suggesting that a CT scan, together with clinical evaluation, may add to increased knowledge, even concerning these lesions (Zimmerman, Bilaniuk, & Gennarelli, 1978).

Cerebral Angiography

If computed tomography is available, cerebral angiography is generally not done to evaluate the effects of head injury. However, computed tomography has certain limitations in its ability to demonstrate isodense lesions and does not fully show the vascular damage that results in many cases of head injury. Often, angiography can identify the exact location and nature of the vascular lesion more accurately. This is particularly true in instances in which an underlying vascular lesion (such as an arteriovenous malformation or aneurysm) is present and may have actually precipitated the accident that caused the head injury. Angiography usually outlines extradural and subdural hematomas, but CT scans also do this very well.

Cerebral angiography should be used to supplement computed tomography in certain instances: if vascular injury is suspected; if the patient shows focal neurological deficits and the CT scan is normal; if the CT findings do not correlate with other aspects of the patient's clinical condition; or if there is reason to suspect that there are isodense lesions that are not visualized adequately on CT scans. Cerebral angiography is limited in its ability to differentiate between an intracerebral hematoma and a cerebral contusion, but this differentiation is achieved readily by CT scanning. In addition, even with skilled clinicians, cerebral angiography carries a small but definite risk of potentially serious complications.

Identification of abnormalities by cerebral angiography is based principally upon evidence of vascular displacement, avascular areas, abnormalities of the time required for the contrast material to pass through the brain, and vascular spasm. Vascular displacement, or abnormal positioning of the vessels, may indicate a supratentorial mass, transtentorial herniation, or an infratentorial mass. However, there may be no shift or displacement of vessels even when mass lesions are present.

Avascular areas usually indicate the presence of a hematoma in patients with recent head injuries, but may also represent infarction. It is often difficult to determine whether the avascular lesion is on the surface or in the brain tissue. Clots at the vertex as well as those in the subfrontal areas are also often difficult to detect. Nevertheless, certain angiographic findings, based on relationships and configurations of vessels and other structures, are reliable indicators of certain lesions.

The time required for contrast fluid to reach venous channels on angiograms provides information regarding reduced cerebral blood flow. Such a reduction may be caused by increased intracranial pressure or systemic hypotension. Vascular spasm, represented as irregular narrowing of segments of the cerebral arteries, is seen in many head-injured patients who have subarachnoid bleeding. Vascular spasm may occur in association with relatively focal cortical contusions, but more often affects the proximal portions of the major cerebral arteries and vessels of the circle of Willis.

Skull X-Rays

Since the advent of CT scanning some researchers have questioned the usefulness of skull x-rays; however, many linear fractures not demonstrated on the CT scan are revealed by x-rays. Although it has little significance concerning immediate management of the patient, the possibility of intracranial hematoma (possibly developing at some time after the head injury), is increased when a skull fracture is present. Thus, a linear skull fracture, demonstrated by x-ray, may indicate the need to consider repeated CT scanning or suggest the need for close clinical observation.

Radionuclide Brain Scans

Radioisotopic imaging is useful in identifying relatively late complications of head injury, such as a chronic subdural hematoma or hydrocephalus. If the subdural hematoma is in a phase during which the density of the hematoma is extremely similar to that of underlying brain tissue, the lesion may be demonstrated quite clearly by the radio-nuclide scan and not well (if at all) on the CT scan. It should also be recognized that contusions of the skull and fractures of the cranial vault may result in abnormal concentrations of isotopes on the peripheral portion of the head and result in inaccurate interpretations.

Echoencephalography

This procedure directs pulses of ultrasound into the cranial cavity. Internal structures can be imaged and positioned by recording the waves (echos) reflected from the skull.

Research on this procedure has shown rather variable and unreliable results. It appears that echoencephalography must be done by a highly skilled and experienced person in order to achieve clinically dependable results. CT scans are much more reliable in identifying mass lesions and providing information about their localization and composition. Since the availability of CT scanning, echoencephalography has not been widely used in assessment of acute head injury.

Pneumoencephalography and Ventriculography

These procedures are not used very frequently to evaluate the effects of acute head injury. In fact, pneumoencephalography is contraindicated when intracranial pressure is increased, a condition common in patients with head trauma. Late effects of head injury, including cerebral atrophy, cyst formation, and asymmetry of the ventricles, may be shown by the pneumoencephalogram.

Ventriculography has been used to outline the ventricular system in patients with head injuries, but provides little information regarding the nature of the lesion responsible for a shift. Ventriculography is contraindicated in head-injured patients with increased intracranial pressure because any introduction of air or other contrast material into the ventricles may produce an additional increase in intracranial pressure.

In some instances computed tomography may not be available and cerebral angiography cannot be obtained quickly for patients who show clinical signs of a possible major intracranial mass lesion. In such cases ventriculography with intracranial pressure measurement may still be important in evaluating the need for immediate surgery.

Electroencephalography

Opinions are varied concerning the value of electroencephalography in evaluating the effects of head injury. Bakay and Glasauer, two neurosurgeons, state explicitly that "Electroencephalography is of little use in the diagnosis of acute head injury or in predicting the outcome" (1980). They emphasize that the EEG often does not correlate with clinical observations, either at the time of initial examination or at later periods. According to these authors, EEGs are frequently inaccurate because the head-injured patient's clinical neurological state is often caused by diffuse damage in the white matter and that such damage is not reflected by electroencephalographic tracings.

Also, in many cases, lesions in cortical areas are masked by tracings originating from other structures. Finally, clinical EEG tracings sample only the upper surfaces of the brain; therefore, basilar contusions are not represented. Although brain contusions are usually associated with definite EEG abnormalities and subdural hematomas cause focal EEG deficits in 50%–80% of the patients, other diagnostic procedures yield far superior information. Cerebral concussions are usually associated with normal EEG tracings. After the acute phase of head injury, however, EEG tracings may represent some of the irreversible effects of brain damage and be useful in assessing the development of post-traumatic epilepsy (Bakay & Glasauer, 1980).

Two other authors, who are neurologists, express a different opinion about the utility of EEG: "The EEG is useful in the investigation of head injury, particularly when serial records are taken at 24-hour intervals during the acute phase and at longer intervals for the follow-up investigation"

(Gilroy & Meyer, 1979). In locations where CT scanning is not available, they recommend that the first EEG tracings be obtained as soon as possible after injury, even though it is difficult to obtain recordings that are free of artifacts when the patient is restless, uncooperative, or receiving intensive care. Following the initial tracings, they suggest that serial recordings should be made at 24-hour intervals if the patient is comatose or stuporous. At least two repetitions of the EEG are recommended at daily intervals, even if the patient has recovered consciousness and the initial record shows evidence of only minor abnormalities.

These authors point out that repeated EEG tracings may identify complications, such as increases in intracranial pressure due to extradural or subdural hematoma or brain edema. They also recommend that another EEG tracing be done about three or four weeks after discharge from the hospital to rule out the development of chronic subdural hematoma. In older persons the EEG may be particularly important in demonstrating impairment of cerebral blood flow associated with increased intracranial pressure, stemming from pre-injury cerebrovascular disease with decreased arterial circulation.

Although the EEG may be normal in cases of mild injury, Gilroy and Meyer emphasize that it is always abnormal in severe head injuries and that there are many features and characteristics of EEG tracings that relate differentially to diagnostic considerations as well as more general aspects of brain pathology in cases of head injury.

Evoked Potentials

There is general agreement that brain evoked potentials may contribute useful information in the evaluation of the head-injured patient. First we will comment on the similarities and differences between EEG tracings and evoked potentials.

The electroencephalogram is a graphic recording of the spontaneous electrical activity of the brain, recorded from the scalp, and is based upon post-synaptic potentials generated in the neuronal cell membranes. Brain evoked potentials are based upon the electrical activity of the same neuronal system that produces the EEG. Thus, injuries to the brain that cause neuronal dysfunction which will alter the EEG are also likely to result in abnormal evoked potential activity.

A basic difference between the EEG and sensory evoked potential is that in the latter procedure a specific controlled stimulus is delivered from the external environment through one sensory system or another which initiates a depolarization wave that travels to the cerebral cortex via a route determined by the sensory avenue stimulated. For example, visual evoked potentials are initiated at the retina and traverse the visual system to the cerebral cortex. The impulses reach the lateral geniculate body (the most caudal part of this system in the brain) and then turn rostrally into the cerebrum via the geniculostriate tract through the temporal and parietal lobes to the occipital cortex.

Abnormalities of visual evoked responses usually indicate impairment at the level of the cerebral hemispheres. Auditory and somatosensory evoked responses, on the other hand, traverse parts of the medulla, pons, midbrain, and diencephalon caudal to the lateral geniculate body and as a result may represent dysfunction at much lower levels than visual evoked responses.

The value in comparisons of this kind stem from the fact that brain stem disorders may be differentiated from hemispheric involvement in comatose patients who have sustained head trauma. For example, if brain stem auditory evoked responses are abnormal in a patient who shows normal visual evoked potentials, the results would tend to implicate the brain stem to a greater extent than the cerebral hemispheres. Conversely, abnormal visual evoked responses, in the presence of normal auditory and somatosensory brain stem potentials, may indicate that the cerebral hemispheres are more seriously involved.

There are many technical problems that can interfere with the validity of evoked potential recordings. A lesion such as a brain contusion does not necessarily result in a functional electrophysiological defect and evoked potentials may be normal. There may be unrecognized impairment of the sensory receptor processes (such as a damaged retina) that may interfere with the procedure. However, when positive results are obtained under careful conditions of recording and multi-modality evoked potentials have been obtained, the results have shown relatively close correlation with parietal, temporal, and occipital lesions as well as differentiation between brain stem dysfunction and involvement of the cerebral hemispheres. Frontal lobe lesions are not as well identified because there is no sensory avenue that leads specifically to this area.

Monitoring Intracranial Pressure

For many years there has been an interest in increased intracranial pressure because it is such a serious source of complication in cases of head injury. The intracranial pressure is generally determined by performing a lumbar puncture, using a water manometer to measure the pressure in the lumbar subarachnoid space. However, this procedure is very difficult to accomplish in many head-injured patients who are extremely restless. Inferences regarding intracranial pressure can be drawn during the initial examination from the type of head injury and the patient's clinical status.

Withdrawal of bloody cerebrospinal fluid may indicate the presence of bleeding within the central nervous system, but this occurs frequently in cases of head injury and, considered by itself, contributes little information to the diagnosis or eventual outcome. There is no way, for example, to know the precise cause or locus of the bleeding merely because blood is found in the cerebrospinal fluid. Therefore, lumbar puncture is generally not indicated in acute head injuries.

However, it is not uncommon for head-injured patients to show a sudden increase in intracranial pressure that may lead to tentorial herniation and additional secondary brain damage. Lundberg (1960) first demonstrated the value of continuous recording of intracranial pressure and this has become a routine procedure in many neurosurgical centers. Intracranial pressure is often monitored because an increase may lead to rapid deterioration of the patient with little warning through clinical signs, and result in herniations of the brain and possible death.

Various methods have been explored to carry out continuous monitoring of intracranial pressure and there is no general agreement on the exact procedure. In many instances a catheter is placed directly into the lateral ventricle, but this involves some risk of infection, particularly when the monitoring procedure lasts more than four days.

VII

POST-TRAUMATIC EPILEPSY

The development of post-traumatic epilepsy constitutes a significant problem for many patients who have sustained a head injury, particularly because it impairs the ability to maintain continuity of consciousness. Patients with epilepsy may, of course, receive warning signals (in the form of an aura) that the seizure is imminent, but there is rarely any way of predicting the exact time of any particular seizure or intervening once the epileptic process has started. There are many activities in normal living that require continuous attention, concentration, and adaptive responses; therefore, the patient who never knows when an epileptic seizure is going to occur is at a serious disadvantage in conducting many kinds of activities.

Much literature has been written about the social stigma associated with epilepsy and it is indeed unfortunate that many people seem to have the attitude that epileptic seizures represent some kind of disorder that goes beyond the usual category of biological dysfunction.

Epileptic patients show a tremendous degree of variability, both in terms of the manifestations of the seizures as well as in any other dimensions, including intelligence and personality factors. It therefore becomes difficult to characterize epilepsy in a meaningful way, and since it is only a manifestation or symptom of some type of disorder of

the brain (including prior trauma), this is not particularly surprising. Post-traumatic epilepsy is a significant problem that has been estimated to involve about 5% of persons with head injuries (Gabor, 1982).

It is generally believed that development of epileptic seizures following head injury is due to the formation of well-localized scar tissue in the brain, but the extent of additional damage due to the head injury may also be a significant interactional factor. Jasper (1970) has pointed out that many pathophysiological changes resulting from head blows may be involved, including vascular lesions and impairment of cerebral circulation, gliosis and formation of meningeal cortical cicatrix, changes in the blood-brain barrier as well as relationships between neurons and glia, and possible disruption of systems which may inhibit the development of uncontrolled electrical activity of the brain in normal subjects. For example, observations have been made that neurons within epileptogenic foci appear to have fewer synaptic endings on their dendrites than those in normal tissue (Westrum, White, & Ward, 1964).

A number of factors predispose an individual to the development of epilepsy following head injury. It is unusual for a patient to develop epilepsy after a closed head injury. The incidence increases in cases in which the dura has been penetrated and becomes even greater when the brain damage has been severe (Caveness, 1976). More specifically, the likelihood of development of late epilepsy is much greater among patients who have had an epileptic seizure during the first week following the injury (Jennett, 1975). Epileptic attacks during the first week are usually of the focal motor type. Partial complex seizures occur only in the later post-injury period. Intracranial and subdural hematomas are also associated with an increased frequency of epileptic attacks, involving about 40% of the cases; epidural bleeding is followed by seizures in only 10% (Gabor, 1982). Depressed skull fractures, particularly with laceration of the underlying brain tissue, frequently cause later epilepsy, with an incidence of up to 60% in severe injuries (Gabor, 1982). In addition, missile injuries (particularly those that are more severe) are followed by epilepsy in 20%–60% of the cases.

The location of the lesion is another factor in the incidence of post-traumatic epilepsy. As with other types of brain lesions that produce epilepsy, traumatic injuries that involve the central part of the hemisphere — particularly the parietal-posterior frontal areas — produce epileptic seizures much more frequently than lesions in the anterior-frontal or occipital areas. Finally, post-traumatic amnesia lasting more than 24 hours, especially in cases of depressed skull fracture, has been associated with an increased incidence of later epilepsy. However, it is possible that the amnesia may merely reflect the more general severity of the brain injury.

The duration of time between the injury and the onset of epilepsy is quite variable. Jennett (1975) noted that 27% of patients who developed epilepsy had their first attack within three months of the injury and that the percentage had risen to 56% by the end of the first year. In a five-year follow-up of patients who had sustained missile injury, 73% had their first seizure within a year of the injury. It must be noted that it is not uncommon for the first seizure to begin long after the injury; Jennett and Teasdale (1981) reported that in 25% of head-injured patients the first epileptic attack began four years post-injury.

Jennett and Teasdale (1981) indicate that seizures characterized by focal motor attacks (common during the first week after injury) are seldom seen during the later period. However, about 40% of later attacks manifest some focal features. An estimated 20% represent partial complex seizures of the temporal lobe type. Petit mal seizures rarely develop after head injury. Approximately 50% of patients who have one or more seizures following a head injury will stop having seizures. In patients who have frequent attacks (10 or more seizures per year) the disorder is likely to continue. This is also true for patients who have had seizures for five years or longer, even though the frequency may be low. According to Gabor (1982), there is a gradual decrease in the frequency of first seizures depending upon time elapsed since the head injury, but in one case (Jennett, 1965) a patient's first seizure began 27 years following his head injury.

Studies of age relationships indicate that children who are under the age of five (particularly less than one year of age) when the head injury is sustained are more likely to have seizures during the first week after injury and less likely to develop late seizures. However, among patients who have had early seizures, persons 16 years of age or older developed late seizures about twice as frequently as those below 16 years of age (an estimated 33%–47%) (Hendrick, Harwood-Hash, & Hudson, 1964).

A recent detailed study of 421 Vietnam veterans has been reported (Salazar, Jabbari, Vance, Grafman, Amin & Dillon, 1985). The subjects in this study had experienced a penetrating brain wound 15 or more years earlier and 53% had post-traumatic epilepsy, with seizures still occurring in about one-half of the victims. The presence of initially large lesions or focal neurological signs had an increased risk of epilepsy. Neither family history nor estimated pre-morbid intelligence had any significant relationship to seizure occurrence.

VIII

A NEUROPSYCHOLOGICAL
MODEL OF BRAIN FUNCTIONS

The localization of functions of the brain (especially the cerebral cortex) has a long history and has been a dominant theme in brain-behavior research. Reitan and Wolfson (1985b) have briefly reviewed the history of such investigations since the early part of the 19th century, when observations were made that lateralized lesions caused motor impairment on the contralateral side of the body.

Broca's investigations of the location of lesions in patients who suddenly lost language functions renewed interest in localization, although there had been no lack of such postulates earlier (Gall, 1810–1819). The discovery by Fritsch and Hitzig in the 1870s that electrical stimulation of certain locations of the cerebral cortex brought about movements on the contralateral side of the body, sometimes even involving contraction of specific muscles, fueled the interest in localization and conceptions of the brain being organized in a highly discrete manner.

The history of these discoveries and contributions, stemming initially from within the framework of neurophysiology and neurology, finally extended into the area of physiological psychology, and is currently represented by behavioral neurology (in the medical tradition) and clinical neuropsychology (in the psychological tradition). This history has been reviewed by Reitan and Wolfson (1985b).

While the localization question was predominant with respect to the independent variable against which behavioral manifestations were compared, the question of lateralized abilities has emerged only more recently. For example, the principal interest 40 to 50 years ago concerned frontal vs. non-frontal lesions (Goldstein, 1942; Halstead, 1947). While there continues to be some interest in the differential effects of anterior-posterior cerebral lesions, discovery of the differential functions of the left and right cerebral hemispheres (in terms of intellectual functions) has led to the current interest and emphasis on left brain-right brain specialization (Reitan, 1955b; Sperry, 1961; Wheeler & Reitan, 1962).

The growing interest in specialized or differentiated functions of the two cerebral hemispheres has been so pronounced that there has been almost implicit agreement on a two-factor theory of brain functions reflected by language and verbal skills (left cerebral hemisphere) and abilities related to spatial, temporal, and manipulatory functions (right cerebral hemisphere). Careful evaluation of thousands of patients with brain lesions has revealed that such a two-factor theory is seriously deficient as a model of human brain-behavior relationships. Reitan conducted these studies on a case-by-case basis, doing neuropsychological examinations independently of complete neurological, neurosurgical, and neuropathological investigations. The information from these independent sources was correlated only after all data had been collected. Since the purpose of these investigations was to determine the reliability of neuropsychological data in relation to independent neurobiological and neuropathological variables, a written report was prepared in each instance in which the implications of the neuropsychological findings for such conclusions were stated.

This approach had special value in leading to the development of a battery of tests that was capable of demonstrating cognitive deficits, regardless of the location of the lesion. The Halstead-Reitan Battery was also found to have significant predictive value in identifying the type of lesion (Reitan, 1962a). Instead of developing a conceptualization based only upon suggestions from the literature or *a priori* notions, the test battery that eventually emerged was a reflection of higher-level brain functions, based on examination of a large number of persons with brain disease or damage. This approach has led to a six-factor theory of brain-behavior relationships that will be described briefly below.

The first factor is concerned with delivery of information to the brain. It might be referred to as a receptive factor utilizing the sensory avenues. Obviously, the brain must receive information from the external environment in order to have any opportunity to process such information. If an individual's sensory avenues were entirely afunctional, there would be no possibility of adaptive interaction between the brain and the environment. Although many types of environmental situations can be described in a limited sensory framework (e.g., a blind or deaf person can still appreciate many significant aspects of the environment but a blind *and* deaf person has a much

more limited capacity for environmental interaction), total sensory deprivation would be catastrophic in terms of brain functions.

In a similar manner, output (response) mechanisms are imperative for normal expression of brain functions. While effector mechanisms refer to both muscular and glandular function, in clinical neuropsychology the emphasis has been on muscular response, including the exquisite muscular phenomena subserving speech. In his theory of biological intelligence, Halstead (1947) identified essentially these same two factors but described them as only a single factor (the Directional factor). Nevertheless, he clearly recognized the necessity for both incoming information and outgoing response for normal expression of brain functions.

The more important considerations concerning clinical neuropsychology are represented by the central processing functions of the brain. Halstead (1947) had conceptualized these functions as being represented by three factors. The first of these, the *Central Integrative Field factor,* was conceptualized as the stored background information of the individual. This factor consisted of organized and integrated memory functions, stored information, and other types of abilities that frequently are measured by intelligence tests. Halstead viewed this factor as being variable and dynamic in nature, under some circumstances being capable of expansion and under others (such as impaired states of consciousness following a head blow) as being constricted.

Halstead represented the basic intellectual function as the *Abstraction factor,* which was responsible for analyzing complex situations into their component parts, identifying their relevance to extensive incoming stimulus material, and utilizing abilities in reasoning and logical analysis.

Finally, Halstead postulated an energy source for brain function, which he referred to as the

Power factor. This factor ran the intellectual "machine," sometimes waxing and waning intraindividually and showing a considerable variability between individuals. Thus, even though two persons might be comparable in terms of input and output capabilities and have similar general backgrounds of information, their intellectual competence and output might differ strikingly depending upon energy levels available for intellectual and cognitive functioning.

The problem with Halstead's conceptualization was that little evidence could be accrued to substantiate the Power factor, even though the concept is appealing in its apparent validity concerning individual differences. Obviously, there may be such a factor that is of great significance for the potential of expressing intellectual and cognitive functioning, but its precise definition and its potential for experimental and operational testing continues to be elusive. This concept has been related to the notion of vigilance, but both the expressive as well as receptive aspects of this factor must be considered. In fact, the available energy to express intellectual functioning may be even more important than alertness and vigilance for incoming information.

The concept of brain-behavior relationships postulated by Reitan and Wolfson (1985a) does not explicitly include a Power factor because of the difficulty in defining, measuring, and experimentally manipulating this potentially important variable. However, it does include the Abstraction and Reasoning factor as the highest level of integrative functioning. In addition, the biological separation of language and speech in one cerebral hemisphere and visual-spatial, temporal and manipulatory skills in the other cerebral hemisphere (which is striking in most individuals even though it may not be totally perfect) strongly suggests these specialized abilities as individual factors.

The model presently proposed begins with input information to the brain through the sensory avenues. The first level of central processing is represented by alertness, attention, registration of incoming information, continued concentration, and relating the incoming information to prior experiences (immediate, intermediate, and remote memory). Persons with brain damage vary greatly in this level of functioning. Some persons with severe and extensive cerebral lesions are so significantly impaired that they do not completely appreciate what is happening in the external world and are therefore obviously unable to understand or analyze what is happening. In clinical examination such patients — who are dull, comparatively unappreciative of stimuli in the environment, and at least partially bewildered by what is going on around them — are sometimes referred to as "obtunded." Clinical experience in neuropsychological examination reveals that such patients tend to do very poorly on almost any task presented to them. Even if the lesion is in the left cerebral hemisphere, the patient may fail to show a very striking differential pattern of performances because all tasks are done so poorly. With careful examination, however, even these patients may demonstrate specific deficits. A great deal depends upon the testing technique, the nature of the test, and the patient's ability to be sufficiently impressed with the task so that an appropriate response can be elicited. Memory falls in a similar category; if the patient is not able to remember past experiences and information and relate incoming information to the memories, the relevance of delivering information to the brain is limited.

It is important to note that the first level of central processing — represented by alertness, attention, concentration, and memory — may show differential impairment, depending upon the specialized content of the task. For example, patients with severely destructive lesions of the left cerebral hemisphere may be considerably less alert in dealing with verbal and language information than in dealing with visual-spatial problems. This occurs because there is a dynamic interaction spreading through the entire neuropsychological behavioral model. The second level of central processing is represented by the third and fourth factors. One of these relates to language, speech, and verbal communicational skills of both a receptive and expressive nature. This factor is largely dependent upon the biological integrity of the left cerebral hemisphere. The other specialized factor, dependent principally upon the right cerebral hemisphere, is concerned with spatial, temporal, and manipulatory skills. Again, the expression of abilities in these areas are dependent on the adequacy of incoming avenues of information as well as response mechanisms. The expression of both language and visual-spatial capabilities are dynamically integrated with adequacy of function at the first level of central processing. If the subject does not have the alertness, memory, or concentrational ability to recommend the input information for left hemisphere or right hemisphere (as appropriate) analysis, the impairment at the first level will be the factor which limits the performances.

The highest level of central processing is represented by abstraction, reasoning, and logical analysis. This factor is essentially similar to Halstead's conceptualization of the Abstraction factor. He considered the Category Test to be the best measure of this factor, and our experience supports this conclusion. It is interesting to note that repeated studies of results obtained with the Category Test indicate that it is remarkably sensitive to cerebral damage, regardless of the location of the lesion. Doehring and Reitan (1962) found that there were no differences in the number of errors found in persons with left cerebral lesions compared to subjects with right cerebral lesions; however, each group performed worse than non-brain-damaged control subjects. Even the pattern of results on individual subtests, reflected as proportions of total errors, were remarkably similar in the two groups with lateralized cerebral lesions.

There has been a presumptive tendency of some neuropsychologists to feel that the Category Test must necessarily reflect impairment of right cerebral functions, presumably because the stimulus material for the test is represented by nonverbal visual-spatial configurations. We strongly recommend, either in the field of clinical neuropsychology or in science more generally, that these questions be approached empirically and that conclusions be based upon actual evidence obtained under scientific conditions, in spite of the fact that it is very tempting for many to believe that one could never have thought of the conclusion had it not been right.

Therefore, the evidence indicates that reasoning, critical analysis of incoming data, formulation of abstractions and principles, and undistorted and logical analysis are general functions of the cerebral cortex. When this level of central processing is significantly impaired, the subject essentially has lost his capability to profit from his experiences in a meaningful and logical way. Individuals with this impairment often appear to be relatively intact; when the disability in this area is prominent and there are no specific disabilities in lower areas of central processing, it is often judged that a "personality" change has occurred. In fact, the "personality" change — often consisting of erratic and ill-considered behavior, deterioration of personal hygiene, a lack of concern and understanding for others in the environment — represents significant changes in the highest level of central processing. Rehabilitation or re-training of brain functions requires a comparative analysis of the dysfunction shown by the individual patient and a model of cognitive re-training that is appropriate and pertinent to the types of neuropsychological deficits that occur (Reitan & Wolfson, in press).

The composition of the Halstead-Reitan Battery fits the neuropsychological model described above in considerable detail, not because it was planned that way but because the tests included in the Battery and their organization were essentially determined by the need to measure appropriate deficits across the entire range of neurological conditions and lesion locations in order to have data that would independently predict the neurological findings. In other words, we needed tests of alertness, attention, and concentration in order to understand the interaction between these functions and the more specific deficits that might occur with lateralized cerebral damage. For example, a patient must have a sufficient degree of ability at the first level of central processing to be able to score adequately on either the Verbal or Performance subtests of the Wechsler Scale even though one cerebral hemisphere may be biologically intact and the other may have a significant and serious lesion.

It is equally important to understand the relationship between the specialized (second level) aspects of central processing and abstraction, reasoning, and concept formation abilities. It is not uncommon to encounter a patient with dysphasia who is so impaired at the third level of central processing that he would be entirely unable to function within normal limits even if the aphasia were completely cured. On the other hand, some patients with significant aphasia do not have striking impairment in abstraction and reasoning abilities and would have a good opportunity for relatively normal functioning if the aphasic difficulties were remediated. In general, the presence or absence of organic language deficits (dysphasia), even if severe, has no more significance for impairment at the third level of central processing than comparable cerebral damage without dysphasia (Reitan, 1960).

There is a dynamic and variable interaction between the levels of central processing for each individual and unless these are understood, one does not have the necessary knowledge and information concerning brain-behavior relationships to initiate a functionally useful program of brain retraining for that patient. Even with such information (based upon the complete Halstead-Reitan Battery) brain re-training is a formidable task and results are variable from one patient to another. We have developed an extensive training program composed of hundreds of individual tasks that can

be used in various ways and in turn are integrated with the results of the Halstead-Reitan Battery (Reitan & Wolfson, in press) and stem directly from them. Preliminary results are very promising (Reitan & Sena, 1983), and are most likely due to the pertinence of the training procedures to the neuropsychological deficits of the subject.

The nature and usefulness of this neuropsychological model can be illustrated by considering its relevance to individual tests. The Speech-sounds Perception Test and the Seashore Rhythm Test serve their principal function in the Halstead-Reitan Battery as measures of alertness, attention, and ability to maintain concentration over time. As the reader is aware, the Speech-sounds Perception Test requires the subject to listen to a tape recording of a nonsense word and, after perceiving the sounds through hearing, to select the matching printed sound from four alternatives on the answer sheet. The Seashore Rhythm Test requires the subject to listen to pairs of rhythmic beats and to record whether the beats in each pair were in the same or difference sequence. Sixty items are included in the Speech-sounds Perception Test and 30 items (of increasing length) are included in the Rhythm Test. Thus, it is necessary for a subject to listen to repeated stimuli and make a rather straightforward judgement. The tests are well-defined, examples are given before the subject begins the test so that he knows exactly what to expect, and the task essentially requires only continued attention to verbal or non-verbal stimuli.

In most cases these tests do not give specific information about the competence of the subject in any particular area of content, although the Speech-sounds Perception Test has been shown to have a correlation of .73 with Verbal IQ (Reitan, 1956a). In addition, persons with left cerebral hemisphere damage make more errors on the Speech-sounds Perception Test than comparable subjects with right cerebral lesions or diffuse damage (Foster, 1982). Although many people have presumed that the Seashore Rhythm Test relates to the functional integrity of the right temporal lobe (presumably because the test involves non-verbal stimuli perceived through the auditory avenue) comparisons of the same groups (Foster, 1982) showed no significant intergroup difference. Since the Seashore Rhythm Test has been explicitly stated to be a right hemisphere indicator, in spite of the fact that there is apparently no data to support this contention, we must emphasize that *experimental results comparing groups with left and right cerebral lesions show no lateralizing significance for this test.* In fact, the principal use of both of these tests in the Halstead-Reitan Battery relates to production of good scores rather than poor performances.

Although each of these measures shows highly significant differences between groups with heterogeneous brain damage and non-brain-damaged control subjects, the importance does not lie in the fact that such differentiations occur. Instead, patients with relatively chronic, static conditions of biological dysfunction of the brain perform relatively better on these tests than patients with acutely destructive lesions. Acute destructive lesions have an impact on brain functions that is quite impairing to overall organizational function, and patients with such lesions frequently demonstrate significant impairment even at the first level of central processing. However, when brain damage has become relatively chronic and stabilized, the first level of central processing (attention and concentration) is often more intact than the second level (specialized functions) or, especially, the highest level (abstraction and reasoning). Therefore, the Speech-sounds Perception Test and the Seashore Rhythm Test frequently have reasonably adequate scores, even though they may fall in the brain-damaged range, and provide information that permits more explicit interpretation of the deficits occurring at the second and third levels of central processing.

It is apparent that the principal requirement of each of these tests relates to attention, alertness, and concentration. The verbal component of the Speech-sounds Perception Test is manifested in some patients with serious lateralized damage involving the left cerebral hemisphere, but the nonverbal content of the Rhythm Test is not sufficient to produce lateralizing implications that are statistically significant. Neither of these tests has a large requirement for abstraction and reasoning skills. Instead, they demand close attention to the specific stimulus material and an immediate judgement in each case, prompt execution of that judgement, and attention to the next stimulus.

We would postulate that the Speech-sounds Perception Test requires some ability at the third level of central processing because the auditory stimulus must be evaluated with respect to four printed alternatives and a judgement must be made to select the correct answer. This test probably does require a minimal element of comparative reasoning, probably exceeding any such requirement in defining words, for example.

We recently completed an unpublished study in which we deliberately evaluated this neuropsychological model by using a verbal test that required a considerable degree of abstraction and reasoning ability (Word Finding Test) and another test that had minimal requirements of this type (the Vocabulary subtest from the Wechsler Scale).

The Word Finding Test consists of 20 items and each item consists of five sentences. In each sentence there is a nonsense word ("grobnik") and the subject's task is to guess the meaning of this nonsense word. In each item there are five trials to guess the meaning of the word and each succeeding sentence offers additional clues. The subject must listen to each sentence, formulate a hypothesis, and record his response. Each successive sentence provides additional information and the subject may change his answer in light of the new information he has received. The meaning is clear to most persons by the fifth sentence in each item. The test score is the number of correct responses.

The Vocabulary subtest was administered in the standard manner according to Wechsler's criteria.

Our postulate was that the Word Finding Test would require scarcely more attention and concentration than the Vocabulary subtest and that both tests were strictly verbal in terms of content. Therefore, the first level of central processing would probably not be a limiting factor with respect to the scores obtained. The second level, because of the verbal content, might well represent a handicap for persons with left cerebral damage. However, persons with right cerebral damage should probably not be significantly impaired at either the first or second level of central processing. Our postulate was that patients with left cerebral damage would perform significantly worse on the Word Finding Test than on the Vocabulary subtest, not because of deficits occurring at the first two levels but instead because the Word Finding Test had the additional requirement of abstraction, logical analysis, and comparison of sentences in order to infer the meaning of the nonsense word from the context.

In terms of predictive results, we felt that patients with right cerebral lesions would have scores on the Vocabulary subtest that were essentially similar to scores obtained by the control subjects. (All three groups were comparable in terms of age and education.) However, because the Word Finding Test had a much greater requirement of abstraction and reasoning (third level of central processing) than the Vocabulary subtest, we postulated that the group having right cerebral lesions would do worse than the control subjects.

The hypotheses were confirmed nearly perfectly. The group with left cerebral lesions performed worse than the group with right cerebral lesions on both the Word Finding Test and the Vocabulary subtest, emphasizing the relevance of the verbal content. The group with right cerebral damage did not perform any worse than the control subjects on the Vocabulary subtest, but scored significantly worse on the Word Finding Test. Finally, in the context of performances for all three groups (demonstrated by T-score transformations of the data) the group with left cerebral lesions generally had lower scores on the Word Finding Test than on the Vocabulary subtest.

We might also consider the Digit Symbol subtest from the Wechsler Scale as it relates to the neuropsychological model. This test has been consistently identified as the most sensitive of the subtests of the Wechsler Scale to cerebral damage, regardless of whether the damage involves the brain diffusely or principally the left or right cerebral hemisphere. Digit Symbol seems to be sensitive regardless of lateralization (Reitan, 1955b), having the lowest mean score of the eleven subtests in each of these three groups.

We would postulate, therefore, that this test permeates the entire neuropsychological model and performances could be limited at any level of central processing. For example, a person might do poorly on Digit Symbol if he were impaired in alertness, attention, concentration to the task, and quickness in performance. This would represent a deficit at the first level of central processing.

The second level might also represent a limitation in performance, regardless of whether the patient had a lesion of the left or right cerebral hemisphere. Patients with left cerebral lesions could be limited in their performances by the requirement to match symbols and numbers (the symbolic aspect of the task); patients with right cerebral damage could be limited by the requirement of drawing unfamiliar spatial configurations.

Finally, the task requires integration of stimuli (numbers and symbols) and it is necessary for the subject to have a certain amount of organizational skill in order to accomplish this transformation (third level of central processing). Thus, on the basis of the neuropsychological model alone, one would predict that Digit Symbol requires adequacy of brain-behavior relationships generally, that the complex nature of the test could limit the performance of the individual brain-damaged subject regardless of the specificity of the impairment, and that patients with either left, right or diffuse cerebral damage would perform worse than control subjects.

The Similarities subtest of the Wechsler Scale is often referred to as a measure of verbal abstraction. This test does not have a significant requirement for attention and concentration capability because each item contains only two words for comparison and these are generally understood without any difficulty. However, the test is strictly verbal in nature and the subject must offer an explanation of how the words in the pair are alike. The presumption is easily made that the words themselves are common knowledge or will be within the vocabulary range of most of the subjects.

The attribution of abstraction to the subtest is based upon the requirement that the subject has to group the words into a single broader category in order to express their similarity. However, we would contend that third level of central processing (abstraction and reasoning) is not a particularly substantial element of this task. It may be more important that the subject be able to define the words and, if such knowledge is available to the subject, it is entirely possible that he would score relatively well on this test. In fact, Wechsler reports coefficients of correlation in three different age groups between Similarities and Vocabulary subtests ranging from .72 to .78, whereas we found correlations between Similarities and the Category Test (an abstraction and reasoning measure) of .54, with a correlation between these latter variables in a group of brain-damaged subjects of only .20.

There may be reason to consider the Similarities subtest of the Wechsler Scale to be more of a test of verbal abilities than abstraction and reasoning skills, and this may explain why this verbal test is a relatively weak (although significant) differentiator between persons with left and right cerebral damage.

The Block Design subtest of the Wechsler Scale has been identified as an excellent indicator of right cerebral damage, particularly in cases with lesions in the posterior part of the hemisphere. This test also has been described as a non-verbal abstraction test. It must be noted that Block Design is not only non-verbal but is explicitly concerned with organization of spatial relationships, a type of function related closely to the status of the right cerebral hemisphere. In addition, Block Design would appear to involve a substantial element of abstraction and organizing ability. Even though the items are presented individually and may not require continued attention and concentration, it appears that Block Design depends heavily upon the specialized functions of the right cerebral hemisphere as well as the general functions of abstraction, reasoning, and logical analysis. It is therefore not surprising that Block Design is effective as a test of adequacy of right cerebral functions.

The four measures in the Halstead-Reitan Battery most sensitive to brain damage generally considered are the Impairment Index, the Category Test, Part B of the Trail Making Test, and the Localization component of the Tactual Performance Test. Considering their relationship to the neuropsychological model, the sensitivity of these tests is hardly surprising.

The Impairment Index derives its sensitivity from being an average score (and therefore presumably being more reliable) as well as being based upon a fairly extensive series of measures that may be adversely affected at any of the three levels of central processing. Therefore, there are many check-points at which the performances of individual brain-damaged subjects might be limited.

The Category Test requires close attention and concentration because the patient must review one item after another, discern any similarities and differences that may be of critical significance, and relate these observations to each other through short-term memory. The Category Test has been referred to as a non-verbal abstraction test and then gratuitously presumed by the uninformed to be a measure of right cerebral functions. There is, in fact, an element of the test that is similar in a sense to Digit Symbol: the subject is required to translate observations of visual-spatial configurations into a numerical representation ranging from one to four as a basis for giving a response. It would appear, then, that both of the specialized (second level) areas of central processing may be involved. Obviously, regardless of ability at the first or second levels of central processing, a heavy requirement falls upon the subject to analyze the nature of the stimulus material, draw reasonable conclusions on the basis of these observations, and apply these conclusions to specific stimulus material in the form of particular responses. The design of the Category Test obviously pervades the entire neuropsychological model and has potential limitation of performances at each level of central processing.

Part B of the Trail Making Test yields a better differentiation between groups of persons with and without cerebral damage than does Part A (Reitan, 1958). Considering how the two parts of this test relate to the neuropsychological model, this finding is not surprising. Part B requires the subject to deal with both numbers and letters (symbolic material that is considerably more complicated than dealing with numbers alone as in Part A). The subject must scan the sheet visually in order to find the next item to which a line is to be drawn (visual-spatial searching) and to keep both the alphabetical and numerical series in mind at the same time with respect to proper organization (analysis and reasoning). Like the Category Test, Part B of the Trail Making Test also obviously pervades the entire neuropsychological model and fulfills the requirements of a generally sensitive test of brain functions.

Finally, the Localization component of the Tactual Performance Test probably derives its sensitivity (at least in part) from the fact that short-term memory processes pervade the higher levels of central processing, even though the subject had not been alerted to this requirement beforehand.

The presumption is again sometimes made that both the Memory and Localization components of this test relate to right cerebral damage because of the visual-spatial nature of the figures involved. The reader should be aware, however, that empirical studies do not support this presumption; clinical investigations have demonstrated that the Memory and Localization components are sensitive to brain damage generally, regardless of whether the right or left cerebral hemisphere is exclusively involved. In addition, these tasks require the subject to organize the relationships of the figures while he/she is taking the test. The general sensitivity of these measures to heterogenous brain damage almost certainly stems from overwhelming requirements at the first and third levels of central processing.

It is obviously a mistake to interpret neuropsychological tests in terms of their apparent or face validity. Some tests are general indicators of cerebral functions, either because of procedural aspects or because they require a number of different types of brain functions in order to produce a correct solution to the task. Other tests, because they are considerably simpler in nature, are indicators of specific cerebral functions and correlate much more closely with localized lesions of the brain (which is true of many of the items in the Luria-Nebraska Battery). The Halstead-Reitan Battery has achieved a practical balance between general *and* specific neuropsychological measures. This did not occur because the Battery was specifically planned that way but instead because these were the testing procedures which would produce the type of data that would permit us to predict the independently established neurological variables for the individual patient.

IX

NEUROPSYCHOLOGICAL
STUDIES OF HEAD INJURY

Early Investigations of Head Injury

Our review of the neuropsychological literature notes that many studies represent interesting but isolated comparisons of persons with and without cerebral lesions. Each of these studies probably makes some kind of contribution to the understanding of brain-behavior relationships, but, unfortunately, few of the studies are within any framework or theoretical conceptualization that is meaningful to the overall abilities subserved by the brain. The fact that one type of ability or measurement shows evidence of deficit in a particular group of brain-damaged patients carries relatively little meaning in comparison with the information conveyed by scores on a number of measures organized into a meaningful conceptualization of brain-behavior relationships, particularly as emerging patterns may relate to independent neurological criterion information.

Because we feel that studies of brain-behavior relationships must be related to a pertinent conceptual framework of neuropsychological functions (in order to be relevant to the individual subject), we will organize our review of the literature according to the neuropsychological model presented above. Because of their frequent clinical use, we will also include a review of the effects of head injury on measures of general intelligence and review studies concerned with the influence of head injuries on personality and emotional aspects of behavior.

Although civilians undoubtedly constitute the majority of head-injured persons (see the chapter on Epidemiology for specific data), many studies of the effects of head injuries have stemmed from World Wars I and II, the Korean Conflict, and military injuries sustained in Vietnam. Studies of brain injury in World War I seem to have been performed more frequently by German researchers than American investigators, probably because the methods of clinical psychology (which were used to evaluate brain-injured soldiers in World War II) were not yet well-developed. The principal investigator of the effects of brain injuries from World War I was probably Kurt Goldstein, whose book, *After-effects of Brain Injuries in War* was based on examination of World War I casualties (although the book was not published until 1942).

Feuchtwagner (1923) reported the results of his examination of gunshot injuries of the brain of 400 soldiers in World War I; however, his evaluation of individual subjects was much more casual and permissive than procedures presently used.

significant deficits on a broad range of neuropsychological functions. The head-injured group of subjects showed a greater degree of improvement from the initial examination to the 12-month testing than from the 12-month examination to the 18-month testing. In addition, the persons who were more severely injured initially showed a greater degree of absolute improvement on the various psychological measures than the subjects who had sustained milder injuries. Nevertheless, those who were more impaired initially continued to demonstrate greater residual deficits 18 months post-injury than the subjects who initially showed mild impairment.

In assessing outcome 18 months after the injury, the groups were divided into those who were judged to have made relatively good recoveries and those who recovered cognitive functions less well. The initial neuropsychological test data was subjected to discriminant analysis to determine the extent to which this data could predict outcome. Although only 34 subjects were included in this study, more than 90% of the cases were correctly placed in either a good outcome or poor outcome group. In a general sense, the severity of initial deficit is a significant determinant of the eventual degree of recovery and residual deficit (in spite of the fact that those with more severe deficits initially show a greater absolute degree of improvement on neuropsychological tests). However, a method for individual prediction, which would seem possible in terms of these results, has not yet been reliably developed (Dikmen, Reitan, & Temkin, 1983).

Following World War II Hans-Lukas Teuber devoted essentially his entire research career to investigation of the psychological effects of penetrating head injuries. He began his investigations in patients who had sustained penetrating brain wounds in World War II and continued his studies with these subjects and head-injured soldiers from the Korean Conflict.

In his earlier investigations Teuber tended to concentrate on various types of perceptual deficits, investigating the effect of head injury on judgement of visual and postural verticality (Teuber & Mishkin, 1954), various aspects of pattern vision (Teuber, Battersby, & Bender, 1949) roughness discrimination (Weinstein, Ghent, & Teuber, 1958), perception of hidden figures (Teuber & Weinstein, 1956), visual field defects (Teuber, Battersby, & Bender, 1960), and a more general review of various types of alterations in perception (Teuber, 1966). He also studied performance types of tasks (Teuber, Battersby, & Bender, 1951; Teuber & Weinstein, 1954) and spatial orientation (Weinstein, Semmes, Ghent, & Teuber, 1956).

Teuber performed studies on memory disorders (Teuber, 1968) and in one investigation focused specifically on anterograde amnesia (Teuber, Milner, & Vaughn, 1968). Some of his investigations concerned the differential effects of right and left cerebral lesions following brain injury (Teuber, 1962) and he devoted considerable attention to what he considered to be the "riddle of frontal lobe damage" (Teuber, 1964). One particular investigation of lateralization and location effects lead to a scholarly consideration of equipotentiality vs. cortical localization in the neuropsychological organization of brain functions (Teuber & Weinstein, 1958). Teuber also evaluated the effects of penetrating brain injury on intelligence (Weinstein & Teuber, 1957).

It is apparent from these extensive investigations that the work of Teuber and his colleagues initiated the modern era of neuropsychological evaluation of head injury. Nevertheless, a limiting factor in his efforts related to his persistent use of cerebral localization as the independent variable against which his experimental data were evaluated. When the majority of Teuber's work was done there was no general recognition of the widespread damage in cases of head injury over and beyond the more focal damage observed by the surgeon. Teuber's presumption that he could use surgical notes as a basis for identifying the brain damage in his subjects undercut the potential for deriving clear expressions of relationships of behavior to the locus of the lesion.

A major early study of somatosensory functions in subjects with penetrating head injuries was conducted by Semmes, Weinstein, Ghent and Teuber (1960). This study used a total of 124 brain-injured subjects and 33 control subjects with nerve injuries of the leg. The authors were remarkably specific in identifying independent variables, considering the fact that the subject material consisted of persons with penetrating brain lesions. The independent variables were identified as (1) unilateral cerebral damage, (2) cerebral damage sparing the sensorimotor area and, (3, 4, & 5) lesions of the sensorimotor area divided according to subsectors (pre-central, post-central and posterior parietal areas). Dependent variables included pressure sensitivity, two-point discrimination, point localization and sense of passive movement. Relationships between the dependent variables were established for damage of both the ipsilateral and contralateral cerebral hemispheres.

The results of the study suggested a somewhat different organization of the dependent variables with respect to the right cerebral hemisphere as compared with the left cerebral hemisphere, a finding that the authors felt contributed to improved understanding of the functional organization not only of the sensorimotor areas but also to the comparative value of associationistic vs. configurational types of psychological theories of perception.

More specifically, the findings suggested that somatosensory functions are more diffusely represented in the right than the left cerebral hemisphere, that deficiencies occur more frequently in the left than the right hand when ipsilateral damage of the sensorimotor area was present, and that the relationship of specific sensorimotor deficits was different for the two hands. Interpretations of the results along these lines, however, required the assumption that damage was equivalent in the two

cerebral hemispheres and the estimate of damage was based only upon observations at surgery with an implicit assumption that the lesions of the brain were no more extensive than those seen at the time of operation. If damage of the two cerebral hemispheres was not equivalent, obviously differences in deficits of the two hands might have been related to differences in both lateralized and possibly diffuse cerebral damage.

Newcombe (1969) also published the results of an extensive investigation of patients with missile wounds of the brain. The subjects in this study were persons who had sustained head injuries in World War II but were not neuropsychologically examined until 1963 to 1966. Thus, approximately twenty years or more elapsed between the time of brain injury and the time of psychological examination. Obviously, these subjects had chronic and static brain lesions and represented a very specialized group. Nevertheless, it would be of interest to determine the very long-term after-effects of head injuries in which there had been definite evidence of cerebral tissue damage.

Newcombe identified 53 subjects with left cerebral lesions and 44 subjects with right cerebral lesions. She subdivided each group into subgroups according to area of damage: frontal, temporal or temporal-parietal, parietal, posterior (including occipital, temporal-occipital, and parietal-occipital). There was also a mixed group of subjects who had lesions involving the frontal-temporal area, the frontal-parietal area, and the frontal-temporal-parietal areas. As would be expected with penetrating missile wounds, the lesions were quite diversified in terms of known areas of cerebral tissue damage. Without question, these patients had extensive involvement and would not qualify well for strict lateralization studies.

Newcombe administered a rather extensive battery of tests but had no particular rationale for the selection. She indicated that she wanted to use a variety of short tests, covering a range of verbal and spatial functions, in order to elicit patterns of impairment. She said that she elected this procedure instead of doing a more intensive investigation.

Newcombe identified some tests as general intelligence measures and these included the Raven Progressive Matrices, the Similarities subtest from the Wechsler Adult Intelligence Scale, and a test of object classification. She also included a number of well-practiced verbal tasks, including the Mill Hill Vocabulary Test and evaluations of reading, writing, oral spelling, arithmetic, verbal fluency, and object naming. Additional verbal tests were included to represent immediate registration, retention, and recall (verbal memory and learning abilities). These tests included measures of digit span as well as random-letter span and selective-noun span, a test of ability to recall letters of the alphabet, sentence repetition abilities, story recall, paired-association word learning, and nonsense syllable learning. Tests in the area of visual pattern identification included a measure concerned with visual pattern matching, recurring recognition of figures based upon visual presentation, and a visual closure test. In addition, she administered tests identified as measures of spatial aptitude. These included cube-counting tasks (taking into account the hidden cubes), the Block Design subtest from the Wechsler Adult Intelligence Scale, and a maze-learning task.

When a variety of tests is used to evaluate brain-behavior relationships, it is generally advantageous to select measures that have previously been shown to reflect the effects of brain damage. Researchers who have had experience in clinical evaluation of individual subjects and correlation of neuropsychological test results with independent neurological, neurosurgical, and neuropathological evidence realize that certain procedures do not provide valid data, even though they might seem to involve brain-related abilities. Nevertheless, many psychologists fail to recognize the importance of validating the procedural adequacy of a particular test and presume that a test having verbal content must necessarily reflect left cerebral damage and a test with non-verbal or spatial content must necessarily reflect right cerebral damage. Even though such a presumption may be reasonable in terms of the content of the test, various conditions may preclude obtaining valid results.

For example, the task may be entirely too difficult and a person with any type of brain lesion would be likely to do poorly. In other instances the task, because of its nature or measurement considerations, may produce a great deal of intra- and inter-individual variability and lead to unreliable results. In some cases, as the one we describe later concerning measurement of finger tapping speed, the apparatus may have inadvertently been improperly designed. Therefore, when an investigator uses tests that have not been validated as measures of brain functions (and thereby do not qualify as neuropsychological tests), it is difficult to interpret the results unless strongly positive evidence emerges.

Newcombe found that on the well-practiced verbal tasks there appeared to be a slight decrease of efficiency in verbal behavior in brain-damaged subjects. However, she felt that comparisons with normative data would be satisfactory and did not use a formally composed control group. Since a psychological test always involves an interaction between the examiner and the subject and many circumstances (both biologically and environmentally based) can affect an individual's performance, a procedure in which a control or comparison group was not deliberately composed and tested by the same examiner provides a hazardous basis for comparisons leading to supposed scientific conclusions.

As might be expected, Newcombe did find that subjects who had dysphasia had mild deficits in reading, writing, spelling, and object naming. However, she also indicated that the only assessment of dysphasic symptoms was done clinically during an initial interview with the subject before the standard testing was actually begun. Thus, this particular finding concerning dysphasia almost certainly represents only a circular procedure (the examiner selected patients with the kinds of deficits that she verified in formal testing).

The tests that were concerned with immediate verbal registration, retention, and recall reportedly showed mild but consistent deficits when compared with normative expectations. The problem with this type of conclusion is that a control group tested under the same circumstances and by the same examiner might also have shown mild but consistent deficits when compared to normative expectations.

The results on measures of visual pattern identification indicated that the group with right hemisphere lesions was probably somewhat worse than the group with left hemisphere damage, especially on the visual closure task.

Finally, on measures of spatial aptitude, the group with right hemisphere damage also performed slightly worse than the left-hemisphere group.

As noted earlier, the extensive damage throughout the brain that customarily occurs in persons with head injuries constitutes a condition that limits the value of attempting to attribute one type of loss to the right cerebral hemisphere and another type of loss to the left cerebral hemisphere. For this purpose it is far better to examine patients with lesions that are more definitely restricted to one hemisphere or the other, rather than to use one group with right hemisphere lesions and an unknown degree of generalized cerebral impairment and another group with left hemisphere lesions and an unknown degree of generalized cerebral impairment. Therefore, limitations in experimental design with relation to the hypotheses proposed for investigation seriously limited the usefulness of Newcombe's (1969) study.

Alertness, Vigilance, and Rate of Information Processing

A considerable number of investigations have studied the question of impairment of alertness, attention, concentration, and rate of information processing. In fact, the Continuous Performance Test was devised specifically for the purpose of evaluating continued attention and concentration in persons with cerebral damage. The results obtained using this test have shown that attention and concentration are impaired in persons with brain injury regardless of the content of the task (verbal stimuli or visual-spatial configurations).

Gronwall and his associates have also studied performances at the first level of central processing in considerable detail in persons who have sustained head injuries. Gronwall and Sampson (1974) investigated a serial audition task given at a pre-determined (paced) rate or at an unpaced rate, discrimination (choice) reaction time, ability to repeat verbal messages correctly which had been given under various listening conditions, ability to perform in the presence of distracting conditions, and ability to perform serial addition of numbers presented under conditions of distraction. Groups were composed of 10 subjects, represented by persons who had sustained severe concussion, mild concussion, and accidents but no concussion. Some of these experiments were conducted only with normal control subjects, who generally were first-year psychology students.

The results indicated that patients who had sustained a concussion generally performed worse during the period they were hospitalized (within 48 hours of admission to the hospital) than when examined again 30 to 40 days after discharge. The results were interpreted as indicating that the subjects showed some initial impairment from which they would recover only in time, even with mild concussion (the criterion being three or less days of hospitalization).

Gronwall and Wrightson (1974) used a similar procedure of requiring the subject to add digits to the preceding digit, with the digits given at a standard rate (paced auditory serial addition task). These researchers found that patients who had suffered concussion were initially unable to process information at a normal rate and recovery to a normal level generally occurred within 35 days. However, they noted that patients who complained of impaired work capability, poor concentration, fatigue, irritability, and headache showed a reduction which persisted for longer periods of time.

Gronwall and Wrightson (1975) used the same serial addition task to compare 20 young adults who had experienced a second concussion with control subjects who had sustained a concussion. While it is difficult to be confident that the severity of concussion was comparable in all instances, those who had experienced two concussions required a longer period of time to recover to normal functional scores.

Gronwall (1977) states that the serial-addition test is not the ultimate and certainly not the only measure of reduction in processing rate after concussion. Nevertheless, he describes this procedure as a test for estimating individual performance during recovery.

Ewing, McCarthy, Gronwall and Wrightson (1980) also studied 10 university students who had recovered from minor head injury sustained one to three years before examination. These researchers used vigilance and memory tests, including the serial addition task. The head-injured subjects performed worse than a matched group of students who had never sustained head trauma. The authors interpret these findings as indicating that adverse cognitive effects of head injury persist long after the incident has occurred, even in persons who had sustained only a minor head injury.

These various studies indicate that impairment of alertness, attention, and concentration occur in victims of head injury, including persons with relatively mild damage. As noted above, Ruesch

(1944) made these same observations many years earlier. It is of interest to see that following a minor head injury, many subjects show a substantial improvement on such measures, often reaching a normal level of performance in about 35 days. Nevertheless, in one of the above studies, persons still continued to show some evidence of deficit when the head injury had been sustained one to three years previously. However, the generality of results based on groups numbering only 10 subjects must be viewed cautiously.

Kløve and Cleeland (1972) investigated the significance of variables, including skull fracture, persistent EEG abnormality, persistent abnormal neurological status, and subdural hematoma in groups of head-injured patients that were comparable with respect to age, education, duration of unconsciousness, and on three of the four variables noted above, but differing on the fourth variable. They used an extensive battery of tests in order to evaluate all levels of central processing. Included were the Speech-sounds Test and Rhythm Test from the Halstead-Reitan Battery, measures of alertness and concentrated attention. They found that skull fracture did not have a significant effect on the neuropsychological measures. However, brain injuries that had resulted in persistent EEG abnormalities or focal neurological findings were generally associated with poorer performances, not only on measures of alertness and concentration but on other neuropsychological variables as well. Their results also indicated that patients who were unconscious for more than three weeks following the injury had neuropsychological deficits that were more consistent and severe than patients with lesser durations of unconsciousness.

This study indicated the value of using an extensive series of neuropsychological measures rather than tests representing only one of the levels of central processing. Obviously, in clinical assessment it is hardly sufficient to base one's evaluation of the patient on a limited sampling of brain functions. Deficits representing the full range of brain-behavior relationships are significant in the complex reactions and performances required in successful adaptation to problems in everyday living.

Using selected measures from the Halstead-Reitan Battery, the Trail Making Test, and the Verbal, Performance, and Full Scale IQ values from the Wechsler Adult Intelligence Scale, Dye, Milby, and Saxon (1979) compared a group of subjects with relatively severe head injuries to a group with mild injuries. The results generally indicated that the brain-damaged groups performed significantly worse than a comparable control group (as has previously been demonstrated and would be expected). However, the head-injured subjects had achieved a relatively chronic status, having been drawn from a population admitted to the hospital during a three-year period before the study began.

Under these conditions, the Speech-sounds Perception Test and the Seashore Rhythm Test, two measures of alertness and concentrated attention, did not show significant differences either in the overall comparisons of brain-injured subjects and the controls or the brain-injured subjects with mild vs. severe injuries. These results are consistent with the hypothesis that these particular measures, representing the first level of central processing in the neuropsychological model described above, may show a degree of recovery with relation to other test findings which indicate achievement of a relatively chronic and static condition of brain functions following injury.

In spite of the evidence that using a number of appropriate tests, and describing brain functions generally and in comparative terms has significant value, studies continue to be reported that involve single tests or measures representing a single area of function. For example, Van Zomeren and Deelman (1978) elected to study reaction time in a group of 57 young males over a two-year period following closed head injury. As one would predict, the results indicated that reaction time is relevant to the impairment experienced following head injury and, in addition, shows improvement over time. It was of interest that choice reaction time related more closely to the severity of brain injury (based on duration of unconsciousness) than simple reaction time, but many prior studies have shown that more complex and difficult tasks, regardless of their particular nature, stress the damaged brain to a greater extent than more simple tasks and thus show greater differences depending upon severity of impairment. Obviously, exactly such a result would have been expected in consideration of the neuropsychological model described above. It is important to recognize, however, that reaction time is a rather limited representation of the behavioral capabilities of human beings and can scarcely be considered an adequate basis for generalization to variables representing other domains of evidence.

Visual-Perceptual Skills and Other Areas of Measurement

It would be much easier to review and evaluate the neuropsychological literature in the area of head injury if research had been done within the framework of a meaningful model of brain-behavior relationships (as is true for much of the research literature in neuropsychology). Most of the studies in the area of head injury are concerned with content areas that seem, in one way or another, to represent the particular interests of individual investigators. It is relatively unusual to find a study in which an extensive and organized battery of tests has been administered, thereby permitting development of an understanding of differential psychological deficits in association with head injury and the primary and secondary damage resulting from it.

Levin, Grossman, and Kelly (1976) tested the ability of patients with closed head injury to recognize various random shapes as a measure of short-term memory. They found that deficits occurred frequently among patients who had specific signs of neurological impairment, particularly when there was evidence of both brain stem and cerebral injury. Skull fracture and EEG abnormalities were not related to short-term memory impairment but patients who had periods of coma with a duration exceeding 24 hours demonstrated an increased incidence of impairment.

The above study prompted the same authors to conduct another investigation, this time using the Facial Recognition Test (1977). The subjects, persons who had sustained closed head injuries, were classified into three groups according to severity and duration of coma. These groups were compared with normative data that had been collected on patients without evidence of cerebral damage.

It was found that patients with more severe head injuries (longer duration of coma) demonstrated less accuracy in Facial Recognition. Again, the evidence suggested that damage of both the cerebral hemispheres and brain stem were factors in producing impaired performances. Patients with evidence of only cerebral involvement, skull fracture, or EEG abnormality were not impaired. The results were interpreted as being consistent with the postulate of Ommaya and Gennarelli (1974), which stated that less severe closed head injuries principally affect peripheral structures of the brain and that more severe blows also involve the deeper (brain stem) structures.

Hannay, Levin and Kay (1981) also studied visual perceptive ability using tachistoscopic exposure of stimulus figures in 42 patients with closed head injury. They compared the results with those produced by 10 normal control subjects. These researchers found that the head-injured patients performed worse than the control subjects, regardless of estimates of their severity of injury. The authors note that their procedure was suited to subjects with a short attention span, so that this factor

would not interfere with the tests of visual perception. They also noted that the tachistoscopic testing was delayed until the patient achieved a normal score on the Galveston Orientation and Amnesia Test (Levin, O'Donnell, & Grossman, 1979).

Obviously, a question could be raised regarding the adequacy of these procedures as a means of focusing the interpretation of the results on visual perception. The authors noted that the control group had a "slightly higher number of years of education" than the patients with closed head injury.

Corkin (1979) also studied visual perception using Thurstone's Hidden Figures Test, comparing veterans of the Korean Campaign who had sustained penetrating head injuries with a group of veterans who had not sustained brain injury. Patients with penetrating head injuries were classified according to laterality of cerebral damage, basing the classification solely on the location of skull defects and intracranial foreign bodies.

No differences were found in the groups with left and right cerebral lesions and Corkin ascribed this result to the fact that there was little leeway in style of performance that was permitted because the subject was required to trace the outlines of the hidden figure as it was represented in a more complex configuration. The possible limitation of manifestation of lateralized differences offered by this rationale completely failed to consider the fact that both receptive as well as expressive deficits may occur differentially in patients with left or right cerebral lesions, and the study represents another instance in which a meaningful neuropsychological model of brain-behavior relationships has been partly ignored. Corkin concluded that more severe deficits were present in patients with larger lesions of the left or right cerebral hemisphere, apparently basing estimates of the size of the lesion only on the presence of hemiparesis and, in patients with left cerebral damage, dysphasia. It should also be noted that these patients were examined approximately twenty years after sustaining brain injuries.

We could continue reviewing additional investigations of visual perception and attempt to evaluate and organize the disparate results and relate them to the many varied conditions of head injury (recognizing that in many of the individual studies the relevant information was largely unknown). However, at this point, it would seem more appropriate to conclude that the many available studies, using quite different tests and procedures, applied to extremely variable groups of head-injured patients, represent an approach to the question that will only very gradually yield any meaningful information with respect to clinical application to individual subjects.

Verbal and Language Functions

There have been many studies of brain-injured subjects who were impaired in their use of language symbols for communicational purposes, but the content of most of the research has been in the investigation of dysphasia. Dysphasia, in turn, has usually been studied in more detail in patients with cerebrovascular disease than in patients with head injury. Wepman, in his book, *Recovery From Aphasia* (1951), evaluated aphasia in soldiers from World War II. This detailed investigation noted that a significant degree of recovery occurred in many of these cases.

As with other significant aspects of neuropsychological functioning, the potential for spontaneous recovery as well as facilitated recovery (retraining of higher-level brain functions) constitutes a very interesting topic and one which will be considered in more detail in the second volume in this series (Reitan & Wolfson, in press). Except for a propensity toward more rapid and complete recovery of language functions after brain injury,

the manifestations of dysphasia appear to be similar to those sustained by patients with other etiological conditions. Therefore, rather than attempt a complete review and consideration of aphasia at this point, the reader is referred to other sources (Goodglass & Kaplan, 1972; Reitan, 1984; Sarno, 1981).

Memory Disorders

Our brief review of the neuropsychological literature indicated that memory disorders have received more published attention as a manifestation of head injury than other areas of cognitive function. Obviously, memory is a very complex type of function and it has been postulated that the neuropsychology of memory may be more affected by the content of memory testing procedures than by memory itself. In other words, a person with a left cerebral lesion will probably be more impaired in tests of verbal memory than in tests relating to spatial configurations. A person who has more severe damage affecting general measures of brain function (such as abstraction, reasoning, and logical analysis) would be expected to perform worse than a person with relatively mild or selected deficits.

Considering the undoubted influence of severity of brain damage and type and location of lesion, it would be surprising to find any highly specific results that characterize memory deficits as such in contrast to other indications of neuropsychological impairment (Reitan & Wolfson, 1984). Nevertheless, one investigator after another describes his investigation as a study of "memory deficit," usually without giving any consideration to the possibility that his results may have been determined by the nature of the testing procedures and the subjects' variable neuropathological conditions (which are notoriously complex and difficult to describe in head-injured persons).

Many studies in this area have attempted to account for severity of damage and, in fact, to compare patients with severe head injuries to subjects with milder brain damage. However, the criterion for this differentiation has almost always depended upon duration of post-traumatic amnesia. This criterion can hardly be considered sufficient among head-injured patients generally, and is clearly inadequate even among patients with closed head injuries.

A number of studies have focused on short-term recognition memory, or the ability to identify stimulus material (usually among a broader array of stimuli) to which the subject has been previously exposed in the recent past. Levin, Grossman, and Kelly (1976) studied this function for recognition of random shapes. They found evidence that when compared with control subjects, patients with head injuries were impaired and the degree of impairment was correlated with the severity of the head injury.

Hannay, Levin, and Grossman (1979) conducted a similar study for recognition of line drawings to which the subjects were previously exposed. In this instance subjects who had mild head injuries (a short duration of post-traumatic amnesia) did not differ from control subjects, but groups of persons with moderate to more severe head injuries showed evidence of impairment.

Brooks (1974) investigated recognition memory of recurring shapes. His results indicated that the subjects with head trauma performed worse than control subjects and that the deficit was related to the duration of post-traumatic amnesia. Brooks used the Continuous Recognition Test developed by Kimura (1963) for additional analysis of recognition memory of recurring shapes, in this instance applying Signal Detection Theory in order to obtain more information regarding the errors made by persons with head injury. This procedure permits identification of deficits relating to impaired memory *per se,* in contrast to a possible

difference between head-injured and control subjects' ability to make a decision.

The results suggested that the deficit in patients with more severe head injuries was in fact due to memory impairment rather than merely to indecisiveness in response or caution in the decision-making process. In a response to the data published by Brooks, Richardson (1979a) also concluded that a response bias, or caution in responding, was not the critical consideration; memory impairment in head injury was the factor responsible for deficits in performance.

These various studies indicate that short-term recognition memory does, in fact, appear to be impaired in patients who have sustained significant head injuries. As will be indicated below, these studies have not taken into consideration the deficits which might be more significant than the memory impairment, and depending upon their possible significance, may actually preclude the clinical significance of the memory loss. In addition, it is difficult to describe the actual severity of brain damage. As would be expected, short-term memory losses were more definite among patients with longer periods of post-traumatic amnesia; if a group had been composed of head-injured patients who had sustained devastating brain injuries, the indications of short-term memory impairment would obviously have been even more pronounced.

Long-term memory appears to have been studied in less detail than short-term recognition memory. The same tendency exists in memory studies generally (over and beyond those concerned with head injury). It is much more difficult to devise acceptable experiments for long-term memory than short-term memory, and such attempts have usually been based upon autobiographical or historical information concerning the individual subject.

Levin, Grossman, and Kelly (1977) conducted an investigation in which evaluation of long-term memory was based upon names of previous television programs. As one might expect, patients who had sustained head injuries did worse than comparable control subjects and the accuracy for memory decreased for programs that were more temporally remote. Again, there would certainly be a question concerning the other aspects of intellectual and cognitive impairment that were responsible for the deficit (over and beyond memory *per se*).

Richardson (1979b) felt that it would be relevant to study memory functions in patients with recent closed head injuries and compare their ability to recall concrete and abstract words with a control group of orthopedic patients. His results indicated that the patients with a head injury performed equivalent to the controls in recalling abstract words, but showed definite deficits in their ability to recall concrete words. He interpreted these findings as indicating impairment of brain-injured subjects in the use of mental imagery as a mnemonic cue in the case of concrete words. He postulated further that this finding has potential significance for understanding the specific types of memory deficits in head-injured persons, that results of this kind may be useful with regard to memory re-training, and that his study indicates the potential for application of the procedures and theoretical interest of experimental psychology to clinical conditions.

Lezak (1979) elected to investigate verbal memory by having patients repeat digits in a forward and backward sequence and evaluate verbal learning by having patients learn lists of common words (as represented in Rey's Auditory-Verbal Learning Test). The author reported results on three groups of eight patients with left, right, or bilateral or diffuse cerebral damage; however, she provided little substantiating or verifying neurological information on the patients. Lezak repeated these examinations over a period of three years. The results demonstrated wide degrees of variability in performance for individual subjects, but

as many researchers have previously demonstrated in numerous studies, the patients showed improvement over time.

Fodor (1972) studied several aspects of memory in patients with head injury, including immediate recall, delayed recall, and recognition memory. She had a particular interest in determining whether recognition memory was facilitated by related information in which the opportunity for coding, or utilization of organization, facilitates recall. The principal conclusion of this study was that patients with estimated pre-morbid normal intelligence were not adversely affected in terms of cognitive and perceptual abilities by head trauma, but they were not as effective in utilizing related stimulus material as subjects in the control group.

In head-injured patients with relatively low IQs (79 or below), there was impairment on the memory measures. These patients also failed to utilize related stimulus material effectively. In fact, they showed evidence of a generalized cognitive disturbance, a finding that would hardly be unexpected considering their IQ values. While studies of memory functions must necessarily compare the "memory" results to measures of other intellectual and cognitive functions, in our opinion this particular study demonstrates that the specificity of memory deficits is diminished when such an attempt is made.

A number of studies have used formal, published tests for evaluating memory and related functions in head-injured patients. Brooks (1972; 1976) and Groher (1977) found that head-injured subjects perform worse than control subjects on the Wechsler Memory Scale. Brooks (1972; 1976) also reported that the deficits shown by the head-injured subjects were related to the severity of injury (as judged by duration of post-traumatic amnesia) as well as to chronological age. However, this investigator again found that skull fracture and persisting neurological signs had no apparent relationship to the test scores.

Groher also used the Porch Index of Communicative Ability (PICA) in his study and performed serial testings at one-month intervals for four months after the initial testing. The head-injured patients showed improvement on both the Wechsler Memory Scale and the PICA, especially the first month after initial testing. However, Groher did the first examination immediately after the patients regained consciousness or as soon as they "demonstrated an ability to tolerate a one-hour testing session." Therefore, it is entirely possible that the results of the initial examination reflected a state of post-injury confusion and contributed to the possibility of greater impairment than would have been shown even a day or two later.

The problem of when to conduct the first examination in studies involving serial evaluation is difficult to determine, but there is much to be said for using a criterion such as discharge from the hospital (or being ready for discharge as far as the head injury is concerned although other injuries may require further hospitalization). In this way the first examination represents a rather stabilized condition of impairment, permitting an assessment of recovery uninfluenced by the confusional period that frequently accompanies gradual recovery of consciousness.

Levin, O'Donnell, and Grossman (1979) have developed a test called the Galveston Orientation and Amnesia Test (GOAT) to evaluate orientation to person, place, and time as well as memory for events preceding and following the injury (anterograde and retrograde amnesia). These researchers studied 52 closed head injury patients and found that the results on GOAT were strongly related to responses to the Glasgow Coma Scale. The GOAT scores were used to assess duration of post-traumatic amnesia. The results indicated that patients who showed evidence of diffuse or bilateral brain injury had a longer period of post-traumatic amnesia than patients with focal lesions. They studied the duration of depressed GOAT scores

(which they define as the duration of post-traumatic amnesia) with relation to long-term outcome, but did not offer a definition of the criteria that were used to evaluate outcome. However, accepting their categories of good recovery (compared with moderate or severe long-term disability), the GOAT results showed a statistically significant relationship. Inspection of the data suggested that amnesia for a period of two weeks or more was a relatively ominous sign concerning eventual recovery, but the number of subjects in each group (good recovery vs. poor recovery) was only 16.

It is apparent from the above brief review of the neuropsychological literature that many selected aspects of neuropsychological behavior have been reviewed under the general category of memory functions. Patients with head injuries have generally been reported to show at least some degree of deficit in memory functions, except in one study (Cronholm & Jonsson, 1957) in which very mildly impaired concussion patients were compared with control subjects. These investigators had the subjects memorize word pairs, tested their recognition of figures, and scored responses of the subjects after having heard a short story. The groups did not differ on these measures.

It certainly would seem that any finding is possible, depending upon the severity of head injury and brain damage. If subjects having very mild head injuries were studied, it appears that many of these investigations of memory would show minimal (if not insignificant) results. As noted above, if patients were selected because they had sustained a very severe head injury (which was the criterion in many of these studies), striking impairment would be expected. It is apparent that some additional criteria over and beyond duration of post-traumatic amnesia is necessary in order to design studies of memory that have more productive and meaningful results.

Finally, the reader who would like to pursue this area may be interested in the publication by

Schacter and Crovitz (1977), which is an extensive review of published research regarding memory function in persons with closed head injury. This review goes well beyond consideration of memory alone, and while focusing on closed head injury, cites results relating to other pathological conditions of the brain as well.

Impairment of Abstraction, Reasoning, and Logical Analysis

There have been relatively few studies oriented directly toward evaluating the highest level of central processing in persons who have a sustained traumatic brain injury. Nevertheless, clinical examination of hundreds of brain-injured persons has convinced us that impairment of abstraction, reasoning, and logical analysis skills are the critical deficits in a patient's unsuccessful attempts to resume occupational duties and other types of activities that represent normal aspects of everyday living.

In fact, as the reader will see in the clinical cases presented in Chapter 10, patients' complaints concerning alertness and attention, reaction time, language, and dealing with spatial relationships occur much less frequently than complaints of a more general nature. The patient frequently describes these general problems as "memory deficits," but after a comprehensive neuropsychological examination they appear to be impairment in the ability to (1) recognize the critical features of complex situations; (2) identify relevant aspects of complex situations in order to solve a problem; and (3) be relevant in everyday behavior. We have found that head-injured patients with impairment in the highest level of central processing are often seriously inefficient in the procedures they use to solve problems, are not able to deal with the many elements that compose most practical problem situations, and neglect the critically important features of situations (such as performing bookkeeping tasks, recognizing an illness, and making

recommendations that affect the lives of other people).

Patients who return to us following a head injury and complain of difficulties of this kind regularly show evidence of significant impairment in abstraction and reasoning abilities (clearly represented by poor scores on the Category Test), find that they were unable to effectively perform their previous occupational and intellectual pursuits, and usually have nowhere to go for assistance in re-training of their brain functions. When we refer patients with these deficits to rehabilitation centers we are often told that the professional personnel can discern no impairment in the subject and, as a result, have no rehabilitation procedures to offer.

A growing number of rehabilitation centers presently have programs for cognitive rehabilitation, but the patient's own diagnosis of his/her deficits (usually, "My memory isn't as good as it used to be") typically serves as the principal basis for prescribing the training activities. We contend that a careful and complete neuropsychological evaluation of each patient is necessary in order to understand the neuropsychological strengths and weaknesses of the individual (at all three levels of central processing) and that a specifically structured set of brain re-training activities (such as the ones included in our REHABIT program) (Reitan & Wolfson, in press) is necessary. It does not require a profound degree of understanding and insight to realize the necessity for identifying all aspects of brain-related functions in order to avoid complications caused by unidentified and unknown areas of deficit. As simple an analogy as the "weak link in a chain" should make this point clear.

In contrast to the tendency of many investigators in this area, Teuber investigated a broad range of cognitive abilities, ranging from simple to complex. Other researchers have also followed this method, using an extensive battery of tests in order to gain insight about the strengths and weaknesses of the individual subject's brain behavior relationships and to evaluate the entire range of functions represented by the brain. Some investigators have focused on measures of intelligence, but such tests have usually been devised to evaluate the intellectual and cognitive abilities of normal subjects, and were not designed as neuropsychological instruments. Nevertheless, the types of tests generally included in comprehensive, individually administered intelligence tests undoubtedly reflect some aspects of abstraction, reasoning, and logical analysis.

We must note in this context, however, that IQ measures are frequently at odds (at least to a degree) with results obtained using measures such as the Category Test, the Trail Making Test, or the Tactual Performance Test. In other words, the brain-related deficits of individual head-injured persons are frequently underestimated by the results on intelligence tests, and in certain critical areas the patient is judged to be much more competent than he/she actually is.

Dikmen, Reitan, and Temkin (1983) compared head-injured and control subjects using the Halstead-Reitan Battery. The Battery includes a large number of tests and represents the various areas and levels of brain-behavior relationships. This study, therefore, had the advantage of permitting comparative estimates of degree of deficit among measurements using testing procedures that range from relatively simple to complex tasks. Previous research has demonstrated that the Halstead-Reitan Battery is sensitive to both the general as well as the specific aspects of cerebral functioning (in contrast to the procedures frequently used by many investigators that were developed to evaluate the abilities of normal subjects and have never been validated in terms of their sensitivity to cerebral damage).

The tests in the Halstead-Reitan Battery have been shown to reflect the differential functions of the left and right cerebral hemispheres as well as

areas within each cerebral hemisphere, and permit the results in studies of head-injured persons to be compared with the types of neuropsychological deficits previously reported in many other conditions of brain damage and disease. In addition, the economy of administering an extensive battery must be considered in relation to the cost of using single testing procedures in various studies. The latter method may have the advantage of focusing attention on specific performances, such as paced attention, visual reaction time, facial recognition, short-term recognition memory of random shapes, short-term recognition memory of line drawings, short-term memory recognition of geometric vs. nonsense figures, etc. An additional consequence of using single testing procedures is to fill the literature with numerous studies which fulfill the well-known academic ethic of "publish or perish."

Dikmen and her colleagues (1983) performed an initial neuropsychological examination on head-injured subjects when they were alert, oriented, and physically well enough to tolerate extensive testing. Each subject was re-examined at 12 and 18 months following the initial testing. The results indicated that patients with brain injury experience a broad range of initial deficits, representing the wide diversity of behavioral performances subserved by the brain. However, higher-level neuropsychological functions — including abstraction, reasoning, complex problem solving, and flexibility in thought processes — appear to be more vulnerable than the lower-level functions of attention, concentration, and simple motor performances (e.g., finger tapping speed and grip strength).

Dikmen and her colleagues have shown that improvement following head injury occurs in both the higher-level and lower-level functions (contrary to Lezak's claim [1979] that improvement occurs on relatively simple tasks but not on complex measures of memory and learning). In general, the spontaneous recovery process continued (at least to a degree) over the 18 months post-injury. It should be noted that patients with more severe initial losses showed a greater degree of improvement during the 18 months post-injury, but also had a greater amount of residual deficit than the patients who had milder initial impairment. This finding was demonstrated with a statistical model that used a deficit-proportional term which assumed that recovery represented a proportion of the initial deficit.

Brooks, Aughton, Bond, Jones and Rizvi (1980) used a fairly extensive battery of psychological tests to evaluate 89 severely head-injured patients. However, they did not use a control group or a research design which allowed evaluation of the degree of impairment that might have been shown by these patients; instead, this investigation was oriented toward establishing relationships among the various psychological tests and the Glasgow Coma Scale. Little relationship was found between these two measures, but the duration of post-traumatic amnesia was significantly related to degree of cognitive performance. In effect, this study once again established the fact that patients with severe head injuries tend to do worse on psychological measures than persons who sustain less severe injuries.

Mandelberg and Brooks (1975) administered the Wechsler Adult Intelligence Scale to severely head-injured subjects and compared their test results with the scores obtained by control subjects. They used a procedure in which additional subjects were examined at specified time intervals following head injury. Ten subjects were examined within three months of the injury, a total of 20 subjects within six months, 30 subjects within 12 months, and the entire group of 40 subjects was completed within 12 months post-injury. These investigators found that head-injured subjects were initially impaired, although the Verbal subtests showed less impairment than the Performance subtests. In addition, recovery occurred more quickly on the Verbal subtests than on the Performance subtests.

Because of the widespread nature of brain damage and the difficulty determining the exact location and severity of the damage in living subjects, results of this kind are difficult to assess in cases of head injury. Numerous studies have shown that the Verbal subtests of the Wechsler Scale are more dependent upon the integrity of the left cerebral hemisphere and that the Performance subtests rely on the integrity of the right cerebral hemisphere (Reitan, 1955b; Kløve & Reitan, 1958; Doehring, Reitan, & Kløve, 1961). Therefore, when patients are selected specifically according to the definitive criteria of left or right cerebral damage, an orderly relationship among lateralization findings and comparative IQ values emerges. Undoubtedly, many additional factors besides brain damage may also affect Verbal-Performance IQ differences, including educational level, occupation, and age. A finding of differences between Verbal and Performance IQ values in a study poorly designed to establish the reasons for these differences scarcely constitutes an adequate basis for a conclusion regarding differences in recovery potential.

Mandelberg (1975) also administered the Wechsler Adult Intelligence Scale to a group of 16 subjects in the latter stages of post-traumatic amnesia and compared their results with 16 other head-injured subjects who were fully conscious. Not unexpectedly, he found that the patients who were still in a state of post-traumatic amnesia performed considerably worse than those who had recovered. Mandelberg established somewhat better comparative scores at a later administration.

Finally, Mandelberg (1976) investigated the relationship of Verbal and Performance IQ values from the Wechsler Adult Intelligence Scale with the duration of post-traumatic amnesia. There was some evidence to relate both of these values to post-traumatic amnesia three months after the injury, but only the Performance IQ showed a relationship at both three and six months post-injury. Data collected at 12 and 30 months post-injury showed no relationship to the degree of post-traumatic amnesia. Recognizing that patients with head injury generally show improvement in time, it is hardly surprising that the initial results would be more closely dependent upon the injury itself with less time for factors such as probable differences in individual recovery rate to obscure correlations with estimated severity of the initial damage.

Investigation of Other Psychological Variables

A number of additional investigations have been done in the area of head injury. In some instances well-designed studies of specific performances have been carried out; in other cases head-injured subjects have been examined with a series of tests organized in no obvious manner.

Weinstein (1954) performed a carefully designed and detailed study of weight judgement with four groups of subjects: (1) persons with penetrating head injuries and somatosensory deficits of the hand; (2) persons with penetrating head injury without somatosensory deficit; (3) patients with peripheral nerve injury of the arm; and (4) persons with peripheral nerve injury of the leg, who served as control subjects. The research indicated that errors in weight judgement are significant in persons with traumatic injury of the brain.

Corkin (1968) performed a careful study of motor functions, and acquisition of motor skills in a patient who had surgery (removal of the anterior hippocampus, the hippocampal gyrus, uncus, and amygdala bilaterally) many years previously for relief of incapacitating non-focal seizures. The question in this case was whether this man, who postoperatively demonstrated a profound anterograde amnesia, would be able to make any progress with practice on a rotary pursuit task, bimanual tracking, and tapping speed. Although the patient was inferior to normal men of his age in both initial and final performances, his scores improved from session to session and it was apparent that in spite

of his memory deficit he was capable of improving his motor skills with practice.

The consistent improvement of scores on the Tactual Performance Test from the first trial to the third trial (regardless of whether the person is classified as a control or a brain-damaged subject) further attests to the potential for improvement of performances even though significant neuropsychological deficits are present (Reitan, 1959b). Reitan (1959c) also demonstrated that either absolute or proportional improvement from subtests five to six on the Category Test was not statistically different in persons with cerebral damage and control subjects. There are many studies to indicate that learning capabilities are impaired in persons who have sustained significant brain trauma, but additional studies indicate that a substantial degree of improvement may be expected on many tasks, even in persons with significant brain damage and neuropsychological deficits.

Emotional and Personality Deviations

There has been a growing number of publications describing the emotional disturbances and deviations in patients who have sustained cerebral disease or damage. However, it generally has been quite difficult to differentiate between intellectual and cognitive losses and their effects on behavior and emotional problems that are not associated with the stresses that accompany neuropsychological deficits. In fact, most persons with cerebral damage probably show some evidence of emotional disorder.

In a study of a heterogenous group of brain-damaged subjects Reitan (1955a) found that the first three clinical scales of the Minnesota Multiphasic Personality Inventory (Hypochondriasis, Depression, and Hysteria) were strikingly elevated and indistinguishable from a comparison group consisting mainly of severely neurotic and paraplegic patients. As noted, the extent to which these emotional problems stemmed from stresses associated with neuropsychological deficit is difficult to answer. In addition, when using instruments such as the Minnesota Multiphasic Personality Inventory, it is important to keep in mind that some of the responses which deviate from normal expectancy are valid symptoms and manifestations of cerebral damage. Therefore, it is reasonable and valid to question whether other normative data and transformational procedures derived from studying psychiatric patients can be applied uncritically to patients with cerebral disease or damage (Reitan & Wolfson, 1985a).

Levin and Grossman (1978) used the Brief Psychiatric Rating Scale to evaluate 70 patients with closed head injury. The subjects were grouped into three categories according to the severity of their injury. These researchers found significant results on this measure, with the more severely injured patients showing more deviant results. The findings were interpreted as reflecting cognitive disorganization, emotional withdrawal, and motor retardation. Neurological measures (which included hemiparesis, dysphasia, and abnormal CT scans) also differentiated the same groups according to severity of behavioral disturbance. In addition, patients who were agitated during the acute post-injury phase also frequently had residual behavioral disturbances. Estimates of differential damage of the two cerebral hemispheres had no relationship to the test results.

Dikmen and Reitan have done a number of studies to investigate the correlates of results on the MMPI with variables related to brain damage. In one investigation laterality (left or right) and caudality (anterior or posterior) of involvement were compared (Dikmen & Reitan, 1974). The results indicated that patients with cerebral lesions, generally considered, showed some evidence of emotional disturbance on the MMPI, characterized particularly by neurotic-like manifestations. Anterior vs. posterior or left vs. right involvement of the cerebral hemispheres had no pervasive effect. In this study, however, the types of brain lesions

included were variable and differed in severity. While such factors may have confounded any differential results related to lateralization or localization, it still appeared definite that any influences resulting from differential localization of cerebral lesions were minimal.

In patients with dysphasia a somewhat different result was obtained. In another study Dikmen and Reitan (1974) compared 15 dysphasic brain-damaged subjects with patients having comparable brain lesions (except for location) and no evidence of dysphasia. A multivariate analysis of the data indicated that the dysphasic subjects obtained higher scores on the nine clinical scales and a univariate analysis showed significantly higher scores on the Pd and Sc scales. The results of this study suggest that aphasia may have fairly general and even specific effects on emotional aspects of adjustment, possibly resulting from the stress induced by both receptive and expressive difficulties that interfere with verbal communication.

Dikmen and Reitan (1977b) also compared the acuteness and chronicity of the head injury to results on the MMPI. Patients were initially given the MMPI when they had recovered normal alertness and were ready for discharge from the hospital (at least in terms of their head injury) and were retested at 12 and 18 months post-injury. Trend analyses of the three evaluations indicated significant progressive reductions in scores on the Hypochondriasis, Depression, Hysteria, Psychasthenia, and Schizophrenia scales. These findings suggested that head-injured patients in general complain of more depression, anxiety, somatic problems, and strange experiences soon after the injury than they do at later periods.

These head-injured patients were also grouped according to the severity of their neuropsychological deficits based on the results of the Halstead-Reitan Battery. On all three of the examinations (initial, 12-month, and 18-month) the patients with more serious neuropsychological deficits also showed evidence of greater emotional difficulties than the subjects who were only mildly impaired. The finding that the patients who continued to demonstrate neurotic-like difficulties over time following the injury had initially more severe neuropsychological deficits is consistent with the findings of Bond (1975) and Goldstein (1942) but conflicts with the results reported by Ruesch, Harris and Bowman (1945) and Lishman (1973). From the findings reported by Dikmen and Reitan (1977a) it would appear that persons with significant initial and residual neuropsychological deficits resulting from head injury experienced the greatest degrees of emotional distress. There has been a tendency clinically to invoke explanations involving "psychogenic mechanisms" when a thorough neuropsychological examination would have provided an improved clinical understanding of the patient's condition.

Finally, Dikmen and Reitan (1977b) performed an extensive study involving 129 subjects with medically documented evidence of cerebral lesions. These subjects were classified into three groups, based on adequacy of performance on a number of variables, including verbal intelligence, performance intelligence, concept formation abilities, sensory-perceptual abilities and motor skills. The purpose of the study was to determine whether differences in MMPI results occurred according to severity of deficits in any or all of these areas. The results indicated that patients with greater impairment of abilities, *regardless of the area of deficit,* showed more deviant scores on the MMPI. Except for adequacy of verbal skills (Dikmen & Reitan, 1974), other variables did not seem to have any specific influence on the level or distribution of MMPI scores. These findings again indicated that the severity of neuropsychological deficit, regardless of the particular type of dysfunction, seemed to be the principal factor causing emotional stress and elevation of MMPI scales.

X

NEUROPSYCHOLOGICAL INTERPRETATION OF INDIVIDUAL HEAD-INJURED CASES

In the history of psychology there has been a great emphasis on development of psychological tests which identify an individual's personal characteristics. As early as 1936 Guilford stated, "Of all the psychometric methods, those coming under the heading of mental tests have overshadowed all others in application and in significance." He went on to say that, "Probably no movement in psychology has been so significant in its social consequences as the mental test movement."

Nevertheless, great consternation has centered around the question of what individual psychological tests actually measure. It is insufficient to merely view the test and its content as a basis for deciding on an answer to this question. After careful consideration Guilford (1936) stated that we must "acknowledge that for the most part we have only vague ideas as to what it is that psychological tests actually measure."

A fundamental reason for the problem in determining what psychological tests measure is that there is a tremendous overlap in the abilities necessary to perform various psychological tests, regardless of whether they appear to be similar or very different in content and requirements. Many years ago Spearman (1927) documented in great detail a general (G) factor which characterizes the performances of individual human beings on psychological tests. His studies indicated quite clearly that to a very great extent the same abilities are required on various tests. Considerations of this kind have led to a great deal of research aimed at identifying and describing human capabilities as they relate to various psychological tests. The basic method used to discover the nature of any particular test has been to establish its intercorrelations with other tests. This procedure presumes that tests which agree very closely with each other in terms of outcome require the same abilities for performances and, as a result, are measures of essentially the same function or skill.

An elaboration of this method of inquiry is represented by the statistical procedure of factor analysis. While Spearman had proposed essentially a two-factor theory (a General or G factor supplemented by a Specific or S factor), Thurstone (1931) introduced a multiple-factor analysis. Thus, instead of initially extracting a postulated general factor based upon the intercorrelations of a number of psychological tests, followed by investigation of residuals to determine whether more specific factors must also be considered, Thurstone's method was directed toward extracting as many factors as required by the intercorrelations among the tests.

Of course, in using factor analysis the presumption is made that the individual tests which load significantly on each of the factors extracted require similar psychological functions for performance. Therefore, the common element of a number of tests, which compose a factor, may be considered as a basis for the fundamental explanation of what each of these tests measure. Obviously, the procedure of factor analysis is considerably more extensive and involved than described above, but it has been used as a method for determining the nature of individual tests and providing an organizational framework for understanding the common and similar elements of a range of tests. For example, Thurstone and many other investigators have attempted to use this approach to identify the factors basic to human abilities or primary mental abilities. In this sense the coefficient of correlation has been established as the basic statistic used to determine what individual psychological tests actually measure.

In spite of the detailed, sophisticated, and extensive research that has been done to identify the nature of individual psychological tests, clinical interpretation still often centers on the apparent content or face validity of the individual test. For example, the Similarities subtest of the Wechsler Scale is frequently referred to as a measure of verbal abstraction abilities because the subject must identify the way in which two words are alike. Similarly, Block Design is referred to as a measure of non-verbal abilities because the subject is required to analyze the figure and reproduce it using component parts (blocks). However, the basic differentiation between the tests relates to their verbal or performance requirement.

What is frequently not recognized is that even though the Similarities subtest is based upon verbal content and even though the Block Design subtest depends on spatial configurations, the common element between these tests presumably would be their heavy dependence upon abstraction and reasoning abilities. Wechsler (1955) reports a correlation ranging from .50 to .55 between Similarities and Block Design for three different age groups. These are statistically significant coefficients, suggesting that there is indeed a common element between these two tests. However, for the same three age groups, Wechsler (1955) also reports a correlation between Similarities and Vocabulary of .72 to .78. The Vocabulary subtest presumably requires minimal abstraction or reasoning skills and instead depends only upon the subject's ability to state the meaning of individual words.

Although these correlations do not establish any basis for presuming that Similarities and Block Design do not have a common element of abstraction and reasoning, they do suggest that Similarities is more closely related to Vocabulary than to Block Design and in turn would raise a question about the extent to which the Similarities score is determined by the subject's knowledge of the meaning of the words involved (vocabulary) rather than upon abstraction and reasoning abilities. Considerations of this kind indicate the difficulty in drawing conclusions about what any particular test measures in comparison with other tests, especially recognizing the strong component of Spearman's G factor that pervades the broad range of mental or psychological tests.

These considerations become even more complicated when one attempts to determine what any particular test measures in both brain-damaged and normal subjects. We performed an unpublished set of correlations based on 50 non-brain-damaged control subjects on the Similarities, Block Design, and Category Tests. The results indicated that Similarities and Block Design had a correlation of .52, a coefficient very similar to that reported by Wechsler (1955). Both subtests correlated significantly with the Category Test, suggesting that each contained a substantial component of abstraction and reasoning (Similarities, .54; Block Design, .40).

The same intercorrelations were computed for 50 subjects with heterogeneous brain damage who were comparable to the controls in age and education. The correlations among the tests, however, were much lower, especially when the Category Test was involved. The r between Similarities and Block Design was .44, but the correlation between the Category Test and Similarities was .20. The correlation between the Category Test and Block Design was .25. Although certain prior results (Reitan, 1956a) suggest that the overall configuration of correlations between various tests for groups with and without brain damage is essentially similar, it continues to be possible that brain damage has a significant effect on intercorrelations.

The next observation concerning these same groups of 50 control and 50 heterogeneous brain-damaged subjects concerns the intercorrelations between subtests of the Category Test. (Intercorrelations between subtests 5 and 6 were omitted because they are based upon the same principal.) The median coefficient between subtests 1 through 5 and 7 (omitting subtest 6) were strikingly low: control subjects, .15, and heterogeneous brain-damaged subjects, .07. Thus, the largest coefficients of correlation were obtained for control subjects, a reduction in coefficients of correlation occurred for 50 heterogeneous brain-damaged subjects, and for both controls and brain-damaged subjects coefficients of correlation were remarkably low between subtests of the Category Test.

It would appear from these findings that the Similarities and Block Design subtests show much more consistency of performance among either non-brain-damaged subjects or brain-damaged subjects than the Category Test. The traditional interpretation of such data might well be that the subtests of the Category Test are essentially unreliable, to a considerable extent their scores are determined by chance circumstances, and as a result they fail to correlate well even with themselves. However, this explanation does not consider the fact that scores for the total Category Test correlate significantly with measures from the Wechsler Scale.

Studies concerned with the validity of the subtest scores of the Category Test diminish the strength of the argument concerning their unreliability. The same 50 brain-damaged and 50 control subjects were compared in terms of the adequacy of their performances. The 50 brain-damaged subjects performed significantly worse than the control subjects on all three of the measures (Similarities, Block Design, and Category Test) but the Category Test differentiated the two groups much more effectively than either the Similarities or Block Design subtests. In fact, each of the individual subtests of the Category Test yielded results which showed a significant difference between the brain-damaged and control groups, and when added into a total score this consistency of performance by the individual tests showed a highly significant difference.

Since one can hardly presume the occurrence of measurements which validly differentiate between a brain-damaged and control group, if the individual measurements were unreliable, one must presume that some type of additional factor is of influence in producing the low coefficients of correlation between individual Category subtests. (One would, in fact, presume that a substantial correlation would be subserved merely by the fact that the tests were given at the same time, under the same conditions, using the same bell and buzzer arrangement for providing information regarding "right" and "wrong" responses, and the general similarity of the procedure.)

In all probability, the difference in obtained coefficients of correlation relates to intrinsic aspects of the testing procedure. When the Similarities and Block Design subtests are given, the procedure requires the examiner to identify and describe the nature of the problem, thereby making the explanation of the tests part of the test instructions. Therefore, the subject (whether brain-damaged or control) knows the exact nature of the problem, what he is supposed to do, and the steps that are necessary for correct solution. However, the procedure used in administering the Category Test is based upon learning theory. It is the subject's task to observe the stimulus material, formulate hypotheses regarding similarities and differences, test these hypotheses in accordance with the bell and the buzzer, and gradually define a principle that can produce correct responses regardless of variability in the stimulus material. In other words, the subject must analyze the problem, use logical analysis, formulate hypotheses based upon his observations, and, only after having been correct in these respects, demonstrate that he understands the nature of the problem and is able to produce correct responses.

Obviously, in a procedural sense the subtests of the Wechsler Scale and the Category Test are extremely different. The Wechsler Scale subtests require the subject to carry out instructions as delivered by the examiner. The Category Test requires the subject to analyze a relatively complex problem, discern its characteristics, and then develop a rational and effective approach to its solution. When these complex, serial elements are involved in the task, intraindividual correlations from one effort to the next seemed to be much less consistent. Nevertheless, it is not at all surprising that the more complex task, requiring analysis of the nature of the problem before its solution is demonstrated, is much more closely related to the integrity of brain functions. The essential point to be made here is that the content of the task, as

manifested by the face validity of stimulus material, is not necessarily the entire basis on which the results should be evaluated.

This point can be made even more effectively by considering experiences we have had in measuring finger tapping speed. It would seem that there is hardly any more simple procedure than to measure how rapidly an individual can tap his finger in a given period of time. The Halstead Finger Oscillation Test uses a specified manual counter having a small arm attached which is depressed by the subject with his index finger as rapidly as possible. The entire configuration of the apparatus is set in a constant position so that the arc covered by the arm moves a standard number of degrees with every tap. These provisions with respect to the procedure and apparatus provide a constant and standard set of conditions for every individual who takes the test, despite the fact that hand-size and finger length may vary from one person to another.

Even though the procedure seemed to work well and to provide a fair test of finger tapping speed from one person to another, we encountered a problem when attempting to evaluate finger-tapping speed with young children. In some instances the child's hand was so small that the child could not reach the tapping arm properly and did not have a fair chance to register the speed of finger movement. We found that it was necessary to develop a new apparatus to use with children aged five through eight years in order to give every child a fair chance to register his finger-tapping speed. We did this by developing a tapping device that required depression of an arm only for a short distance in order to trip a switch that registered the movement.

In addition, use of this new apparatus required an electronic registration of the number of depressions (taps), as contrasted with the mechanical depression required with the apparatus for older children and adults. (We had observed that the mechanical counter sometimes skipped ten points, going from a registered count of 20 to 31 on a single tap.) Realizing that there was nothing more simple than measuring finger tapping speed, we felt that it might be advantageous to bypass the manual tapping device and use only the electronic tapping procedure, even though our preliminary observations had definitely indicated that the electronic counter yielded a greater number of taps, per unit of time, than the manual apparatus. We reasoned that we could compensate for this with a standard linear adjustment.

Despite the reasonable considerations involved and the presumption that one tapping apparatus would most certainly yield results that were comparable to another tapping apparatus, we were duly cautious and collected data with both tapping tests on the same subjects over an extensive period of time. We observed that results seemed to be quite consistent in many cases, with the electronic apparatus getting somewhat greater speeds. However, to our surprise, in occasional cases we observed striking disparities. The manual counter, requiring discrete finger movements, sometimes showed striking deficits with one hand or the other whereas corresponding deficits with the electronic counter were not present.

We finally became aware that the manual counter much more consistently represented deficits on the side that was contralateral to the damaged cerebral hemisphere. This did not happen in every case, but in many instances a relatively adequate score was achieved with the electronic tapper regardless of the fact that the contralateral cerebral hemisphere had a lesion which reduced finger tapping speed on the manual counter. We finally realized that persons with lateralized cerebral damage severe enough to cause impairment of rapidity of discrete movements of the contralateral index finger (as required on the manual tapper) did not necessarily cause the same impairment in the subject's ability to use the electronic counter; the patient was often able to

"jiggle" his way to a fairly respectable score when discrete finger movements were not required.

Procedural considerations may obviously be equally as important as the apparent test content and requirements in specific measurements. In fact, as we have repeatedly emphasized, a test battery for evaluation of brain-behavior relationships must be much more sophisticated in its organization than merely representing scores for individual subjects on tests that are interpreted with respect to what they appear to measure (face validity). Procedural considerations in collection of data may influence the obtained measurements. Of course, it is also necessary to use complementary methods of inference in order to understand how the results apply to the individual subject (Reitan, 1967b).

Despite these careful bases for developing a test battery for evaluation of the unit of value (namely, the individual human being), many neuropsychologists persist in the belief that the only scientifically valuable information relates to comparisons of groups of subjects. The notion behind this type of thinking is that science requires generalization, and generalization cannot be based upon an N of 1. Instead, scientific conclusions must represent what generally happens under specified conditions.

The contention stemming from this position is that any accurate conclusions about the individual subject must necessarily represent only a fortuitous or "chance" occurrence. Obviously, such a contention must be inaccurate or there would be no chance for specific diagnosis of any medical or neurological condition. In fact, it is possible, through accruing the right kind of evidence, to conclude that certain highly specific conditions are present to support a specific diagnostic conclusion and that other conditions definitely are not. Therefore, in some cases, it is possible to specify the points of information or evidence that rule in a particular conclusion and rule out all others.

For example, Koplick's spots are specifically diagnostic of measles. Our problem in neuropsychology, if we are to be relevant with our description of the individual subject, is to discern the array of evidence that is sufficient to draw specific conclusions regarding brain-behavior relationships for the individual person. Those who eschew this kind of procedure in favor of group comparisons and statistical tests of significance as the only appropriate method of science also disclaim the value of the individual human being with regard to application of scientific knowledge.

However, the methods of science as related to individual evaluation and diagnosis in neuropsychology await precision. At the present time our only approach is to provide illustrations of interpretations of neuropsychological data in individual cases. There is no doubt that such interpretations can be made and that the uniqueness of the individual subject can be described, at least in part (Reitan, 1962a; Reitan & Wolfson, 1985a). The requirement is that the neuropsychological test data be sufficient to predict specific characteristics of the individual, independently obtained, and have no procedural overlap with the neurological and history data. If the procedure is merely a matter of learning the history and what other diagnostic procedures have shown, and then repeating such hearsay (as if supported by the neuropsychological test data), the errors of individual case illustration have only been repeated. If our conclusions are based only on what we know independently from neuropsychological examination, the criterion derives only from independent and "blind" prediction of other established points of information.

For example, neuropsychological data concerning the effects of head injury are totally useless as far as the individual subject is concerned unless they have been established as sufficient to make predictions of independently obtained information. If the patient has independent evidence of a right anterior temporal lobe contusion, neuropsychological test data should be evaluated in terms of its specific relevance in identifying such a condition. This is the standard to which we have subjected the results of the Halstead-Reitan Battery in evaluating brain-behavior relationships for the individual subject. Of course, after evaluating the test results and determining their significance, responsible procedure requires that they be correlated with other clinical findings and the patient's complaints. The following case examples should be read critically, evaluating the potential of the neuropsychological test data to reflect the specific characteristics of the patient's neurological findings.

It may be interesting to note that many years ago using this procedure of individual prediction resulted in the observation that head injury routinely caused not only specific indications of cerebral lesions but generalized impairment as well. Before the accrual of evidence indicating that persons with significant head injuries had generalized as well as focal lesions (resulting from tension and shearing effects, displacement of brain structures, and cerebral edema), such conclusions were routine when using the Halstead-Reitan Battery. These findings resulted first from the Battery having been developed to reflect impairment of brain functions generally, regardless of the location of an identified focal lesion, and second, from knowledge of interpretation based upon individual evaluation of thousands of cases using a test battery that had been devised and validated to reflect both the strengths and weakness of brain functions in individual patients.

We learned many years ago (Reed, 1963) that lesions which developed from within the skull (e.g., strokes and intrinsic tumors) yielded much sharper differences between Verbal and Performance IQ values, depending upon the cerebral hemisphere involved, than traumatically-induced brain lesions (even though the neurosurgeon had indicated that the lesion involved only one cerebral hemisphere). Thus, in patients with craniocerebral trauma (including persons with closed head injuries), it is common to find evidence of more neuropsychological deficit involving one hemisphere than the other, but in nearly every case there are significant indications of generalized damage.

We invite the reader to consider the neuropsychological test data on the following patients in careful detail with relation to the history information and independent neurological findings, in order to develop a full appreciation and understanding of the neuropsychology of head injury as applied to the individual case.

CASE #1

Name: W.C.

Age: 30

Education: 12

Sex: Male

Handedness: Right

Occupation: Mechanic and
             Restaurant owner

Background Information

W.C. worked as a mechanic and also owned a small pizza restaurant. He had been in good health until he was involved in a moving vehicle accident at the age of 30. He was a passenger in the front seat and was thrown through the windshield, sustaining an extensive laceration of the right frontal area.

W.C.'s wife, who was with him when the accident occurred, reported that he did not begin to regain consciousness until approximately three hours after the injury and did not recognize her for the first hour he was conscious. He was confused for several hours after being admitted to the hospital but gradually began to recognize others, communicate verbally, and regain his orientation. He was hospitalized for four days, discharged, stayed at home for two days, then sought admission to another hospital where he remained for 18 days.

The patient reported experiencing headaches which felt like a severe pressure inside his head. W.C.'s wife also noticed that he seemed to be somewhat confused, frequently repeated himself verbally, and did not seem to be aware of this behavioral change himself. He also was described as having distinct personality changes: being much more irritable than before, having temper outbursts, and being easily upset by circumstances which previously did not bother him, such as the behavior of his two small children. This vague, generalized impairment continued and at the time of neuropsychological examination (two and one-half months after the injury) the patient had not yet felt that he was able to return to work.

Neurological Evaluation

W.C. reported that the feeling of pressure in his head became more pronounced when he moved about and was often accompanied by spells of mild dizziness. He denied any difficulty with his speech or auditory function, but said that his vision frequently blurred and had interfered with activities such as reading the newspaper.

Neurological examination was essentially within normal limits but the neurologist noted that the patient was intellectually impaired. W.C. had difficulty understanding simple directions and perseverated in carrying out various tasks. His alertness was diminished and he seemed somewhat confused generally. Although both pupils reacted to light the left was slightly larger than the right. Extraocular muscular function was intact and the visual fields were not constricted. All other aspects of the neurological exam, including electroencephalograms done three weeks and two months post-injury were within normal limits. Because of his complaints and the neurologist's observations that related to impaired alertness and confusion, W.C. was referred for neuropsychological examination.

Neuropsychological Examination

W.C. had a great number of complaints on the Cornell Medical Index Health Questionnaire. He said that he was often troubled with bad spells of sneezing and his nose was continually stuffed up, he had pains in the heart or chest area, often had severe toothaches and bleeding of the gums, usually felt bloated after eating, suffered from severe stomach pains, had severe pains in the arms or legs, and pains in his back made it impossible for him to work. He also reported that he frequently suffered from severe headaches, had pressure or pain in his head which made his life miserable, often had spells of severe dizziness and frequently felt faint, and had constant numbness or tingling in parts of his body as well as twitching of the face, head or shoulders. He said that he had great difficulty sleeping, usually was tired and exhausted when he arose in the morning, and often got spells of complete exhaustion or fatigue.

The patient also had a number of emotional complaints, including getting mixed up completely when he had to do things quickly, finding that his work fell apart when he was watched by a superior, feeling misunderstood by others and easily upset by criticism, and finding that people often annoyed and irritated him. He also reported that sudden noises made him jump or shake badly, that he became scared at sudden movements or noises at night, and was often awakened from his sleep by frightening dreams. W.C. felt that these problems had become more pronounced since the head injury.

Results on the Minnesota Multiphasic Personality Inventory also suggested that this man had significant emotional problems. The elevations on the Hypochondriasis and Hysteria scales, with a considerably lower score on the Depression scale, might raise a question of an emotional basis for the patient's somatic complaints. The elevation on the Schizophrenia scale suggests that W.C. might

be somewhat withdrawn and have difficulty establishing close emotional relationships with others in his environment.

The absence of objective findings on the neurological examination, in conjunction with the evidence of emotional problems in adjustment, would bring up the question of whether the post-injury problems reflected underlying emotional tension. (Many patients with similar histories are referred for psychiatric or clinical psychological evaluation). Fortunately, the neurologist who referred W.C. for neuropsychological testing was aware of the value of neuropsychological evaluation and felt that such an examination should be done to determine the course of treatment.

The test results indicate that W.C. had developed intellectual abilities within the average range but currently showed signs of significant generalized impairment of neuropsychological functions that particularly affected higher-level functions involved in abstraction, reasoning, and the capability to deal with complex problems.

The patient earned a Verbal IQ (101) almost exactly at the Average level (exceeding 53% of his age peers) and a Performance IQ (89) 12 points lower, in the upper part of of the Low Average range and exceeding about 23%. The Verbal subtest scores indicate that the patient performed a little poorly on Information (8) and Vocabulary (7), but most of the values were approximately at the average level. It would seem likely that W.C. probably was never particularly good in school and may not have been oriented toward intellectual or verbal activities.

The Performance subtests were more suggestive of impairment of brain functions. Compared to other subtest scores the Digit Symbol (7) subtest and the Picture Arrangement subtest (3) were poorly done and raise the possibility of right anterior temporal lobe dysfunction.

As we have often stated, the Wechsler Scale was not designed to provide a complete evaluation of brain-behavior relationships, either in terms of

THE HALSTEAD-REITAN
NEUROPSYCHOLOGICAL TEST BATTERY

Patient **W.C.** Age **30** Sex **M** Education **12** Handedness **R**

WECHSLER-BELLEVUE SCALE

VIQ	101
PIQ	89
FS IQ	95

Information	8
Comprehension	9
Digit Span	11
Arithmetic	10
Similarities	9
Vocabulary	7

Picture Arrangement	3
Picture Completion	8
Block Design	8
Object Assembly	11
Digit Symbol	7

HALSTEAD'S NEUROPSYCHOLOGICAL TEST BATTERY

Category Test 86

Tactual Performance Test

Dominant hand:	6.4
Non-dominant hand:	5.8
Both hands:	3.1

Total Time	15.3
Memory	5
Localization	3

Seashore Rhythm Test

Number Correct **14** 10

Speech-sounds Perception Test

Number of Errors 14

Finger Oscillation Test

Dominant hand:	45	45
Non-dominant hand:	43	

Impairment Index 0.9

TRAIL MAKING TEST

Part A: **35** seconds
Part B: **312** seconds

MINNESOTA MULTIPHASIC PERSONALITY INVENTORY

		Hs	77
		D	53
?	50	Hy	64
L	46	Pd	46
F	60	Mf	59
K	48	Pa	50
		Pt	52
		Sc	73
		Ma	55

REITAN-KLØVE TACTILE FORM RECOGNITION TEST

Dominant hand: **9** seconds; **0** errors
Non-dominant hand: **10** seconds; **0** errors

REITAN-KLØVE SENSORY-PERCEPTUAL EXAM

				Error Totals	
RH ___ LH ___	Both H:	RH **1** LH ___		RH **1** LH ___	
RH ___ LF ___	Both H/F:	RH **4** LF ___		RH **4** LF ___	
LH ___ RF ___	Both H/F:	LH ___ RF ___		RF ___ LH ___	
RE ___ LE ___	Both E:	RE ___ LE **2**		RE ___ LE **2**	
RV ___ LV ___	Both:	RV ___ LV ___		RV ___ LV ___	

REITAN-KLØVE LATERAL-DOMINANCE EXAM

Show me how you:

throw a ball	**R**
hammer a nail	**R**
cut with a knife	**R**
turn a door knob	**R**
use scissors	**R**
use an eraser	**R**
write your name	**R**

Record time used for spontaneous name-writing:

Preferred hand	**12** seconds
Non-preferred hand	**29** seconds

Show me how you:

kick a football	**R**
step on a bug	**R**

TACTILE FINGER RECOGNITION

R 1 ___ 2 ___ 3 ___ 4 **1** 5 **1**   R **2 / 20**
L 1 ___ 2 ___ 3 **1** 4 ___ 5 ___   L **1 / 20**

FINGER-TIP NUMBER WRITING

R 1 **1** 2 **1** 3 **3** 4 **3** 5 **4**   R **12 / 20**
L 1 **3** 2 **3** 3 **1** 4 **1** 5 **1**   L **9 / 20**

REITAN-INDIANA APHASIA SCREENING TEST

Form for Adults and Older Children

Name: _____ W. C. _____ Age: __30__

Copy SQUARE	Repeat TRIANGLE
Name SQUARE	Repeat MASSACHUSETTS "Massachusses"
Spell SQUARE	Repeat METHODIST EPISCOPAL "Method Epicopol"
Copy CROSS	Write SQUARE
Name CROSS	Read SEVEN
Spell CROSS	Repeat SEVEN
Copy TRIANGLE	Repeat/Explain HE SHOUTED THE WARNING.
Name TRIANGLE	Write HE SHOUTED THE WARNING.
Spell TRIANGLE	Compute 85 – 27 =
Name BABY	Compute 17 X 3 =
Write CLOCK	Name KEY
Name FORK	Demonstrate use of KEY
Read 7 SIX 2	Draw KEY
Read MGW	Read PLACE LEFT HAND TO RIGHT EAR.
Reading I	Place LEFT HAND TO RIGHT EAR
Reading II	Place LEFT HAND TO LEFT ELBOW

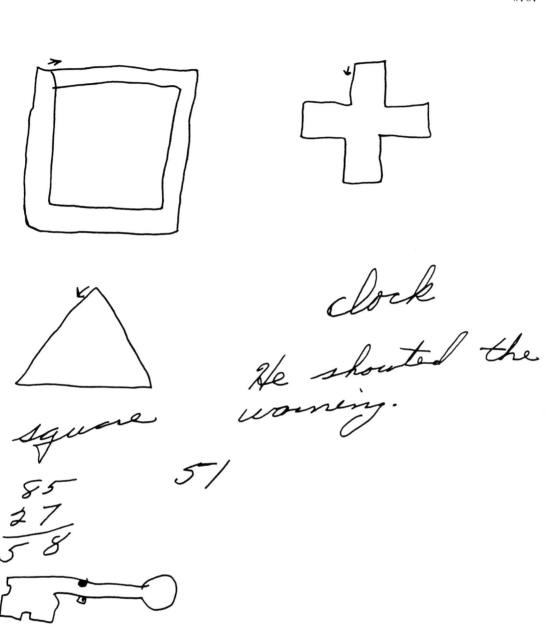

clock

He shouted the warning.

square

51

$$\begin{array}{r} 85 \\ 27 \\ \hline 58 \end{array}$$

content or methodological aspects of approach; however, in this case the 12-point difference between Verbal and Performance IQ values would be consistent with early reports (Wechsler, 1955) that Performance IQ is more susceptible to cerebral damage than Verbal IQ. The reader should be aware that this finding is true in instances of relatively stabilized diffuse cerebral damage but is not true for patients with acutely destructive lateralized cerebral lesions. Therefore, one of the basic problems in using the Wechsler Scale for identification of brain damage is that the results vary according to the particular type or condition of brain damage that is present. Without prior independent knowledge of the type or condition of brain damage that exists, interpretation of the Wechsler results becomes permissive.

In this instance, for example, the lower Performance IQ is consistent with (but not indicative of) cerebral damage. The low score on Picture Arrangement may be due to right anterior temporal lobe damage, but it is entirely conceivable that a low score on Picture Arrangement may be caused by other factors and additional confirming information would be necessary to be able to use the Picture Arrangement score diagnostically. In the evaluation of brain-behavior relationships the Halstead-Reitan Battery provides a framework within which interpretation of the Wechsler scores takes on significant additional meaning.

Scores on the four most sensitive indicators in the Halstead-Reitan Battery were all in the impaired range. The patient earned an Impairment Index of 0.9 (about 90% of Halstead's tests had scores in the brain-damaged range), performed very poorly on the Category Test (86), did even worse on Part B of the Trail Making Test (312 sec), and had a deficient score on the Localization component (3) of the Tactual Performance Test. Considering the fact that the Wechsler subtest scores suggest an adequate earlier development of intellectual functions, the scores on the four most sensitive measures must be considered a significant

indication of impaired brain functions (Reitan, 1985).

Lateralizing findings were also present. Although the Lateral Dominance Examination indicated that W.C. was strongly right-handed, right-footed, and right-eyed, his finger tapping speed was only slightly faster with his right hand (45) than his left (43) and he made some errors on the right side in tests of bilateral simultaneous tactile stimulation. He had some difficulty perceiving a stimulus to his right hand when it was given simultaneously with a stimulus to the left hand, but showed more striking evidence of impairment when the right hand was in competition with the left face.

The subject had somewhat more difficulty in finger-tip number writing perception on the right hand (12 errors) than the left (9 errors) but the findings predominantly indicated generalized dysfunction involving each cerebral hemisphere. Finally, the patient had difficulty enunciating METHODIST EPISCOPAL. Omitting the last syllable from METHODIST and the "S" in EPISCOPAL are types of responses given by persons with left cerebral lesions. Therefore, we see that W.C. had tactile-perceptual, motor, and language responses which indicate left cerebral hemisphere dysfunction.

Indicators of right hemisphere impairment were also present. The patient had a distinct tendency to fail to perceive an auditory stimulus to the left ear when stimuli were given to both ears simultaneously. He also performed somewhat slowly on the complex psychomotor tasks required by the Tactual Performance Test when using his left hand (5.8 min) compared with his right (6.4 min).

Also note the definite indication of right cerebral dysfunction in W.C.'s attempt to copy the key: He added notches to the stem (apparently as an afterthought) but the notches deviated in the same direction rather than being complementary. The patient also had some difficulty trying to achieve symmetry in the teeth, but the major deficit of the key is related to the notches in the stem. W.C. was not completely successful in making the arms of the cross symmetrical. He drew an inner and outer boundary on the square but many people (including control subjects) do this and our customary procedure is to tell the patient that an inner line is not necessary.

In summary, the test results were unequivocal in indicating cerebral damage. Although the lateralizing findings were not sufficiently strong to postulate a focal lesion of either cerebral hemisphere, they were entirely consistent with a hypothesis of generalized cerebral damage. It would seem likely that the lower Performance IQ (compared to the Verbal IQ) is also a sign of diffuse cerebral damage.

In retrospect we also would postulate that the low Picture Arrangement score indicates right temporal lobe dysfunction, particularly in light of the patient's tendency toward imperception of a stimulus delivered to the left ear with bilateral simultaneous auditory stimulation and the somewhat poor performance with the left hand (compared with the right) on the Tactual Performance Test.

It would be difficult to judge which cerebral hemisphere was more significantly impaired, but in the context of the overall test results such a judgement is not required. There is little usefulness in attempting to reach conclusions that have limited practical implications and are probably not subject to confirmation by independent validational findings. The important information to be gained from this set of test results is that this man is significantly and seriously impaired in higher-level aspects of brain functions. He becomes confused easily and is impaired in his ability to deal with tasks that require him to keep more than one element in mind at the same time (demonstrated by his score on Part B of the Trail Making Test). He has similar but more general difficulties with situations requiring him to define the nature of the problem based on his observations, analysis, and logical thinking (shown by his performance on the Category Test).

The patient's failure to return to work is probably caused more by his impairment in these higher-level functions than his specific deficits. Nevertheless, deficits in visual-spatial problem-solving skills — demonstrated especially in W.C.'s attempt to copy the key — would be a major disadvantage to a mechanic.

The neuropsychological impairment, associated with brain damage almost certainly sustained at the time of the head injury but unrecognized by the neurological examination, was clearly manifested by the neuropsychological test results. Findings of this kind are encountered frequently and when a patient is confused or seems to be intellectually impaired following a head injury she/he should certainly be referred for neuropsychological examination, even if no objective evidence of deficit is revealed by the neurological examination.

Neuropsychological remediation of cognitive deficits, or brain retraining, is a rather recent development. W.C. serves as a good example of a head-injured patient in whom training with RE-HABIT would certainly be indicated. We would recommend beginning the cognitive rehabilitation program with simple tasks on Track C, which focuses on relatively pure abstraction and reasoning problems. As the patient regains ability in "learning how to learn," it would be advisable to broaden the content of the training material. We would move to Track D to effect an integration between abstraction and reasoning requirements and the visual-spatial and manipulatory deficits. Even though W.C. performed the Tactual Performance Test within normal time limits, his drawings of the geometric figures and the key in the Aphasia Test demonstrated definite difficulty in dealing with spatial relationships.

It appears that W.C. needs fundamental training in visual-spatial and manipulatory skills and, considering his definite impairment in abstraction and reasoning abilities, must relearn these skills and integrate them with basic problem-solving abilities. Such integration of abstraction and reasoning is also necessary in tasks involving language and verbal content. In fact, the full range of brain retraining is necessary in patients who show specific involvement of both the left and right cerebral hemispheres in the context of generalized impairment of brain functions.

In this case, because there was such pronounced impairment in W.C.'s reasoning and logical analysis skills, we would begin at that level to facilitate his ability to progress with the more specific content of the other Tracks. It would be important to initiate such training as early as possible in order to link the gains made by training with the improvement that will occur with spontaneous recovery. From a clinical point of view it is encouraging for the client to note improvement in his capabilities, regardless of whether they are the result of specific training exercises or spontaneous recovery. From a research point of view it might be desirable to dissociate these two effects, but their interaction and facilitating influence have a very beneficial clinical effect upon the patient's motivation and morale.

CASE #2

Name: R.B.

Age: 37

Education: 12

Sex: Male

Handedness: Right

Occupation: Truck Driver

Background Information

Two and one-half months before this neuropsychological examination R.B. became involved in an argument with a neighbor. During the course of the argument the neighbor struck R.B. from behind with a blunt object and rendered him unconscious for several minutes. After regaining consciousness the patient was able to walk home, with a gait which his wife described as being very unsteady. He continued to be obviously impaired for the next several hours and was brought to a major medical center and hospitalized.

R.B. was confused and complained of a headache when admitted to the hospital. Shortly after being admitted he again lost consciousness for about 12 hours. He later had no memory of the injury or of being transported and admitted to the hospital. He showed evidence of decreased hearing in the right ear and complained of peculiar sensations and abnormal odors. The patient gradually improved, his headache lessened, and by the fifth day of hospitalization he was no longer confused. However, he was unable to stand with his eyes closed (Romberg sign) and the hearing loss and abnormal olfactory sensations were still present. Nevertheless, he was considered to be well enough to be discharged from the hospital and arrangements were made for follow-up medical examinations.

Neurological Examination

Two months after the injury R.B.'s headache had disappeared and he had no difficulty walking, though he did note that he would sometimes feel dizzy after exertion. The deafness of the right ear persisted and the patient still complained of sensing peculiar odors. He also reported that his attitude toward others had changed since the accident; he now felt that he was more friendly and understanding. In addition, he had discontinued drinking alcoholic beverages because they did not taste the same and he felt the intoxicating effects much more quickly than he had before the injury. Except for the severe hearing loss in the right ear and loss of olfaction bilaterally, the neurological examination (including the EEG and laboratory studies) within normal limits. Results of the audiometric examination confirmed the right-sided hearing loss and suggested a neural origin.

Neuropsychological Evaluation

Neuropsychological examination was done two and one-half months after the injury. The Cornell Medical Index Health Questionnaire revealed relatively few complaints but did indicate that R.B. had a hearing loss, often felt faint, and had spells of severe dizziness. The patient denied any other problems and clinically his main complaint was loss of his sense of smell.

The patient earned a Verbal IQ (114) in the middle part of the High Average range (exceeding about 82% of his age peers) and a Performance IQ (107) in the upper part of the Average range (exceeding about 68%). The Verbal subtest scores indicated that R.B. performed somewhat below his usual level on Information (9) and Digit Span (7). Digit Span is usually low among hospitalized persons, including control subjects. We would infer that the relatively low Information score may relate to a lifestyle characterized by minimal amounts of reading and limited intellectual pursuits.

The Performance subtests would raise a question about impairment of brain functions, particularly because of the low score on Digit Symbol (7). The Block Design (9) score might suggest specific impairment of the right cerebral hemisphere, but this would obviously be an over-interpretation if based only on the results of the Wechsler Scale.

Despite IQ values that generally exceeded about 77% of his age peers, the patient performed somewhat poorly on each of the four most sensitive indicators in the HRNTB. The Impairment Index (0.9) indicates a consistent impairment on most of Halstead's tests. In fact, the only score among those contributing to the Impairment Index that fell within the normal range was the Total Time of the Tactual Performance Test (15.3 min), but even this measure approached the cut-off score of 15.7 minutes. R.B. did not perform particularly poorly on the remaining three measures (among the four most sensitive indicators), but his scores on each were within the brain-damaged range. These results, especially considering the adequate IQ values, strongly suggest that R.B. had experienced at least a mild degree of brain damage (Reitan, 1985).

The Sensory-perceptual Examination was done essentially without error. Because of the patient's deafness in his right ear it was not possible to test for bilateral simultaneous auditory perception. However, R.B. made no mistakes in tests using tactile or visual stimuli and performed perfectly in tactile finger recognition and within the normal range in finger-tip number writing perception.

Note, though, that results of other tests of lateralized functions deviated from normal expectancy. The patient had no particular problems on the Aphasia Screening Test except in pronouncing METHODIST EPISCOPAL and possibly in right-left orientation. His addition of a syllable in pronouncing EPISCOPAL is typical of many persons with left cerebral damage (Wheeler & Reitan, 1962). R.B. did not actually make an error when asked to place his left hand to his right ear, but he initially showed some confusion and it was apparent to the examiner that the subject had to stop and think carefully before being able to respond correctly.

If R.B.'s other test scores had been within the normal range, these findings by themselves would probably not be sufficient to implicate the left cerebral hemisphere; however, in the context of the patient's performances on the four most sensitive indicators, these results appear to be genuine manifestations of mild left cerebral dysfunction.

Indicators of right cerebral hemisphere dysfunction were more distinct. The patient was just a little slow in finger tapping speed with his left hand (38) compared with his right (45) and showed a distinct deficit with his left upper extremity in grip strength. He also required almost as much time to do the Tactual Performance Test with his left hand on the second trial (5.9 min) as he did with his right hand on the first trial (6.0 min). His potential for improvement when using both hands documents the specificity of the mild deficit with the left upper extremity.

However, the reader may also have noted that each of these tests may have been limited by motor dysfunction of the left upper extremity and wonder whether these deficits could be a reflection of peripheral (rather than central) impairment. The positive findings on the general indicators greatly enhance the likelihood that these left-sided deficits are related to brain damage. We see that the mild impairment of motor functions with the left upper extremity is supported by the general indicators as

THE HALSTEAD-REITAN
NEUROPSYCHOLOGICAL TEST BATTERY

Patient **R.B.** Age **37** Sex **M** Education **12** Handedness **R**

WECHSLER-BELLEVUE SCALE

VIQ	114
PIQ	107
FS IQ	111

Information	9
Comprehension	13
Digit Span	7
Arithmetic	15
Similarities	14
Vocabulary	12

Picture Arrangement	12
Picture Completion	9
Block Design	9
Object Assembly	11
Digit Symbol	7

TRAIL MAKING TEST

Part A: **27** seconds
Part B: **96** seconds

STRENGTH OF GRIP

Dominant hand: **61.0** kilograms
Non-dominant hand: **51.5** kilograms

REITAN-KLØVE TACTILE FORM RECOGNITION TEST

Dominant hand: **15** seconds; **0** errors
Non-dominant hand: **15** seconds; **0** errors

REITAN-KLØVE SENSORY-PERCEPTUAL EXAM

RH___ LH___	Both H: RH___ LH___	
RH___ LF___	Both H/F: RH___ LF___	} NO
LH___ RF___	Both H/F: LH___ RF___	ERRORS
RE___ LE___	Both E: RE___ LE___	— NOT DONE
RV___ LV___	Both: RV___ LV___	RT. EAR DEAF.
___ ___	___ ___	} NO
___ ___	___ ___	ERRORS

TACTILE FINGER RECOGNITION

R 1___ 2___ 3___ 4___ 5___ R **0** / **20**
L 1___ 2___ 3___ 4___ 5___ L **0** / **20**

FINGER-TIP NUMBER WRITING

R 1 **1** 2___ 3___ 4___ 5___ R **1** / **20**
L 1 **2** 2___ 3___ 4___ 5___ L **2** / **20**

HALSTEAD'S NEUROPSYCHOLOGICAL TEST BATTERY

Category Test 52

Tactual Performance Test

Dominant hand: **6.0**
Non-dominant hand: **5.9**
Both hands: **3.4**

Total Time	15.3
Memory	5
Localization	3

Seashore Rhythm Test

Number Correct **24** 8

Speech-sounds Perception Test

Number of Errors 15

Finger Oscillation Test

Dominant hand: **45** 45
Non-dominant hand: **38**

Impairment Index **0.9**

REITAN-KLØVE
LATERAL-DOMINANCE EXAM

Show me how you:

throw a ball	**R**
hammer a nail	**R**
cut with a knife	**R**
turn a door knob	**R**
use scissors	**R**
use an eraser	**R**
write your name	**R**

Record time used for spontaneous name-writing:

Preferred hand	**5** seconds
Non-preferred hand	**15** seconds

Show me how you:

kick a football	**R**
step on a bug	**R**

REITAN-INDIANA APHASIA SCREENING TEST

Form for Adults and Older Children

Name: _____R. B._____ Age: __37__

Copy SQUARE	Repeat TRIANGLE
Name SQUARE	Repeat MASSACHUSETTS "Massachusses"
Spell SQUARE	Repeat METHODIST EPISCOPAL "Methodist Episticopol"
Copy CROSS	Write SQUARE
Name CROSS	Read SEVEN
Spell CROSS	Repeat SEVEN
Copy TRIANGLE	Repeat/Explain HE SHOUTED THE WARNING.
Name TRIANGLE	Write HE SHOUTED THE WARNING.
Spell TRIANGLE	Compute 85 − 27 =
Name BABY	Compute 17 X 3 =
Write CLOCK	Name KEY
Name FORK	Demonstrate use of KEY
Read 7 SIX 2	Draw KEY
Read MGW	Read PLACE LEFT HAND TO RIGHT EAR.
Reading I	Place LEFT HAND TO RIGHT EAR OK, but briefly confused.
Reading II	Place LEFT HAND TO LEFT ELBOW

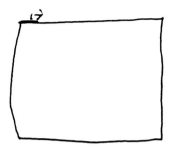

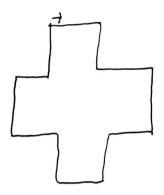

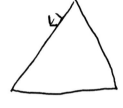

Clock   Square

He Shouted a warning.

```
  85
- 27
―――
  58
```

51

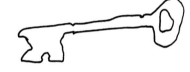

probably being related to impaired right cerebral functions, just as the general indicators supported the interpretation of the very mild left cerebral findings.

We also find that the types of errors this man made in his drawings of figures are characteristic of persons with mild right cerebral damage. Although the deficit in visual-spatial relationships was demonstrated most clearly in the drawing of the cross, the patient also made errors in drawing the square and triangle, finding it necessary to compensate as he proceeded and finally closed the figure. The drawing of the key can probably be considered to be within normal limits.

Because of their relative mildness we would not label these errors in drawing as constructional dyspraxia; however, they definitely deviate from normal expectancy, characterize the type of deficits seen in persons with mild right cerebral damage, and are significant in the interpretation of the overall results. In fact, the score on Block Design (9) may also be part of this total picture of mild impairment.

In summary, even though the overall impairment is mild, this particular configuration of test results can hardly be considered representative of a normal brain and the consistency of the findings constitutes a major basis for this conclusion. The results are suggestive of mild generalized cerebral dysfunction and there seems little doubt that the right cerebral hemisphere is more involved than the left. The relatively mild nature of the lateralizing signs and the adequate scores on many of the tests rule out the presence of a strictly focal lesion or a progressive pathological condition. The results are strongly indicative of an insult to the brain and specifically consistent with a hypothesis of a closed head injury. Convincing indications of generalized impairment (contrast the four most sensitive indicators with the IQ values) and evidence of lateralizing signs that involve each cerebral hemisphere are present. It is likely that this man will show continued improvement in the future, since only two and one-half months have elapsed since the injury was sustained.

CASE #3

Name: P.G.

Age: 28

Education: 9

Sex: Male

Handedness: Right

Occupation: Prison inmate

Background Information

Approximately three years before the current evaluation P.G. was struck on the head with an iron pipe. He was knocked unconscious but the exact duration of unconsciousness could not be determined. It was known, however, that he was stuporous for at least several days and was transferred from a local hospital to a major medical center for a more thorough evaluation. At that time the patient had significant expressive aphasia; he was not able to talk but could follow simple commands. When he was transferred he still had a large area of swelling over the left posterior parietal region.

Neurological Examination

Neurological examination revealed that the patient had a right facial weakness, a left pupil that was larger than the right pupil, and elevation of the left optic disc. Eight days after the injury P.G. had not shown any improvement and, in fact, had evidence of increasing papilledema. The patient was taken to surgery and it was discovered that he had a small subdural hematoma over the right cerebral hemisphere and an intracerebral hematoma in the left frontal area. The cerebral cortex in this area appeared to be contused and about 15 cc of hematoma was aspirated from the frontal lobe at a depth of about 1 cm. Following this procedure P.G. showed gradual and uneventful improvement.

About three months after the injury the patient began having epileptic seizures which were only partially controlled with medication. The clinical purpose of this present neurological evaluation was to achieve better seizure control and we had an opportunity to examine P.G. neuropsychologically at that time.

Neuropsychological Evaluation

This man showed a striking 40-point difference between Verbal (80) and Performance (120) intelligence levels. He performed quite poorly on the Digit Span (0) and Arithmetic (3) subtests of the Wechsler Scale and his scores were also somewhat below average on Information (7), Comprehension (9), and Vocabulary (8). Considering the fact that the patient had only a ninth-grade education, it seems likely that his Verbal intelligence was probably never well developed; nevertheless, a complete inability to perform the Digit Span subtest suggests that P.G. has experienced some type of impairment. The low Arithmetic score might possibly be related to lack of academic training, but it would also seem that some impairing factor had influenced this score as well.

P.G. did quite well on the Performance subtests, scoring above the average level on each subtest except Digit Symbol, although even on this subtest he earned a score of 10. Even though Digit Symbol had the lowest score of the Performance subtests, we would be disinclined to use this finding to substantiate a hypothesis of cerebral damage. The clinical basis for this interpretation centers on whether the score in question represents a normal performance for the individual involved; in this case it seems likely that an average score on Digit Symbol might well represent a normal performance for P.G.

In summary, the Wechsler results suggest that this man probably never had a particularly good educational background and, in addition, shows specific deficits on the Digit Span (and possibly Arithmetic) subtest. Although these results would not be inconsistent with left cerebral damage, they would hardly be an adequate basis for assuming that left cerebral damage was present (despite the 40-point difference in favor of the Performance IQ).

The four most sensitive indicators in the HRNTB showed variability in level of performance. The Impairment Index, 0.4, is a borderline value. Part B of the Trail Making Test (107 sec) was done rather poorly, suggesting impaired cerebral functions. The Category Test (37) and the Localization component of the Tactual Performance Test (8) were performed quite adequately. Thus, these results suggest that the patient does not have severe impairment of adaptive abilities and, considered independently, would hardly be sufficient to conclude that brain damage was present.

The next step in the analysis of the test results involves consideration of lateralizing findings. Although definitely right-handed, the patient's finger tapping speed was not quite as fast with his right hand (45) as his left (46) and he required slightly more time on the Tactile Form Recognition Test with his right hand (14) than his left (10). These findings involve both a motor (expressive) and tactile (receptive) deviation from normality and may have significance for left cerebral damage.

Results on the Aphasia Screening Test contributed further evidence of impairment. When asked to name the TRIANGLE, the patient responded "diamond." This particular response

sometimes occurs among normal subjects and, by itself, cannot be used as an unequivocal indication of dysnomia. However, P.G.'s attempts to spell TRIANGLE definitely deviated from normal expectancy and did not represent the type of errors customarily seen in persons with low education. Therefore, we have to conclude that this spelling of TRIANGLE definitely raises the possibility of left cerebral damage.

Probably even more convincing evidence of cerebral dysfunction was derived from P.G.'s response when he was asked to read 7 SIX 2. He failed to recognize that SIX represented either a word or a number and this type of error is frequently observed as a subtle manifestation of left cerebral dysfunction. The patient was not quite exact in his enunciation of MASSACHUSETTS and METHODIST EPISCOPAL, but the mistakes he made are the kind frequently seen among control subjects and have no significance for impaired brain functions.

Finally, when the patient attempted to write HE SHOUTED THE WARNING he made an error characteristic of brain-damaged persons in writing SHOUTED. Whether this is called dysgraphia or spelling dyspraxia may be open to question, but P.G.'s difficulty in using letters to form the word strengthened the hypothesis of left cerebral damage derived from spelling TRIANGLE. It is apparent from the patient's script that he has had the prior educational experience necessary to write simple words; therefore, lateralizing findings of significance for the left cerebral hemisphere included (1) somewhat slow finger tapping speed with the right hand; (2) mild slowness in tactile form recognition with the right hand; and (3) mild but definite errors on the Aphasia Test involving the use of language symbols for communicational purposes. Based on these findings we would conclude that this man shows evidence of mild dysphasia.

Other test results suggested mild impairment of right cerebral functions. Probably the most definite of these was seen in tactile finger localization.

THE HALSTEAD-REITAN
NEUROPSYCHOLOGICAL TEST BATTERY

Patient ____P.G.____ Age __28__ Sex __M__ Education __9__ Handedness __R__

WECHSLER-BELLEVUE SCALE

VIQ	80
PIQ	120
FS IQ	99

Information	7
Comprehension	9
Digit Span	0
Arithmetic	3
Similarities	11
Vocabulary	8

Picture Arrangement	13
Picture Completion	13
Block Design	15
Object Assembly	12
Digit Symbol	10

TRAIL MAKING TEST

Part A: __39__ seconds
Part B: __107__ seconds

STRENGTH OF GRIP

Dominant hand: __55__ kilograms

Non-dominant hand: __45__ kilograms

REITAN-KLØVE TACTILE FORM RECOGNITION TEST

Dominant hand: __14__ seconds; __0__ errors

Non-dominant hand: __10__ seconds; __0__ errors

REITAN-KLØVE SENSORY-PERCEPTUAL EXAM

			Error Totals	
RH ___ LH ___	Both H: RH ___ LH ___	RH ___ LH ___		
RH ___ LF ___	Both H/F: RH _1_ LF ___	RH _1_ LF ___		
LH ___ RF ___	Both H/F: LH ___ RF ___	RF ___ LH ___		
RE ___ LE ___	Both E: RE ___ LE ___	RE ___ LE ___		
RV ___ LV ___	Both: RV ___ LV ___	RV ___ LV ___		
___ ___		___ ___		
___ ___		___ ___		

TACTILE FINGER RECOGNITION

R 1__ 2__ 3__ 4__ 5__   R __0__ / 20

L 1__ 2 _1_ 3 _1_ 4 _1_ 5__   L __3__ / 20

FINGER-TIP NUMBER WRITING

R 1 _2_ 2 __ 3 __ 4 _2_ 5 __   R __4__ / 20

L 1 _2_ 2 __ 3 _1_ 4 __ 5 _1_   L __4__ / 20

HALSTEAD'S NEUROPSYCHOLOGICAL TEST BATTERY

Category Test   37

Tactual Performance Test

Dominant hand:	4.4
Non-dominant hand:	3.3
Both hands:	2.0

Total Time	9.7
Memory	8
Localization	8

Seashore Rhythm Test

Number Correct ____15____   10

Speech-sounds Perception Test

Number of Errors   12

Finger Oscillation Test

Dominant hand:	45	45
Non-dominant hand:	46	

Impairment Index   0.4

REITAN-KLØVE
LATERAL-DOMINANCE EXAM

Show me how you:

throw a ball	R
hammer a nail	R
cut with a knife	R
turn a door knob	R
use scissors	R
use an eraser	R
write your name	R

Record time used for spontaneous name-writing:

Preferred hand	__6__ seconds
Non-preferred hand	__14__ seconds

Show me how you:

kick a football	R
step on a bug	R

REITAN-INDIANA APHASIA SCREENING TEST

Form for Adults and Older Children

Name: _____ P. G. _____ Age: __28__

Copy SQUARE	Repeat TRIANGLE
Name SQUARE	Repeat MASSACHUSETTS "Massachusses"
Spell SQUARE	Repeat METHODIST EPISCOPAL "Methodist Epistopol"
Copy CROSS	Write SQUARE
Name CROSS	Read SEVEN
Spell CROSS	Repeat SEVEN
Copy TRIANGLE	Repeat/Explain HE SHOUTED THE WARNING.
Name TRIANGLE "Diamond"	Write HE SHOUTED THE WARNING.
Spell TRIANGLE "T–R–I–G–U–L–A–R"	Compute 85 – 27 =
Name BABY	Compute 17 X 3 = "41"
Write CLOCK	Name KEY
Name FORK	Demonstrate use of KEY
Read 7 SIX 2 "7 times 2." Examiner asked him to try it again. Then OK.	Draw KEY
Read MGW	Read PLACE LEFT HAND TO RIGHT EAR.
Reading I	Place LEFT HAND TO RIGHT EAR
Reading II	Place LEFT HAND TO LEFT ELBOW

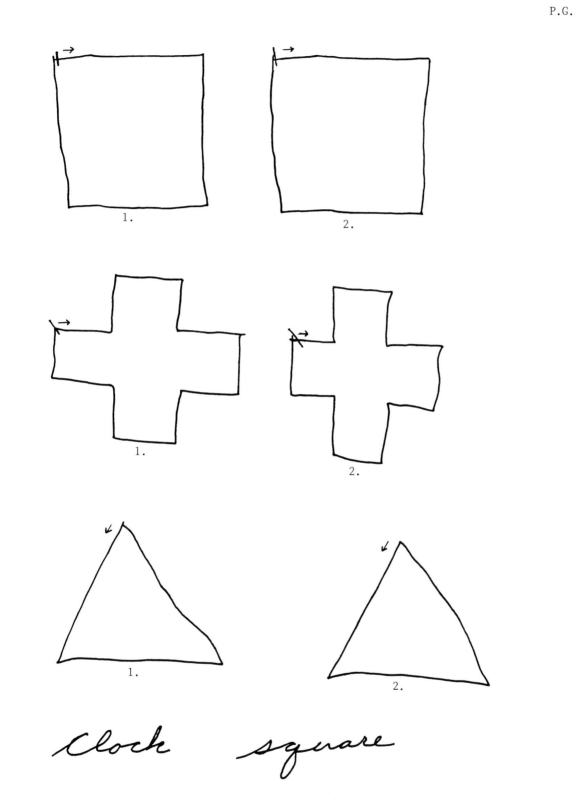

1.

2.

1.

2.

1.

2.

clock   square

He showed the warning

$$
\begin{array}{r}
85 \\
-27 \\
\hline
58
\end{array}
$$

41

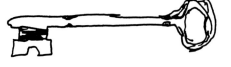

As shown by his performance with his right hand, the patient demonstrated that he had the basic abilities to do this task without error; however, he made three mistakes in 20 trials with the left hand. His grip strength was somewhat reduced in his left upper extremity (45 kg) compared with his right (55 kg) but this finding is probably not as convincing as the evidence of mild left finger dysgnosia. On the Tactual Performance Test the patient was also a little slow with his left hand (3.3 min) compared with his right (4.4 min) but we would classify this as the least significant of the three possible indicators of right cerebral dysfunction. Taken together, however, they do suggest that the right cerebral hemisphere is probably mildly impaired.

One might also raise a question about P.G.'s drawings of simple figures. The second attempt to draw the cross represents the instance in which the patient came closest to demonstrating brain-related deficiencies, but considering the variation shown by normal subjects, attribution of right cerebral damage on the basis of these drawings would be questionable.

At this point one can summarize the test results on P.G. by noting that there was strong evidence of left cerebral damage and mild evidence of right cerebral damage. These lateralizing results fell in the general context of a moderately poor score on Part B of the Trail Making Test, bilateral impairment in finger-tip number writing perception, and a 40-point disparity between Verbal and Performance IQ values. Even if limited educational background was responsible for lowered Verbal IQ, it would appear that left cerebral damage was also a contributing factor.

In summary, the test results suggest that this man has mild diffuse brain damage involving the left cerebral hemisphere to a greater extent than the right. There is certainly no basis for postulating a focal or progressive lesion of either cerebral hemisphere. In fact, the test results would be compatible with a relatively stabilized condition of the brain in a biological sense.

P.G.'s findings are quite characteristic of the long-term residual deficits of persons with head injuries. It is entirely likely that this man: (1) was considerably more impaired immediately after the injury was sustained than he was at the time of this testing; (2) has made an excellent recovery during the three years since the injury; and (3) is unlikely to show any further spontaneous recovery. Actually, considering the evidence of brain damage, it is surprising that P.G. performed as well as he did.

The right subdural hematoma may not have caused much deficit, but the intracerebral hematoma of the left frontal area was associated with definite cerebral cortical damage. In addition, the blow to the head must have been quite substantial and we would have expected the patient to demonstrate evidence of more generalized cerebral damage. This case serves as an interesting example of the potential for spontaneous unassisted recovery of brain functions and demonstrates the manifestations of mild residual deficits.

CASE #4

Name: W.B.

Age: 52

Education: 11

Sex: Male

Handedness: Right

Occupation: Factory worker

Background Information

W.B. had completed 11 grades in school and was working as an unskilled factory worker when he suffered a head blow in a moving vehicle accident. He was semi-conscious when admitted to the hospital and remained in a state of impaired consciousness for nine days before gradually beginning to regain his orientation. However, he still had periods of confusion and his memory for events pre- and post-accident was severely impaired.

Neurological Examination

Upon admission to the hospital W.B. was completely disoriented but able to move all four extremities spontaneously. He had a 4-inch laceration that extensively damaged the soft tissue overlying the skull in the left parietal-occipital area. Although the left external auditory canal was filled with blood, only a small laceration could be observed. There did not appear to be any leakage of cerebrospinal fluid. The pupils were equal and reacted to light; extraocular movements were intact and funduscopic examination was normal.

W.B. did not respond to verbal commands but did withdraw from painful stimuli. Gross examination suggested that the cranial nerves were intact, deep tendon reflexes were equal and slightly hyperactive, and bilateral Babinski signs were present. Bilateral cerebral angiograms done on the day of admission were within normal limits and an echoencephalogram revealed no midline shift. An electroencephalogram done nine days after the injury (when the patient was beginning to show normal orientation and communication) was within normal limits.

Neuropsychological testing was performed seven weeks after the injury. At that time the patient was fully conscious and showed no evidence of localizing findings on the neurological examination. However, the neurosurgeon felt that W.B's mental recovery was slow and showed significant intellectual impairment.

The patient himself had few complaints except that he felt that his memory was poor. His responses on the Cornell Medical Index Health Questionnaire revealed no particular complaints; he even denied that he had ever been knocked unconscious. Thus, it appeared that the validity of the results were questionable. The patient was not able to complete the Minnesota Multiphasic Personality Inventory.

Neuropsychological Evaluation

W.B. earned Verbal, Performance, and Full Scale IQ values in the Borderline range or the lower limit of the Low Average range of intelligence. The patient's IQ values exceeded only 4%–9% of his age peers. The results on the Verbal subtests do not provide much information to suggest that the patient had ever had intelligence levels that were in the normal range. Even his Information score (7), which was the highest of his Verbal subtest scores, was a full standard deviation below the average. His Vocabulary score (4) was two standard deviations below the average. It is possible that W.B. had experienced deficits in Verbal intelligence that consistently affected all of the Verbal subtests of the Wechsler Scale, but the more likely explanation is that he was never very bright.

The Performance subtest scores, on the other hand, do suggest the possibility of some impairment. The patient performed very poorly on Picture Arrangement (1) and Object Assembly (1) and it would seem possible that he might have had better abilities in the past. As is often the case, from the Wechsler scores alone it is difficult to confidently infer the premorbid intellectual level and draw conclusions regarding brain damage.

The patient performed very poorly on the four most sensitive indicators in the HRNTB. Even if W.B. had not had average intelligence in the past, the defective scores on these four measures suggest that he almost certainly has experienced brain-related impairment of cognitive functions. In light of these poor performances it is not surprising that the neurosurgeon felt that W.B.'s intellectual functions were impaired. It is likely that the physician was responding more to the indication of impaired alertness (demonstrated by the scores on the Category Test and Part B of the Trail Making Test) than the patient's verbal communicational skills.

Lateralizing indicators — specific pathognomonic signs as well as comparisons of performances on the two sides of the body — were also present. These types of findings definitely confirm the hypothesis of cerebral damage, which was initiated by the Wechsler scores, more strongly suggested by results on the four most sensitive measures, and definitively confirmed with the evidence indicating involvement of both cerebral hemispheres.

The patient showed definite abnormalities on the Aphasia Screening Test. His inability to name the TRIANGLE is probably a manifestation of dysnomia, although one cannot draw this conclusion definitely because W.B. did not offer an incorrect name. His confusion in spelling TRIANGLE may be at least partly related to his educational background, but the particular errors he made (insertion of the "I" and "A" after the "G") suggests that he was confused in a way that is typical of persons with left cerebral damage.

W.B.'s next error was in reading MGW. It is possible that the patient confused the letters, but it is equally likely that impaired vision may have caused him to mistake the "G" for an "O." The patient also had mild difficulty enunciating. In MASSACHUSETTS he substituted a "CH" sound for the "S" sound. He had more distinct difficulty repeating METHODIST EPISCOPAL. Omission of the "T" at the end of METHODIST is not significant, but confusing the sounds involved in EPISCOPAL is strongly suggestive of left cerebral damage.

Also note the patient's impaired ability to write SQUARE. It is not uncommon for persons with limited educational backgrounds to have difficulty writing the letter "Q"; however, when W.B. printed the word it appears that he may have perseverated with a letter resembling another "S." In this instance it is difficult to differentiate between effects of a limited education and impairment of the left cerebral hemisphere.

When asked to read SEVEN the patient named the letters individually before saying the word. It would appear that he has some difficulty interpreting the symbolic significance of printed letters and needed every possible cue in order to be able to read correctly. He also had a little difficulty in computing 85 − 27 = ; he first recorded "68" as his answer and then corrected it to "58." Again, it is difficult to be certain that this error reflects left cerebral damage rather than poor educational training.

Next, the patient showed evidence of mild right-left confusion when he was asked to place his left hand to his left elbow. Even though he spontaneously corrected his error, mistakes of this kind are made much more commonly by persons with

THE HALSTEAD-REITAN
NEUROPSYCHOLOGICAL TEST BATTERY

Patient _____ **W.B.** _____ Age __**52**__ Sex __**M**__ Education __**11**__ Handedness __**R**__

WECHSLER-BELLEVUE SCALE

VIQ	80
PIQ	76
FS IQ	74

Information	7
Comprehension	5
Digit Span	4
Arithmetic	4
Similarities	3
Vocabulary	4

Picture Arrangement	1
Picture Completion	3
Block Design	4
Object Assembly	1
Digit Symbol	3

TRAIL MAKING TEST

Part A: __**111**__ seconds
Part B: _____ seconds
(Discontinued: 423 seconds at G)

STRENGTH OF GRIP

Dominant hand: __**30.0**__ kilograms
Non-dominant hand: __**23.5**__ kilograms

REITAN-KLØVE TACTILE FORM RECOGNITION TEST

Dominant hand: __**62**__ seconds; __**1**__ errors
Non-dominant hand: __**54**__ seconds; __**0**__ errors

REITAN-KLØVE SENSORY-PERCEPTUAL EXAM

					Error Totals	
RH ___ LH ___	Both H:	RH ___ LH **1**		RH ___ LH **1**	
RH ___ LF ___	Both H/F:	RH **1** LF ___		RH **1** LF ___	
LH ___ RF ___	Both H/F:	LH ___ RF ___		RF ___ LH ___	
RE ___ LE ___	Both E:	RE ___ LE **3**		RE ___ LE **3**	
RV ___ LV ___	Both:	RV ___ LV ___		RV ___ LV ___	

TACTILE FINGER RECOGNITION

R 1 __ 2 **1** 3 **4** 4 **2** 5 **2**   R **9** / 20
L 1 __ 2 **1** 3 3 4 __ 5 __   L **4** / 20

FINGER-TIP NUMBER WRITING

R 1 **2** 2 **2** 3 **2** 4 __ 5 **1**   R **7** / 20
L 1 **1** 2 **1** 3 **1** 4 **1** 5 **2**   L **6** / 20

HALSTEAD'S NEUROPSYCHOLOGICAL TEST BATTERY

Category Test _____ **117** ___

Tactual Performance Test

Dominant hand:	**15.0 (2 blocks)**
Non-dominant hand:	**15.0 (1 block)**
Both hands:	**15.0 (1 block)**

Total Time	**45.0 (4 blocks)**
Memory	**0**
Localization	**0**

Seashore Rhythm Test

Number Correct __**16**__ _____ **10**

Speech-sounds Perception Test

Number of Errors _____ **39**

Finger Oscillation Test

Dominant hand:	**47**	**47**
Non-dominant hand:	**38**	

Impairment Index __**1.0**__

REITAN-KLØVE
LATERAL-DOMINANCE EXAM

Show me how you:

throw a ball	**R**
hammer a nail	**R**
cut with a knife	**R**
turn a door knob	**R**
use scissors	**R**
use an eraser	**R**
write your name	**R**

Record time used for spontaneous
name-writing:

Preferred hand	**7** seconds
Non-preferred hand	**21** seconds

Show me how you:

kick a football	**R**
step on a bug	**R**

REITAN-INDIANA APHASIA SCREENING TEST

Form for Adults and Older Children

Name: ___W. B._____ Age: __52__

Copy SQUARE	Repeat TRIANGLE
Name SQUARE	Repeat MASSACHUSETTS "Massatuchess"
Spell SQUARE	Repeat METHODIST EPISCOPAL "Methodiss Episdeole"
Copy CROSS	Write SQUARE Had difficulty writing the "q".
Name CROSS	Read SEVEN "S-E-V-E-N--Seven"
Spell CROSS	Repeat SEVEN
Copy TRIANGLE	Repeat/Explain HE SHOUTED THE WARNING.

Name TRIANGLE
    "Part of a cross, but not
    like it."
	Write HE SHOUTED THE WARNING.

Spell TRIANGLE "T-R-I-A-N-G-I-A-L-E"	Compute 85 – 27 =
Name BABY	Compute 17 X 3 =
Write CLOCK	Name KEY
Name FORK	Demonstrate use of KEY
Read 7 SIX 2	Draw KEY
Read MGW "M-O-W"; spontaneously corrected.	Read PLACE LEFT HAND TO RIGHT EAR.
Reading I	Place LEFT HAND TO RIGHT EAR
Reading II	Place LEFT HAND TO LEFT ELBOW Placed left hand to right elbow; immediately corrected.

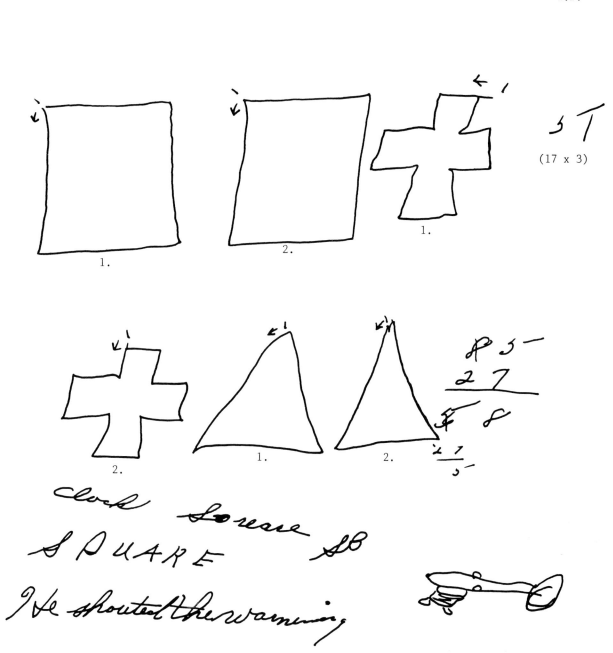

1.

2.

1.

2.

1.

2.

5 T

(17 x 3)

R 5
2 7
—
8

clock Louise SB

SQUARE

He shouted the warning

left than right cerebral damage (Wheeler & Reitan, 1962). Thus, although his errors were not pronounced and probably would not be classified as dysphasic, the Aphasia Screening Test yielded results which definitely indicated left cerebral hemisphere dysfunction. W.B's mistakes can be recognized as being quite typical of persons with left cerebral damage and the errors certainly represent mild impairment of the ability to use language symbols for communicational purposes.

The Aphasia Screening Test has the advantage of using standardized stimulus material and when the neuropsychologist has had extensive experience with many patients he/she can recognize the types of errors that characterize left or right cerebral damage, even if the deficits are not severe enough to merit a diagnosis of dysphasia. In fact, there is a gradual gradation of difficulty in dealing with verbal symbolic material for communicational purposes, extending from mild (but real) evidence of left cerebral damage to types of deficits customarily recognized by aphasiologists.

This man's drawings showed evidence of right cerebral hemisphere damage. His first attempt to draw the cross demonstrated imbalances of the extremities that certainly raise a question about mild constructional dyspraxia. The second cross was better, but the drawing of the key had unequivocal significance. The most striking manifestation relating to constructional dyspraxia was the notches on the stem of the key near the teeth. The fact that the patient made these notches in the same direction instead of complementary is a near-certain indication of brain-related impairment.

Again, one might question whether a diagnostic statement of constructional dyspraxia could be applied on the basis of these drawings. As we have noted earlier, this is a clinical judgement and should not be permitted to cloud recognition of the fact that the patient had types of difficulties dealing with simple spatial relationships that are characteristic of persons with right cerebral damage.

The patient showed other lateralizing findings based upon comparisons of performances on the two sides of the body. Probably the most reliable indication of left cerebral damage was W.B.'s greater difficulty on the Tactile Finger Recognition Test with his right hand (9 errors) than his left (4 errors). He also required more time with his right hand (62 sec) in tactile form recognition than with his left hand (54 sec) and made one error when using his right hand. Finally, in one instance, he failed to appreciate a stimulus to his right hand when given simultaneously with a stimulus to the left face.

The fact that the patient performed very poorly on the Speech-sounds Perception Test (39 errors) falls in the same category as a number of the other test results that relate to verbal material; it is difficult to discern the extent to which this score relates to poor general intelligence and education, although the score is probably a valid reflection of cerebral damage (at least to some extent).

Some of the lateralizing indicators also implicated right cerebral damage, including slow finger tapping speed with the left hand (38) compared with the right (47) and reduced grip strength in the left upper extremity (23.5 kg) compared with the right (30.0 kg). The patient also showed evidence of misperception on the left side in tests of bilateral simultaneous sensory stimulation. The deficits occurred particularly with auditory stimulation, in which W.B. failed to recognize the stimulus to the left ear in three of four instances when stimuli were given bilaterally. The patient also had a tendency to fail to perceive a stimulus to his left hand when given simultaneously with a competing stimulus to the right hand.

One might be tempted to attribute the patient's poor performance with his left hand (second trial) on the Tactual Performance Test to right cerebral dysfunction; however, the major conclusion to be drawn from the pattern of performances on the TPT is that W.B. had significant difficulty on each trial. In fact, he did not do any better on the third trial (using both hands) than using only the left hand alone. Therefore, the results on this measure do not provide convincing evidence of lateralized cerebral damage; instead, they suggest that the patient's ability to perform complex and difficult tasks is significantly and seriously impaired.

In summary, W.B.'s test results represent significant generalized impairment of neuropsychological functions dependent upon the condition of the brain. Although there is no doubt that this man has dysfunction of each cerebral hemisphere, the results do not suggest the presence of any specific focal lesion. Even though W.B. may never have been particularly intelligent, the evidence of neuropsychological deficit is quite apparent and definite.

Neuropsychological testing was done only seven weeks after the injury was sustained. Although W.B. was probably on a recovery course and will continue to improve, it is likely that the final consequences of his cerebral damage will be sufficiently severe and permanent to cause him serious adaptational problems in the future. We also should note that this man was 52 years old when he was injured and there is some reason to believe, at least from clinical observation, that older persons have more difficulty than younger persons in regaining neuropsychological functioning following a head injury.

CASE #5

Name: C.H.

Age: 57

Education: 8

Sex: Female

Handedness: Right

Occupation: Cook

Background Information

C.H. was the assistant head cook at a university medical center cafeteria when she sustained a severe head injury in a moving vehicle accident. She first received emergency medical treatment at the scene of the accident and was then admitted to a major medical center. Physical examination at that time showed considerable trauma to the soft tissues of the scalp as well as lacerations requiring emergency suturing.

Upon admission to the hospital the patient was stuporous and did not speak. She responded in a generalized and rather purposeless manner to painful stimulation and at times became very restless. It was possible to determine that C.H. had some weakness of the right limbs and face and a fracture of her right clavicle. Pupillary size was unequal with the right pupil larger than the left. Although ocular movement to the right was observed, C.H. did not move her eyes to the left of midline. Babinski signs were present bilaterally. Cerebral angiograms showed a shift of structures from left to right with evidence of a left subdural hematoma.

Surgery was performed and acute subdural hematomas were found and removed from both parietal areas. More extensive surgery was performed on the left cerebral hemisphere with repair of extensive contusion and laceration of the frontal and temporal lobes.

Neurological Examination

C.H. remained stuporous and her right hemiparesis became more profound during the first few post-operative days. Gradually, after about one week, she began to resume speaking and recover movement in her right limbs. She continued to improve during the month that she was hospitalized.

According to her neurosurgical evaluation at that time C.H. was ambulatory and speaking well, her wounds had healed, there was no evidence of intracranial hypertension, and she had completely recovered her motor functions. However, the neurosurgeon felt that she had significant post-traumatic mental impairment manifested by memory lapses, obstreperousness, and confusion. The neurosurgeon, who was a clinical specialist in the area of head injury and well-known for his publications in this area, felt that the patient would make a good recovery "in the mental sphere" and that the overall prognosis was fairly good.

Neuropsychological Evaluation

Neuropsychological examination was done almost exactly one month after the injury. Many of the tests could not be administered because of the patient's severe impairment. Repeated instructions and practice were necessary on Part A of the Trail Making Test and when the patient finally took the test she required 241 seconds to complete it. C.H.

was not able to understand the instructions well enough to even do the sample of Part B.

Repeated efforts were made to communicate the instructions of the Category Test but with essentially no success. The patient was not able to coordinate her verbal response with depressing the lever. For example, she would say "three" and pull lever one. Because she was making consistent errors in Subtest II and obviously did not understand what was involved, the test was discontinued.

We were able to obtain responses for motor and sensory-perceptual tasks as well as certain other well-defined procedures, but the patient was not able to make any progress on tasks that required a continued performance supported by her own initiative. Although C.H. was able to converse in simple terms and did not appear to be as impaired as the testing indicated, in nearly every formal testing situation she demonstrated that she had great difficulty understanding instructions and was not able to carry out any but the simplest procedures.

As noted, many of the tests could not be administered. We did give the Wechsler Scale, but the patient was able to earn very little credit. For example, the scaled scores of 2 and 3 on Information and Comprehension corresponded with raw scores of 1 and 3, respectively. C.H. was able to repeat six digits forward and three backwards on the Digit Span subtest, earning her a score of 6. On the other subtests the patient was not able to earn very much additional credit.

The Finger Oscillation Test and Strength of Grip measurement yielded information that was helpful in comparing the status of the two cerebral hemispheres. Although definitely right-handed, this woman performed worse on each of these tasks with her right hand than her left.

The Sensory-perceptual Examination showed only minimal impairment. The patient made no mistakes on any of the tests of unilateral or bilateral sensory stimulation. She made three errors on her right hand in Tactile Finger Recognition. In testing her left hand we were not able to obtain reliable results; the patient always moved her finger immediately after the stimulus was delivered and seemed unable to avoid this type of response. We attempted to have her open her eyes after each trial and use her other hand to point to the finger she thought was touched but because that finger was already moving she had a special cue.

We were able to examine the patient for fingertip number writing perception on each hand; surprisingly she had almost no difficulty with this task, making only one error in 20 trials on each side. These findings, in the context of the extremely limited performances on more complex tests, suggest that the patient did not have specific structural involvement of the parietal lobe in either cerebral hemisphere. We would presume that the bilateral parietal hematomas represented bleeding in the subdural space rather than direct tissue damage to the underlying cerebral cortex in these areas. Note, however, that the patient did show definite evidence of motor impairment, especially of the right upper extremity; this finding probably correlates with the contusion and laceration of cerebral cortical tissue observed in the frontal lobe.

Because the surgical procedure had also revealed extensive tissue damage in the left temporal lobe, we would expect C.H. to show impairment in dealing with language symbols for communicational purposes (dysphasia). Recall that C.H. gave the impression of having relatively normal language abilities in casual conversation. It is not uncommon for a patient who has pronounced expressive dysphasic deficit to communicate reasonably well under permissive circumstances but demonstrate serious deficits when required to respond to the type of specific stimulus material found in the Aphasia Screening Test.

When asked to name the SQUARE C.H.'s response was entirely inappropriate. Her spelling of SQUARE was correct except that she omitted the "E," an error that may be related to her rather limited educational background. She was able to

THE HALSTEAD-REITAN
NEUROPSYCHOLOGICAL TEST BATTERY

Patient _____ **C.H.** _____ Age __**57**__ Sex __**F**__ Education __**8**__ Handedness __**R**__

WECHSLER-BELLEVUE SCALE

VIQ	**70**
PIQ	**72**
FS IQ	**63**

Information	**2**
Comprehension	**3**
Digit Span	**6**
Arithmetic	**0**
Similarities	**1**
Vocabulary	**1**

Picture Arrangement	**1**
Picture Completion	**0**
Block Design	**1**
Object Assembly	**0**
Digit Symbol	**0**

TRAIL MAKING TEST

Part A: __**241**__ seconds
Part B: Could not do.

STRENGTH OF GRIP

Dominant hand: __**16.5**__ kilograms
Non-dominant hand: __**18.5**__ kilograms

REITAN-KLØVE TACTILE FORM RECOGNITION TEST

Dominant hand: __**0**__ errors
Non-dominant hand: __**0**__ errors

REITAN-KLØVE SENSORY-PERCEPTUAL EXAM — No errors

Error Totals

RH___LH___	Both H: RH___LH___	RH___LH___
RH___LF___	Both H/F: RH___LF___	RH___LF___
LH___RF___	Both H/F: LH___RF___	RF___LH___
RE___LE___	Both E: RE___LE___	RE___LE___
RV___LV___	Both: RV___LV___	RV___LV___

TACTILE FINGER RECOGNITION

R 1 **1** 2 **1** 3 **1** 4___ 5___   R **3** / **20**
L 1___ 2___ 3___ 4___ 5___   SEE DESCRIPTION IN TEXT

FINGER-TIP NUMBER WRITING

R 1___ 2___ 3___ 4___ 5 **1**   R **1** / **20**
L 1 **1** 2___ 3___ 4___ 5___   L **1** / **20**

HALSTEAD'S NEUROPSYCHOLOGICAL TEST BATTERY

Category Test   <u>Discontinued</u>

Tactual Performance Test

Dominant hand: <u>Could not do.</u>
Non-dominant hand: <u>Could not do.</u>
Both hands: <u>Could not do.</u>

         Total Time _____
         Memory _____
         Localization _____

Seashore Rhythm Test

Number Correct <u>Could not do.</u>   _____

Speech-sounds Perception Test

Number of Errors <u>Could not do.</u>   _____

Finger Oscillation Test

Dominant hand: __**18**__   **18**
Non-dominant hand: __**29**__

Impairment Index _____

REITAN-KLØVE
LATERAL-DOMINANCE EXAM

Show me how you:
throw a ball	**R**
hammer a nail	**R**
cut with a knife	**R**
turn a door knob	**R**
use scissors	**R**
use an eraser	**R**
write your name	**R**

Record time used for spontaneous name-writing:
Preferred hand	**13** seconds
Non-preferred hand	**26** seconds

Show me how you:
kick a football	**R**
step on a bug	**R**

REITAN-INDIANA APHASIA SCREENING TEST

Form for Adults and Older Children

Name: _____C. H._____ Age: __57__

Copy SQUARE	Repeat TRIANGLE
Name SQUARE "Four." Examiner questioned. "Six - - looks like a five."	Repeat MASSACHUSETTS "Mach-chusett"

Spell SQUARE
    "S-Q-U-A-R"
	Repeat METHODIST EPISCOPAL
	    "Matisdis Dispico"

Copy CROSS	Write SQUARE
Name CROSS	Read SEVEN
Spell CROSS	Repeat SEVEN
Copy TRIANGLE	Repeat/Explain HE SHOUTED THE WARNING. Explanation: "I don't know. It's all filled out. When you get it all filled out."
Name TRIANGLE "Curve - curves like they use a razor with." When told TRIANGLE by examiner, patient said, "Yes, curve."	Write HE SHOUTED THE WARNING.
Spell TRIANGLE "T-R-I-A-L"	Compute 85 - 27 = Added on first attempt. 34 - 13 given by examiner. Patient called it a "+" and attempted to multiply.
Name BABY	Compute 17 X 3 =Patient needed to write problem on paper. Given 12x2 and patient answered "42". When given 3x2 patient wrote
Write CLOCK Drew the clock first. Wrote only when again requested. Then said, "That's a curve, picture of a clock."	Name KEY 42x3 on paper and attempted to multiply.
Name FORK	Demonstrate use of KEY
Read 7 SIX 2 "Six -- 7 and then a 6 and a 2."	Draw KEY "Don't know whether I can draw it or not."
Read MGW	Read PLACE LEFT HAND TO RIGHT EAR.
Reading I	Place LEFT HAND TO RIGHT EAR
Reading II "This is the Friday - Friday - A-M-W-L - F-A-M-O-I-L -- W-I-N-N-E-L -- off the dog show."	Place LEFT HAND TO LEFT ELBOW Placed left hand to right elbow.

C.H.

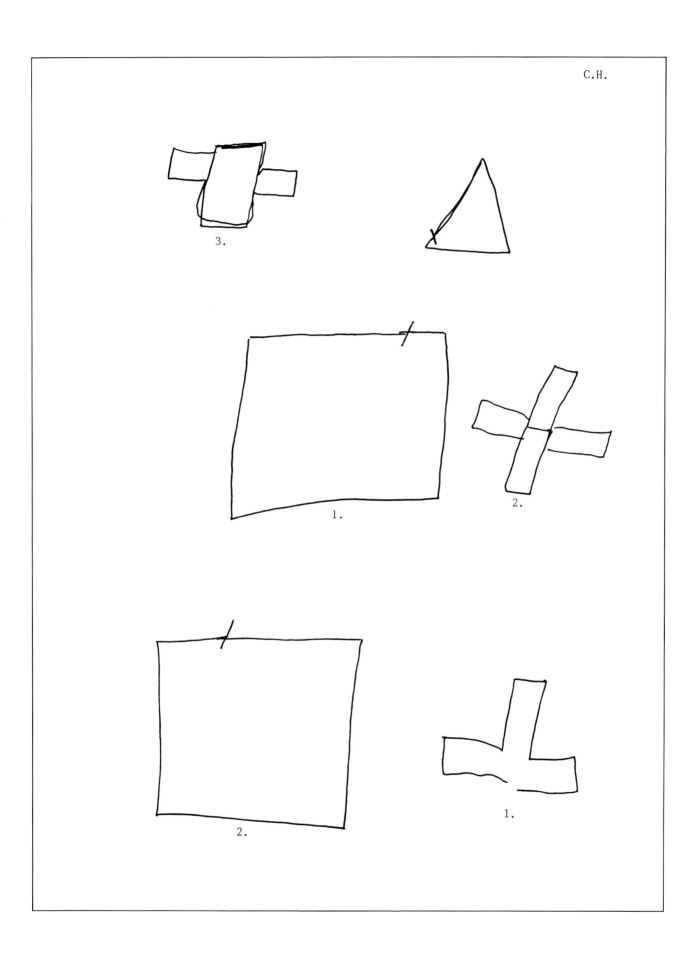

3.

1.

2.

2.

1.

he shouted a Warning

Square

(1)
$$\begin{array}{r} ^1\;8\,5 \\ 2\,7= \\ \hline 1\,1\,2 \end{array}$$

(2)
$$\begin{array}{r} 8\,5 \\ 2\,7 \\ \hline 6\,8 \end{array}$$

$$\begin{array}{r} 3\,4 \\ -\,1\,3 \\ \hline 3\ 1 \\ =2\ 3 \\ \hline 2\,6\ 1- \end{array}$$

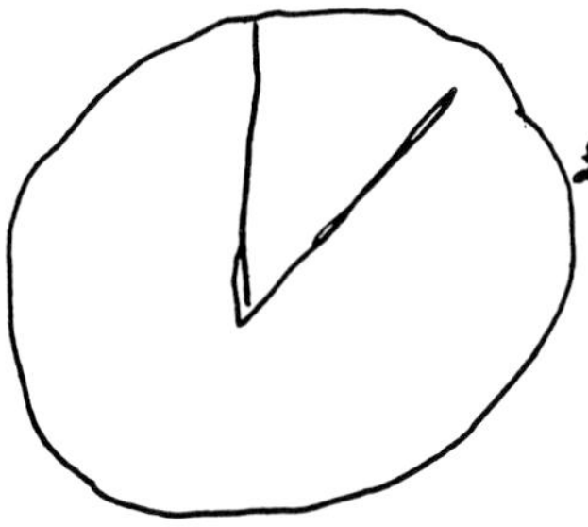

Clock

$$\begin{array}{r} 2 \\ -\,1 \\ \hline 1 \end{array}$$

$$\begin{array}{r} ^i\,7 \\ 3 \\ \hline 4\,2 \end{array}$$

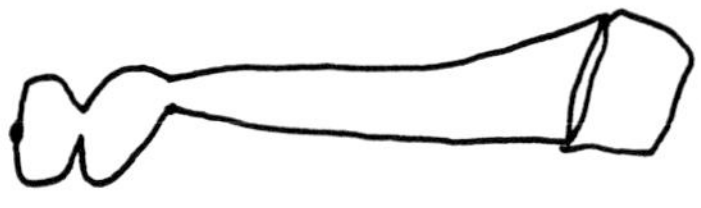

$$\begin{array}{r} 4\,2 \quad (3 \times 2) \\ 3 \\ \hline 1\,4 \end{array}$$

name and spell CROSS correctly, but when asked to name the TRIANGLE she said, "Curve-curves like they use a razor with." The examiner finally told C.H. the name of the figure and the patient responded by saying "Yes, curve." Finally, C.H. had to be told repeatedly that the name was TRIANGLE and she made an effort to spell it but became confused toward the end of her attempt.

The patient named the BABY correctly but when asked to look at the picture of the CLOCK and write the name she responded by attempting to draw the stimulus picture. Following this effort the examiner again asked her to write the name and she responded by saying, "That's a curve-picture of a clock." It is apparent that she was perseverating with the word "curve," a type of response that is not uncommonly seen in persons with severe impairment of expressive naming functions. We see that C.H. was able to write "clock" legibly. She named the FORK correctly but had difficulty with 7 SIX 2, responding first to the SIX and then to the entire configuration.

The patient was able to read individual letters and the simpler reading item but became entirely confused when attempting to read HE IS A FRIENDLY ANIMAL, A FAMOUS WINNER OF DOG SHOWS. She was not able to get any of this item correctly read, obviously confusing FRIENDLY as "FRIDAY." She apparently was not able to read certain of the other words and made an attempt by reading individual letters. Even the latter part of the sentence contained errors such as "off" for OF, an insertion of "the," and "show" for SHOWS. We would suspect that the patient demonstrated additional evidence of verbal perseveration in her identification of individual letters, ending each series with the letter "L."

C.H. also showed fairly typical evidence of central dysarthria, a finding much more common in persons with left cerebral lesions than right (Wheeler & Reitan, 1962). The criterion here relates to omission, addition, or transposition of syllables rather than merely slurring of the sounds involved. The patient demonstrated such difficulties with both MASSACHUSETTS and METHODIST EPISCOPAL.

The patient offered a poor explanation of the sentence HE SHOUTED THE WARNING but her response was so inappropriate that it is difficult to evaluate. There are several possible explanations for her response: (1) she simply did not understand the meaning of the sentence; (2) she was not able to verbally communicate her understanding of the meaning; or (3) she was so generally confused that the sentence had no meaning at all to her. Nevertheless, note that she was able to write the sentence quite satisfactorily. (It is not uncommon, particularly for persons with rather limited educational backgrounds, to substitute "a" for "THE.")

The patient had great difficulty even with simple arithmetical computations. In her first attempt to solve $85 - 27 =$ she added the numbers. In her second attempt she subtracted, but made an error that might be attributable to poor educational background. The examiner pursued the question of possible dyscalculia further by writing another problem for the patient ($34 - 13$). In this instance the patient was not given any verbal instructions that the problem involved subtraction. She proceeded by attempting to multiply, although she did not do this correctly.

The patient was not able to make any progress doing 17×3 mentally and needed to write the problem on the paper. She did not solve the problem correctly, but was apparently making an attempt to multiply. She was asked to do 12×2 mentally and she answered "42." The examiner then decided to give her a very simple problem and asked her to solve 3×2 by writing the problem down on the paper. The patient wrote "42×3" on her paper and attempted to multiply but her answer of 16 indicates that she had little understanding of the numerical relationships involved. These demonstrations provide clear evidence of dyscalculia, both in terms of impaired ability to understand numerical relationships as well as the arithmetical procedures of addition, subtraction, and multiplication.

The patient also showed her confusion when she was asked to place her left hand to her left elbow; she responded by placing her left hand to her right elbow. It is difficult to discern whether this error is a definite indication of right-left confusion (a left hemisphere sign) or a manifestation of generalized confusion. However, it is the kind of mistake that is made much more commonly by persons with left cerebral lesions than persons with generalized or right cerebral damage (Wheeler & Reitan, 1962).

Finally, C.H. had great difficulty copying simple spatial configurations. Even her drawings of the square showed confusion in dealing with spatial form, manifested particularly by drawing lines of unequal length and having to compensate when closing the figure. Difficulty with the cross, however, was more obvious. C.H. became confused trying to achieve symmetry of the extensions, showing definite signs of constructional dyspraxia.

In summary, the Aphasia Screening Test showed distinct impairment in (1) simple naming of objects (dysnomia); (2) simple spelling (spelling dyspraxia); (3) appreciation of the symbolic significance of individual letters (visual letter dysgnosia); (4) understanding the symbolic significance of configurations of letters that form words (dyslexia); (5) enunciation of words (central dysarthria); (6) understanding and comprehending verbal communications through the auditory avenue (auditory verbal dysgnosia); (7) understanding numerical relationships and arithmetical processes (dyscalculia); (8) right-left differentiation; and (9) the ability to construct simple spatial configurations (constructional dyspraxia). The patient also showed a definite tendency toward perseveration of verbal responses, a finding characteristic of tissue damage in the language area of the left cerebral cortex.

It is apparent from the above analysis of the neuropsychological data that considerable emphasis was placed upon results of the Aphasia Screening Test in deriving positive evidence of cerebral damage. The signs of dysphasia, coupled with the distinct indications of constructional dyspraxia, were sufficient to implicate each cerebral hemisphere. The impairment of the right upper extremity in both grip strength and finger tapping speed suggested more serious damage of the left cerebral hemisphere, although the patient performed poorly in finger tapping speed on both hands.

The relative absence of sensory-perceptual deficits suggests that the structural aspect of the brain lesion(s) did not involve the posterior parts of the cerebral hemispheres, although traumatic injuries, regardless of location, tend to cause less deficits on these tasks than intrinsic tumors or vascular occlusions (Hom & Reitan, 1982). The severe general nature of C.H.'s deficits, particularly involving higher-level and more complex tasks, was clearly demonstrated by both the Verbal and Performance IQ values as well as the fact that the patient was so severely impaired that she was not even able to take many of the tests.

The severity of C.H.'s impairment, manifested on both general and specific indicators of brain function, conflicts somewhat with the neurosurgeon's conclusion that the patient had shown a very good recovery (except for "mental deficits") and particularly that she had achieved complete recovery of motor functions. Further, the neurosurgeon noted that the patient was "speaking well." The reader can see, however, that the neuropsychological evaluation demonstrated that the patient had motor deficits and serious manifestations of speech and language dysfunctions. In fact, the severity of her impairment caused us to have grave reservations concerning her prognosis for recovery (Dikmen & Reitan, 1976). The reason for the disparity in opinions in this case probably related to the fact that in casual encounters the patient made a clinical impression of being fairly capable and formal testing was necessary to reveal her deficits.

This case illustrates that neuropsychological evaluation can make a very valuable clinical contribution. Unless the patient's deficits are identified, a realistic approach toward rehabilitation cannot be properly instituted, the consequences of the deficits on performances in everyday life cannot be correctly evaluated, and estimates of prognosis cannot be made with any degree of accuracy.

CASE #6

Name: C.B.

Age: 26

Education: 12

Sex: Male

Handedness: Left

Occupation: Storekeeper

Background Information

At the age of 25 C.B. was involved in a moving vehicle accident and sustained a severe head injury. His prior medical history included the usual childhood diseases as well as an attack of pertussis as an infant and an episode of infantile convulsions. He recovered from these illnesses uneventfully and apparently developed normal cognitive functions.

The head injury caused immediate unconsciousness and upon admission to a local hospital the patient was in a decerebrate state, had trouble breathing, and had an elevated body temperature. He remained in a decerebrate condition for an extended period of time and had pronounced spasticity of his upper and lower extremities. Bilateral burr holes revealed no evidence of intracranial bleeding.

The patient's state of impaired consciousness continued for several months then gradually began to show some improvement. Five and one-half months after the injury C.B. started to recognize his surroundings and was able to follow simple commands; however, he could not feed himself and required assistance with almost every activity that he did. He was transferred to a major medical center for further evaluation and treatment.

Neurological Evaluation

At the time C.B. was transferred the general physical examination was essentially within normal limits although he showed obvious neurological deficit. Extraocular movements were adequate except that C.B. could not move his eyes beyond the midline toward the left side. His gait appeared to be somewhat ataxic but this was actually difficult to determine because of his extreme spasticity. Despite the spasticity, he was able to move his upper and lower extremities on command. He had flexion contractures of both elbows and wrists and his body was held in a decorticate position most of the time.

The patient was not able to perform the finger-to-nose test but the heel-to-knee test was done well. He also had fair muscle strength of his upper extremities. Deep tendon reflexes were hyperactive on the left side and Babinski and Hoffmann signs were present bilaterally. It was not possible to conduct a reliable sensory examination. Bilateral carotid angiograms and a right vertebral angiogram done six months after the injury revealed no midline shift or displacement of vessels.

C.B. received physical therapy and speech therapy during the 23-day period that he was hospitalized but showed very little improvement in any respect. A decision was made to discharge him from the hospital because it appeared to the patient's mother and physicians that the home environment might be more stimulating in a social sense. It was clear from the findings that this patient had suffered very severe deficits even though it was not possible to identify specific areas of brain damage.

Neuropsychological Evaluation

Neuropsychological examination was done 16½ months after the injury. The patient still had great difficulty with spasticity in his muscular performances. His speech, which was usually a whisper, was slow and deliberate and lacked many consonants, especially at the end of words, a condition referred to as "smudging." However, after spending some time learning to understand his speech, it was possible for the examiner to do the Verbal subtests of the Wechsler Scale. C.B. had very little difficulty understanding the examiner's verbal communication.

It is entirely likely that the patient's severe spasticity of his upper extremities was a significant factor in limiting the adequacy of his performance on certain motor tests. Since some patients with brain trauma have these types of speech and motor difficulties, we felt that it would be useful to include an example of such a case in order to illustrate the value of neuropsychological assessment in these circumstances.

C.B. had been left-handed before his injury but presently showed signs of mixed dominance, doing some unimanual tasks with his right hand and some with his left. However, he wrote with his left hand, had originally been left-handed, and in our examination we treated him as a left-handed person.

When approached by the examiner the patient smiled in a very friendly manner, seemed eager to respond and cooperate, and was obviously elated when his verbal responses were understood. Because he tired quite easily, the testing session was extended over two days. We deliberately scheduled the Wechsler Scale for the second day to give the examiner more time to become accustomed to the patient's speech.

It was apparent that C.B.'s spastic movements were inhibiting his performances on the Performance subtests and probably reduced his scores. He also had great difficulty making progress on the Tactual Performance Test (especially with his left upper extremity) and it is possible that this limited progress had a secondary influence on the Memory and Localization scores. C.B.'s motor difficulties were obviously shown on the Aphasia Screening Test by the attempts to draw figures and write. Although these problems might have slowed his progress on the Trail Making Test, it was the examiner's impression that C.B. needed to think deliberately and carefully as he went along and that this was the principal limiting factor.

Slight modifications in the testing procedure were made in order to evaluate C.B. The patient had difficulty writing "S" for SAME and "D" for DIFFERENT on the Seashore Rhythm Test and suggested to the examiner that he leave the space blank if the pair of beats were different and make a short, rough line if they were the same. On the Speech-sounds Perception Test C.B. was able to make a rough pencil mark to indicate his response. On the Picture Completion subtest he attempted to give a verbal response but also pointed with his finger to make sure that the examiner understood his response. In some instances he actually spelled out his response with his finger on the table when the examiner had difficulty understanding him. Thus, it was possible to adapt the testing procedures in a number of respects and gain useful results.

In patients with motoric (response) limitations, it is often difficult to determine the extent to which the deficits are due to central processing dysfunctions and the amount caused by lack of motor control. Many patients with response limitations (such as those with cerebral palsy) have significant central processing deficits as well as

THE HALSTEAD-REITAN
NEUROPSYCHOLOGICAL TEST BATTERY

Patient __C.B.__ Age __26__ Sex __M__ Education __12__ Handedness __L__

WECHSLER-BELLEVUE SCALE

VIQ	99
PIQ	86
FS IQ	93

Information	13
Comprehension	8
Digit Span	7
Arithmetic	9
Similarities	9
Vocabulary	11

Picture Arrangement	8
Picture Completion	15
Block Design	5
Object Assembly	8
Digit Symbol	2

TRAIL MAKING TEST

Part A: __195__ seconds
Part B: __263__ seconds

STRENGTH OF GRIP

Dominant hand: __18__ kilograms

Non-dominant hand: __9__ kilograms

REITAN-KLØVE TACTILE FORM RECOGNITION TEST

Dominant hand: __18__ seconds; __0__ errors

Non-dominant hand: __20__ seconds; __0__ errors

REITAN-KLØVE SENSORY-PERCEPTUAL EXAM — No errors

					Error Totals	
RH___LH___	Both H:	RH___LH___		RH___LH___		
RH___LF___	Both H/F:	RH___LF___		RH___LF___		
LH___RF___	Both H/F:	LH___RF___		RF___LH___		
RE___LE___	Both E:	RE___LE___		RE___LE___		
RV___LV___	Both:	RV___LV___		RV___LV___		

TACTILE FINGER RECOGNITION

R 1___ 2___ 3___ 4 __3__ 5___   R __3__ / 20

L 1___ 2___ 3___ 4 __1__ 5 __1__   L __2__ / 20

FINGER-TIP NUMBER WRITING

R 1 __3__ 2___ 3___ 4___ 5 __1__   R __4__ / 20

L 1 __1__ 2 __1__ 3 __1__ 4___ 5 __2__   L __5__ / 20

HALSTEAD'S NEUROPSYCHOLOGICAL TEST BATTERY

Category Test	74

Tactual Performance Test

Dominant hand:	10.0 (No blocks)
Non-dominant hand:	10.0 (6 blocks)
Both hands:	10.0 (6 blocks)

	Total Time	30.0 (12 blocks)
	Memory	2
	Localization	0

Seashore Rhythm Test

Number Correct	28	2

Speech-sounds Perception Test

Number of Errors	6

Finger Oscillation Test

Dominant hand:	16	16
Non-dominant hand:	19	

Impairment Index	0.7

MINNESOTA MULTIPHASIC PERSONALITY INVENTORY

		Hs	67
		D	51
?	50	Hy	62
L	53	Pd	48
F	46	Mf	39
K	61	Pa	50
		Pt	42
		Sc	51
		Ma	40

REITAN-KLØVE LATERAL-DOMINANCE EXAM

Show me how you:

throw a ball	R
hammer a nail	R
cut with a knife	L
turn a door knob	R
use scissors	L
use an eraser	L
write your name	L

Record time used for spontaneous name-writing:

Preferred hand	63	seconds
Non-preferred hand	49	seconds

Show me how you:

kick a football	R
step on a bug	R

REITAN-INDIANA APHASIA SCREENING TEST

Form for Adults and Older Children

Name: _____ C. B. _____ Age: __26__

Copy SQUARE	Repeat TRIANGLE "Tria-a-a-ngo"
Name SQUARE	Repeat MASSACHUSETTS "Massachusess"
Spell SQUARE	Repeat METHODIST EPISCOPAL "Methodist Epistical"
Copy CROSS	Write SQUARE
Name CROSS	Read SEVEN
Spell CROSS	Repeat SEVEN
Copy TRIANGLE	Repeat/Explain HE SHOUTED THE WARNING. Explanation - "Danger;railroad"
Name TRIANGLE	Write HE SHOUTED THE WARNING.
Spell TRIANGLE	Compute 85 – 27 =
Name BABY	Compute 17 X 3 =
Write CLOCK	Name KEY "Hee"
Name FORK "For"	Demonstrate use of KEY
Read 7 SIX 2	Draw KEY
Read MGW	Read PLACE LEFT HAND TO RIGHT EAR.
Reading I	Place LEFT HAND TO RIGHT EAR
Reading II	Place LEFT HAND TO LEFT ELBOW

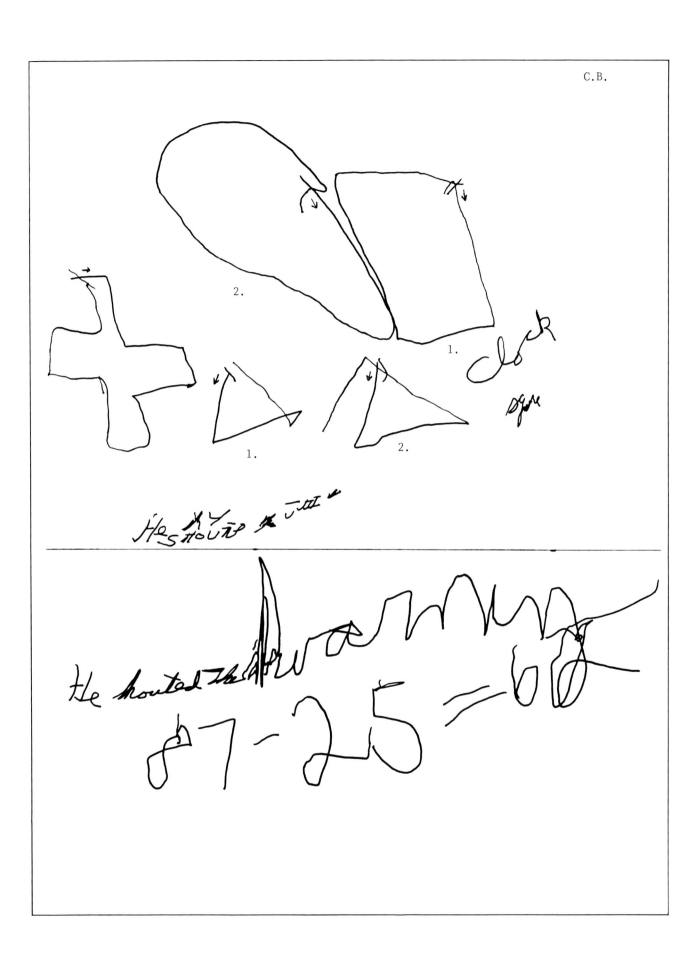

$$85 - 27 = 38$$

51

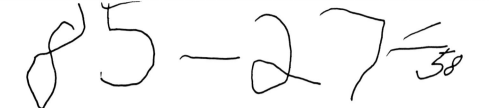

motor dysfunction; others have equivalent response limitations but few, if any, higher-level deficits. Therefore, it is important to be able to answer questions of this kind when planning the patient's therapy.

C.B. earned a Verbal IQ (99) almost exactly at the Average level, exceeding about 47% of his age peers. It is possible that he had experienced a mild degree of impairment on certain subtests, but this would be difficult to discern from the distribution of scores.

The Performance subtests showed evidence of probable deficit, but impairment of motor functions with the upper extremities may also have been contributory. Almost certainly the poor Digit Symbol score (2) was mainly a reflection of the patient's difficulty in using a pencil to make the symbols. Therefore, the Performance IQ of 86 is probably not an entirely valid expression of the Performance intelligence of this man.

The patient showed definite impairment of brain functions on the four most sensitive indicators in the HRNTB. The Impairment Index of 0.7 included measures of primary and complex motor functions (Finger Oscillation Test and Tactual Performance Test). In addition, as noted above, the Memory and Localization components of the Tactual Performance Test may have been influenced by the difficulty placing the blocks.

Because of these considerations, the Impairment Index should be analyzed in terms of the results on the Category Test (74), the Seashore Rhythm Test (28 correct), and the Speech-sounds Perception Test (6 errors). The impaired score on the Category Test probably indicates a significant deficit in the area of abstraction, reasoning, and logical analysis skills. It is important to note, however, that when C.B. was required only to pay attention to well-defined stimulus material and maintain concentration over time (Speech-sounds Perception and Rhythm Tests) he was able to do quite well. The poor score on Part B of the Trail Making Test (263 sec) probably was not limited to

any significant degree by impaired motor functions and therefore supports the Category Test as a reflection of impairment of flexibility in thought processes. It is also likely that the low score on the Localization component of the Tactual Performance Test (0) indicates some impairment of higher-level functions, but, as mentioned above, may have been influenced by his motor difficulties.

Despite his difficulties in speaking, the patient was able to communicate essentially correct responses on the Aphasia Screening Test. His problems with motor control were obvious in his attempts to write and draw. As noted, it was necessary for the examiner to listen carefully in order to understand the subject's speech. He made certain errors, particularly in trying to enunciate the "K" sound; he responded to the picture of the fork as "FOR" and named the key as "HEE."

C.B.'s writing, although done with great difficulty, appeared to be basically correct. Some question might be raised about his writing of "SQUARE"; although the writing is cramped, it appears that each letter was appropriately formed.

It was difficult for the examiner to be sure of the adequacy of responses in repeating TRIANGLE, MASSACHUSETTS, and METHODIST EPISCOPAL; it appeared that C.B. elongated some of the vowel sounds but enunciated correctly.

The only questionable performance that may be brain-related would be the patient's drawing of the key. It is difficult to differentiate between impaired motor control and a deficit in representing the spatial configuration, but this key suggests that C.B. may have had some visual-spatial problems.

This patient's motor deficits were very pronounced and appeared to have lateralizing significance in some instances. For example, on the Tactual Performance Test C.B. performed quite poorly with his left hand (10 min, 0 blocks) compared with his right (10 min, 6 blocks) and, despite being left-handed, was somewhat slow in finger tapping speed with the left hand (16) compared with the right (19). Conversely, his grip strength was distinctly greater in his left upper extremity (18 kg) than his right (9 kg).

Although the principal observation was one of generalized impairment of motor capabilities, the lateralizing findings were sufficiently pronounced to question the integrity of each cerebral hemisphere, with the right cerebral hemisphere appearing to be slightly more involved than the left.

Sensory-perceptual deficits were relatively mild and equally distributed on the two sides. The somewhat increased time results on the Tactile Form Recognition test (LH-18 sec; RH-20 sec) may have been due to difficulty in pointing to the correct figure. Since C.B. made no errors on this test the results are not necessarily indicative of impaired cerebral functions. However, the mistakes made on tests of Tactile Finger Recognition and Finger-tip Number Writing Perception exceeded the expected limits for normal subjects and suggested the presence of mild, bilateral impairment of brain functions.

A review of all of the test results indicates that motor problems, manifested particularly by spasticity of the upper extremities, were the most prominent difficulties experienced by this subject. Aside from these deficits, the rest of the test results are essentially in line with expectations for a person who has sustained a severe closed head injury. Scores on several of the Verbal subtests of the Wechsler Scale indicate that the patient had previously developed relatively normal intelligence. Certain findings that have lateralizing significance suggested more involvement of the right than left cerebral hemisphere (although grip strength particularly implicated the left cerebral hemisphere).

The overall results, including the measures of tactile function, would suggest generalized cerebral involvement with the right cerebral hemisphere possibly more dysfunctional than the left.

This conclusion would be consistent with an interpretation of the drawing of the key as demonstrating some degree of deficit in dealing with spatial relationships.

The good scores on the Seashore Rhythm Test and the Speech-sounds Perception Test strongly suggest that, in a biological sense, the brain's condition is relatively stabilized rather than progressively deteriorating. Under these circumstances it would seem likely that the extreme spasticity is a function of damage to elements of the motor system below the level of the cerebral cortex and constitute a problem that is separate from the indications of higher-level deficits (much as is seen in some instances of cerebral palsy).

Findings on the Minnesota Multiphasic Personality Inventory were essentially within normal limits. The relative elevation on the Hypochondriasis Scale is probably reflecting the realistic physical problems and symptoms of the patient rather than any type of psychiatric disorder. In total, the neuropsychological evaluation (except for the motor control problems) is similar to expectations in cases of severe closed head injury sustained some time before the examination. However, expressive (response) deficits must be considered part of the total picture for the individual; if speech and movement are significantly impaired as expressions of central processing, the overall manifestation of brain functions will certainly be affected.

Finally, it is interesting to note that the extended initial period of coma and impaired consciousness did not appear to result in neuropsychological deficits that were necessarily more severe than those seen in many persons who regain consciousness much more quickly. It is possible, and perhaps likely, that the long period of impaired consciousness and the motor dysfunction were both due to damage at levels below the cerebral cortex and that cortical (and perhaps cerebral) damage was no more pronounced than in many other cases with severe closed head injury.

CASE #7

Name: H.B.

Age: 35

Education: 12

Sex: Female

Handedness: Right

Occupation: Bookkeeper

Background Information

H.B. was in an automobile accident when she was 34 years old and suffered severe trauma, including multiple broken ribs, a punctured lung, considerable blood loss, a head injury with a broken nose, and many cuts and bruises. She was unconscious for an undetermined period of time.

H.B.'s recovery was relatively uneventful except for severe headaches that persisted after she was discharged from the hospital. Computed tomography done to investigate the cause of the headaches was within normal limits.

The patient returned to work as the bookkeeper for her husband's business but found that she was not able to work as well as she had before the injury. She made many mistakes, neglected important details and generally performed unsatisfactorily. The poor quality of her work was a serious point of contention between H.B. and her husband and affected their entire relationship.

H.B. also had a number of other symptoms of emotional distress that were not present before the injury: she now experienced excessive fatigue, reduced ability to understand situations, impaired reflexes, feelings of fear when she attempted to drive, episodes of depression, forgetfulness, insomnia, fear of being in crowds or even going shopping, panic reactions for no apparent reasons, anxiety over financial matters, feelings of personal insecurity and increased dependence on others, and difficulty controlling her emotions, including frequent outbursts of anger. Previously her home life with her husband and three children had been relatively satisfactory but she now described the situation as "traumatic."

Neurological Examination

The neurosurgeon who had treated H.B.'s head injury performed a neurological examination and reported the results to be essentially within normal limits. He did note, however, that before her injury the patient had won many prizes for her floral arrangements; since the accident she had lost her ability to arrange flowers. At this point, 10 months after the injury, H.B. sought evaluation by a local neuropsychologist who administered the Halstead-Reitan Battery and the Minnesota Multiphasic Personality Inventory. The results are presented below.

Neuropsychological Examination

The test results indicate that H.B. performed poorly on a number of measures in the Halstead-Reitan Battery (despite her average intelligence levels). She showed deficits on tests requiring logical analysis, abstraction and reasoning abilities and tasks that involved visual-spatial relationships and manipulatory skills. The findings are quite characteristic of persons with closed head injuries who have residual deficits. The patient also showed indications of emotional difficulties and expressed feelings of tension, anxiety and depression.

The patient earned a Verbal IQ (110) in the lower limit of the High Average range (exceeding about 75% of her age peers) and a Performance IQ (91) that was 19 points lower, in the lower limit of the Average range (exceeding about 27%). These values yielded a Full Scale IQ (102) almost exactly at the Average level (exceeding 55%). Although her Vocabulary score (14) was well above average, the general distribution of subtest scores suggests that H.B. has probably not led a particularly active life in an intellectual or cultural sense.

The patient consistently performed worse on the Performance subtests than the Verbal subtests. Her highest score on any of the Performance subtests matched her lowest score on any of the Verbal subtests and showed a significant lack of overlap. This finding definitely suggests that H.B. may have experienced some impairment of Performance intelligence. Additional test results, to be described below, support the hypothesis that the impairment H.B. demonstrated on the Performance subtests is related to damage of the right cerebral hemisphere.

This woman had difficulty on brain-sensitive tests, earning an Impairment Index of 1.0 (100% of these tests had scores in the brain-damaged range). She had particular problems on a task that required her to use logical analysis and abstraction abilities. We would predict that it would be extremely difficult for this woman to see how things fit together, formulate reasonable hypotheses to explain her observations, and draw meaningful conclusions. The measure reflecting these deficits was the Category Test, one of the most sensitive measures to the biological integrity of the cerebral hemispheres. Undoubtedly these cognitive deficits (reflected by her score of 83 errors) have very practical implications relating to H.B.'s efficiency of behavior.

The patient also performed very poorly on the Tactual Performance Test, a measure that requires manipulatory performances under unique and somewhat difficult conditions. H.B.'s scores on the TPT indicate that she has a great deal of difficulty adapting to unfamiliar situations. In other words, her ability to deal with new types of problems is severely undercut. Although these are subtle kinds of losses they are significant in their implications of inefficiency in everyday living.

Note, though, how well H.B. performed on tasks that were well-defined (despite her problems on many of the other tests). She showed that she was able to focus her attention on specific stimulus material and maintain attention over time (Speech-sounds Perception Test). She was also rather quick and alert when she knew exactly what she was supposed to do (Trail Making Test).

H.B.'s major difficulty occurred on tasks that required her to define the nature of the problem, make relevant observations, and draw meaningful conclusions on the basis of these observations. The type of impairment H.B. demonstrates almost certainly indicates that she will probably not be able to exercise very good judgment in analyzing complex situations and deciding upon the best and most appropriate course of action. It is likely that these deficits underlie her forgetfulness and impaired efficiency in doing the bookkeeping for her husband's business.

Results on the Minnesota Multiphasic Personality Inventory also showed some deviation from normal. The findings indicated that the patient did not have any significant impairment in basic aspects of affective integrity, but she does show some signs of depression, anxiety, tension, and concern over her bodily functions. Although results of this kind could be associated with the evidence of impaired brain functions described above, such findings are also seen in persons who have no indications of neuropsychological deficit.

As noted, the test findings are perfectly characteristic of persons who have sustained craniocerebral trauma. In many respects, the patient's performances were done relatively well. The most striking evidence of higher-level impairment was found in the areas of complex manipulatory skills and abstraction, reasoning, and logical analysis

THE HALSTEAD-REITAN
NEUROPSYCHOLOGICAL TEST BATTERY

Patient __H.B. (I)__ Age __35__ Sex __F__ Education __12__ Handedness __R__

WECHSLER-BELLEVUE SCALE

VIQ	110
PIQ	91
FS IQ	102

Information	9
Comprehension	17
Digit Span	10
Arithmetic	4
Similarities	11
Vocabulary	14

Picture Arrangement	9
Picture Completion	8
Block Design	7
Object Assembly	6
Digit Symbol	9

TRAIL MAKING TEST

Part A: __34__ seconds
Part B: __69__ seconds

STRENGTH OF GRIP

Dominant hand: __22__ kilograms

Non-dominant hand: __21__ kilograms

REITAN-KLØVE TACTILE FORM RECOGNITION TEST

Dominant hand: __19__ seconds; __0__ errors

Non-dominant hand: __16__ seconds; __0__ errors

REITAN-KLØVE SENSORY-PERCEPTUAL EXAM

			Error Totals	
RH ___ LH ___	Both H: RH ___ LH ___		RH ___ LH ___	
RH ___ LF __1__	Both H/F: RH ___ LF __3__		RH ___ LF __4__	
LH ___ RF ___	Both H/F: LH ___ RF ___		RF ___ LH ___	
RE ___ LE ___	Both E: RE ___ LE ___		RE ___ LE ___	
RV ___ LV ___	Both: RV ___ LV ___		RV ___ LV ___	

TACTILE FINGER RECOGNITION

R 1___ 2___ 3___ 4___ 5___ R __0__ / 20

L 1___ 2___ 3___ 4___ 5___ L __0__ / 20

FINGER-TIP NUMBER WRITING

R 1__2__ 2__1__ 3___ 4___ 5___ R __3__ / 20

L 1__2__ 2___ 3___ 4___ 5___ L __2__ / 20

No aphasia, but cross and key drawings
suggest mild constructional dyspraxia.

HALSTEAD'S NEUROPSYCHOLOGICAL TEST BATTERY

Category Test		83

Tactual Performance Test

Dominant hand:	16.9	
Non-dominant hand:	13.8	
Both hands:	10.0	

Total Time	40.7
Memory	5
Localization	3

Seashore Rhythm Test

Number Correct	22	10

Speech-sounds Perception Test

Number of Errors	8

Finger Oscillation Test

Dominant hand:	49	49
Non-dominant hand:	35	

Impairment Index __1.0__

MINNESOTA MULTIPHASIC
PERSONALITY INVENTORY

		Hs	72
		D	71
		Hy	68
L	56	Pd	45
F	53	Mf	52
K	51	Pa	56
		Pt	58
		Sc	55
		Ma	50
		Si	64

REITAN-KLØVE
LATERAL-DOMINANCE EXAM

Show me how you:

throw a ball	R
hammer a nail	R
cut with a knife	R
turn a door knob	R
use scissors	R
use an eraser	R
write your name	R

Record time used for spontaneous name-writing:

Preferred hand	6	seconds
Non-preferred hand	18	seconds

Show me how you:

kick a football	R
step on a bug	R

abilities. The overall findings indicated right cerebral damage as well as generalized cerebral impairment.

Measures of lateral dominance indicated that H.B. was definitely right-handed. Taking this into account, she performed quite poorly in finger tapping speed with her left hand (35) compared with her right (49). She also had definite difficulty perceiving a tactile stimulus to the left side of the face when given simultaneously with a stimulus to the right hand.

On a complex manipulatory task (Tactual Performance Test) she had a little more difficulty with her left hand (13.8 min) compared to her right (16.9 min) than would be expected, but the significance of these findings related to generalized (rather than lateralized) impairment. The patient also demonstrated mild constructional dyspraxia in her attempt to copy simple spatial configurations. These findings all point toward right cerebral dysfunction and are supported by the evidence of impaired Performance Intelligence.

As commonly seen in persons with craniocerebral injuries, H.B. also showed some mild left hemisphere deficits. For example, her grip strength was somewhat low in the right upper extremity (22 kg) compared to the left (21 kg) and she had slightly more difficulty in tactile form recognition with her right hand (19 sec) than her left (16 sec). To summarize up to this point, the overall results point toward generalized cerebral damage with the right cerebral hemisphere more dysfunctional than the left.

It is very likely that this woman is not able to function anywhere nearly as efficiently as she did in the past, particularly in instances in which she must deal with complex situations involving multiple elements. Furthermore, she almost certainly will have difficulty with tasks requiring analysis of circumstances, identification of the essential nature of the problem, the ability to use good judgement in considering all aspects of a situation, and overall efficiency of performance. And as we have

observed, the patient also showed impairment on tasks that require complex manipulatory procedures and the ability to adapt to rather novel and unique kinds of problem situations.

The Minnesota Multiphasic Personality Inventory also suggested that H.B. feels some degree of tension, apprehension, anxiety, and mild depression. It is entirely likely that these difficulties stem (at least in part) from the cognitive impairment she has experienced, although it must always be remembered that many people who have no evidence of brain damage also have emotional problems of this kind. In this case it would be advisable for the patient to receive psychological counseling to relieve the feelings of insecurity and apprehension that she probably experiences.

At this point, the principal need of this woman relates to retraining of higher-level brain functions. We would strongly recommend use of REHABIT, with special emphasis on Track C to redevelop basic abilities in abstraction and reasoning. We would then use Tracks D and E to integrate these skills with visuospatial performances.

The local neuropsychologist who had tested H.B. was not prepared to provide cognitive rehabilitation but did attempt to counsel her for her emotional problems of adjustment. However, the patient continued to have significant problems and finally went to a fairly distant medical center for further neuropsychological evaluation. We were able to review a report of the results obtained in this examination, done approximately 32 months after the injury.

This examination was based upon the Luria-Nebraska Neuropsychological Battery and the Minnesota Multiphasic Personality Inventory. According to the psychologist who did this evaluation, the results of the Luria-Nebraska Neuropsychological Battery indicated no evidence of brain impairment with "all of her scaled scores falling within the normal range." Despite these good scores, the examiner noted that the patient had difficulty with tasks that required persistent or concentrated effort and that she took an abnormal amount of time and required more than the usual amount of energy to finish various tests.

The major portion of this report, however, was based upon the MMPI. The neuropsychologist noted that H.B. seemed to be a conventional and moralistic person who was rather rigid and inflexible in her problem-solving abilities. The report went on to say that, "She is very critical of herself and quite dissatisfied. She is significantly depressed and anxious and has little insight into her own behavior. She is suspicious of others and likely easily hurt and offended. She is a ruminative person who probably expends a great deal of time thinking and worrying about her difficulties. She is a passive-dependent person who feels inadequate and helpless and has difficulty expressing her feelings. She tends to deny unacceptable feelings, especially anger and hostility.

"She has a high need for achievement and may be overly sensitive to perceived losses and changes in functioning. She will feel guilty when she falls short of her goals and will tend to blame herself for her problems. She is quite unable to work at this time and has a low stress tolerance. Her depression is secondary to the trauma of the accident. The accident, appears, from history, to be the major contributing factor to her anxiety and present adjustment difficulties. On the basis of these symptoms, it would be expected that the patient would show a high level of disability."

Following this examination H.B. returned home, re-contacted the local neuropsychologist who had initially examined her, and asked to have further consultation. At this time she was referred to the Neuropsychology Laboratory in Tucson for a repetition of the Halstead-Reitan Neuropsychological Test Battery. Even though the patient had shown significant evidence of impairment when the Halstead-Reitan Battery was first administered,

the local neuropsychologist believed that the patient had shown a great deal of improvement during the 23 months that had elapsed since his examination. In any case, it seemed important to determine whether H.B.'s problems related strictly to emotional reactions to the accident or whether her adjustmental difficulties and emotional problems might stem from impairment of higher-level brain functions.

The Halstead-Reitan Battery was readministered one month after the Luria-Nebraska Battery had been given. When the patient appeared for the examination and recounted her difficulties they were quite similar to those reported initially. Her headaches had been treated with some degree of success and were no longer as severe as they had been originally. However, her emotional problems (including depression, panic states, inefficiency in performance, and inability to work as a bookkeeper) were still present.

In fact, we learned that these problems had been exacerbated by the evaluation done one month ago. H.B.'s husband had never been understanding or tolerant of her emotional problems and, since the most recent psychological examination had demonstrated no evidence of brain-related impairment, the tension between H.B. and her husband had become considerably more pronounced and at this point the patient felt that her marriage was seriously threatened. In discussing this aspect of the situation, H.B. revealed much more information than was included in the written report based on the Luria-Nebraska Battery and the Minnesota Multiphasic Personality Inventory quoted above. H.B. informed us that the neuropsychologist, deciding that her problems were emotionally based, had explored with her some of the difficulties she had been having with her husband and had concluded that the fundamental problem was one of impaired sexual adjustment resulting from neurotic reactions to the accident.

The overall pattern of test results on the second examination with the Halstead-Reitan Battery changed somewhat since the initial evaluation; H.B. showed improvement in some areas and more difficulties in others. Nonetheless, the overall findings continued to demonstrate residual deficits associated with craniocerebral trauma.

Approximately 10 months had elapsed between the date of the head injury and the initial neuropsychological examination. Our studies have indicated that improvement after craniocerebral trauma frequently continues for as long as 18 months or more (Dikmen & Reitan, 1976). Therefore, compared to the results of the initial examination, we would expect that the patient might show some additional improvement in certain areas.

H.B. increased her Verbal IQ six points to 116, a score in the High Average range (exceeding about 86% of her age peers). Her Performance IQ showed a 10-point increase (to 101), a value just above the Average range and exceeding about 53% of her age peers. These scores reflect a slightly greater increase than might be expected on the basis of positive practice-effect and probably represent a mild degree of improvement since the time of the initial examination.

The patient had previously demonstrated significant and serious impairment on a number of brain-related tasks, particularly those requiring abstraction, reasoning, and logical analysis skills. Although H.B. showed some improvement in this area, she continued to have a number of difficulties.

We can summarize H.B.'s performances by saying that she (1) still had some impairment on tasks that required her to use logical analysis and reasoning abilities; (2) was not as bright and quick as normal persons in dealing with tasks that involved multiple elements; (3) had some impairment in her ability to focus on certain types of specific stimulus material and maintain efficiency of performance; (4) had mild difficulty dealing with spatial configurations (reflected both in her drawings of simple objects as well as in some of the Performance subtests

of the Wechsler Scale); and (5) showed deficits in being able to continue working on tasks that were difficult and frustrating for her.

It appears that the impairment shown by this woman manifests itself in a lowered level of frustration tolerance. In addition, direct assessment of the patient's emotional status (Cornell Medical Index Health Questionnaire) indicates that she has many complaints about her bodily functioning and somatic condition as well as a number of emotional problems that may be quite serious in nature. She presently indicated that she has constant noises in her ears, pains in the heart or chest area, difficulty breathing, frequent leg cramps, frequent upset stomachs and severe itching, frequent severe headaches, and spells of severe dizziness.

H.B. said that she often feels faint, has spells of complete exhaustion or fatigue, is worn out by every little effort, is constantly too tired and exhausted even to eat, has great difficulty sleeping, and believes that she suffers from severe nervous exhaustion. She states that she wears herself out worrying about her health, that severe pains and aches make it impossible for her to work, and the way things are at present she seems always to be ill and unhappy.

In her self-assessment H.B. also had quite a number of emotional complaints. She reported that she is frightened by strange people and places, always gets directions or orders wrong, finds that her work falls apart when she is under any kind of stress, is indecisive, usually feels unhappy and depressed, often cries, feels that life looks entirely hopeless, and often wishes she were dead and away from it all. She says that little things get on her nerves and make her angry, that she must constantly try to control herself, that she is constantly keyed up and jittery, and often becomes suddenly scared for no good reason. From these responses it is apparent that H.B. feels much more physical and emotional stress than most people.

Similar findings occurred on the Minnesota Multiphasic Personality Inventory. The results definitely

THE HALSTEAD-REITAN
NEUROPSYCHOLOGICAL TEST BATTERY

Patient ___H.B. (II)___ Age __37__ Sex __F__ Education __12__ Handedness __R__

WECHSLER-BELLEVUE SCALE

VIQ	116
PIQ	101
FS IQ	110

Information	12
Comprehension	17
Digit Span	10
Arithmetic	7
Similarities	15
Vocabulary	15

Picture Arrangement	11
Picture Completion	12
Block Design	7
Object Assembly	7
Digit Symbol	10

TRAIL MAKING TEST

Part A: __52__ seconds
Part B: __91__ seconds

STRENGTH OF GRIP

Dominant hand: __23__ kilograms

Non-dominant hand: __21__ kilograms

REITAN-KLØVE TACTILE FORM RECOGNITION TEST

Dominant hand: __8__ seconds; __1__ errors

Non-dominant hand: __9__ seconds; __0__ errors

REITAN-KLØVE SENSORY-PERCEPTUAL EXAM — No errors

			Error Totals
RH ___ LH ___	Both H: RH ___ LH ___	RH ___ LH ___	
RH ___ LF ___	Both H/F: RH ___ LF ___	RH ___ LF ___	
LH ___ RF ___	Both H/F: LH ___ RF ___	RF ___ LH ___	
RE ___ LE ___	Both E: RE ___ LE ___	RE ___ LE ___	
RV ___ LV ___	Both: RV ___ LV ___	RV ___ LV ___	
___ 1		___	
___ 1		___	

TACTILE FINGER RECOGNITION

R 1 __ 2 __ 3 __ 4 __ 5 __ R __0__ / 20

L 1 __ 2 __ 3 __ 4 __ 5 __ L __0__ / 20

FINGER-TIP NUMBER WRITING

R 1 _3_ 2 __ 3 _1_ 4 __ 5 __ R __4__ / 20

L 1 _2_ 2 _1_ 3 __ 4 __ 5 __ L __3__ / 20

HALSTEAD'S NEUROPSYCHOLOGICAL TEST BATTERY

Category Test	46

Tactual Performance Test

Dominant hand:	10 (4 in)
Non-dominant hand:	10 (4 in)
Both hands:	10 (7 in)

Total Time	30.0
Memory	3
Localization	1

Seashore Rhythm Test

Number Correct __22__ | 10

Speech-sounds Perception Test

Number of Errors | 4

Finger Oscillation Test

Dominant hand:	50	50
Non-dominant hand:	50	

Impairment Index __0.7__

MINNESOTA MULTIPHASIC
PERSONALITY INVENTORY

		Hs	66
		D	94
?	0	Hy	82
L	56	Pd	64
F	66	Mf	45
K	46	Pa	79
		Pt	86
		Sc	81
		Ma	53
		Si	77

REITAN-KLØVE
LATERAL-DOMINANCE EXAM

Show me how you:

throw a ball	R
hammer a nail	R
cut with a knife	R
turn a door knob	R
use scissors	R
use an eraser	R
write your name	R

Record time used for spontaneous name-writing:

Preferred hand	7 seconds
Non-preferred hand	17 seconds

Show me how you:

kick a football	R
step on a bug	R

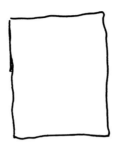

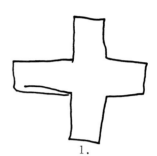

1.

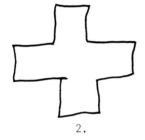

2.

clock

square

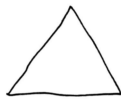

He shouted the warning.

$$\begin{array}{r} 85 \\ -\ 27 \\ \hline 58 \end{array}$$

51

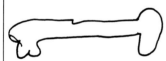

suggested that the patient is quite depressed, generally anxious and apprehensive, feels insecure and uncertain about her abilities, and is having some difficulty in relating to other people in her environment. Compared to the results on the initial testing these MMPI scores indicate that the patient's emotional stability has deteriorated. These adverse changes are almost certainly related to the difficulties she has encountered as a result of her head injury.

The test findings on the second examination were quite compatible with the type of residual impairment seen in persons with craniocerebral trauma. Despite IQ values that generally exceeded about 75% of her age peers, H.B. earned a Halstead Impairment Index of 0.7 (indicating that approximately 70% of these tests had scores in the brain-damaged range). The Impairment Index was somewhat better on the second testing primarily because of practice-effects on some of the measures (e.g., the Category Test).

Although measures of lateral dominance indicated that the patient was definitely right-handed, her finger tapping speed was no faster with her right hand than her left (though not seriously deficient with either hand). In the context of the other test results this finding might point toward some impairment of left cerebral functions.

H.B.'s poor performance on the Tactual Performance Test (a complex and difficult manipulatory task) manifested her limited ability to deal with a stress-producing procedure. Note that she performed no better with her left hand than her right, a finding suggesting the presence of right cerebral damage. Her mild difficulty copying simple spatial configurations (constructional dyspraxia), together with the reduced scores on some of the Performance subtests of the Wechsler Scale, also indicates right cerebral dysfunction.

As expected in cases of craniocerebral trauma, we found evidence of generalized cerebral damage with findings implicating damage of each cerebral hemisphere. Thus, although the patient showed a mild degree of improvement since the initial examination, the overall results continue to indicate the type of impaired brain functions that are quite consistent with residual effects of a prior head injury.

In order to be successful, approaches to rehabilitation must necessarily be based upon an understanding of the patient's deficits. H.B. continued to have serious deficiencies in the area of abstraction, reasoning, and logical analysis. It undoubtedly is much more difficult for her now than before her injury to perform complex tasks that require concentration and organization. Note that she complained of difficulty in trying to do her husband's bookkeeping without making serious mistakes; based on the present neuropsychological test results, this is exactly the kind of problem we would predict that she would have. Although there is no doubt that she was more seriously impaired in the past than she is presently, she continues to show cognitive deficits.

H.B. should definitely receive cognitive retraining using the REHABIT program. She probably does not need a great deal of training with Track A, but considering her deficits, Tracks B, C, D, and E would be appropriate.

The second major recommendation for H.B. relates to her strong need for psychological counseling. At present her own emotional resources are seriously undermined and she needs considerable support. It would be extremely important that this psychological counseling be undertaken by someone familiar with the neuropsychological difficulties that the patient experiences, because these problems are probably the basis for the undercutting of her self-confidence. Therefore, she needs an opportunity to engage in therapy with a psychologist who has an understanding of neuropsychology so that she can be given support and understanding concerning her neuropsychological deficits as they relate to her problems in everyday living. In addition, it is apparent that she needs counseling from a psychologist who has experience working with persons who have emotional difficulties. A clinical psychologist with training in neuropsychology would be the ideal therapist.

Finally, a question must be raised regarding the disparity between the neuropsychological results obtained with the Luria-Nebraska Battery and the Halstead-Reitan Battery. Questions regarding the clinical similarities and differences between the batteries cannot be fully answered on the basis of one case, but some obvious differences exist which may be noted.

Luria's approach to evaluation of brain-behavior relationships used the methods of behavioral neurology rather than clinical neuropsychology. The similarities and differences in the methodology of these areas has been reviewed in detail (Reitan & Wolfson, 1985b). In brief, behavioral neurology depends upon clinical observation of specific deficits (such as aphasia, agnosia, and apraxia); clinical neuropsychology evaluates not only specific types of deficits but also assesses complex cognitive abilities through the use of psychological measurements based upon scaled distributions.

We would postulate that Luria's assessment of the clinical status of this patient would have been mostly negative. Although H.B. manifested evidence of mild constructional dyspraxia, she had no aphasia, agnosia, or profound dyspraxia. Her deficits were demonstrated principally on tests that yielded scaled measurements of complex and fairly difficult tasks rather than on performances of relatively simple, discrete behaviors.

In assessing brain-behavior relationships it is important to realize that patients with focal, acutely destructive cerebral lesions (the patients often seen by neurologists as immediate medical problems) frequently manifest specific deficits; however, patients with chronic, static brain damage causing adjustmental (rather than medical) problems frequently have very few specific deficits, despite their compromised general neuropsychological functions. (The reader may wish to refer to

Reitan & Wolfson [1985a] for a discussion of the complementary value of general and specific indicators of brain function and how both types of measures were integrated into the Halstead-Reitan Neuropsychological Battery.)

The methods of behavioral neurology, sometimes referred to in clinical neuropsychology as the "sign" approach (Reitan & Wolfson, 1985a) have been shown to produce negative findings in about *half* of a heterogenous group of patients with definitive diagnoses of cerebral disease or damage (Wheeler & Reitan, 1962). As noted above, the negative findings occur most frequently in persons with chronic, static cerebral damage rather than in patients having recent strokes or rapidly developing intrinsic tumors (Hom & Reitan, 1982; Hom & Reitan, 1984).

In this case, the differences between the specific techniques of behavioral neurology and the general assessment procedures in clinical neuropsychology (and the probability of false-negative and false-positive conclusions) probably represents the basis for the conflicting findings in the Luria-Nebraska Battery and the Halstead-Reitan Battery. Although Golden (1981) has tried to extend and quantify the approach and procedures adopted from Luria, the original approach is still represented by behavioral neurology and many of its testing procedures involve specific and simple performances.

Patients with acutely destructive, focal cerebral lesions (such as strokes and intrinsic tumors) often show positive findings in tests of specific deficits but persons with chronic, static, generalized brain damage (such as the type resulting from craniocerebral trauma) frequently fail to demonstrate any positive results unless there are concurrent focal lesions (such as those produced by penetrating missiles). Since H.B. had few specific deficits, one would expect false-negative results from testing procedures derived largely from behavioral neurology.

CASE #8

Name: D.C.   Sex: Male

Age: 25   Handedness: Right

Education: 20   Occupation: Student

Background Information

D.C., a 25-year-old graduate student, sustained a head injury while playing football. Although others who observed the game felt that he did not lose consciousness, the patient himself reported that he was stunned and dazed and may have been unconsciousness for about 15 minutes. He said that his memory of events was vague for several hours following the injury. The morning after the accident D.C. had a moderately severe headache that was aggravated by moving his head from side to side or stooping over. He gradually showed improvement but sought medical evaluation because of the continuing headaches and diplopia of vertical gaze.

Neurological Examination

The physical and neurological examinations were essentially normal except for the above-mentioned findings and evidence of papilledema. The patient entered the hospital for a more complete evaluation and the original neurological findings were confirmed. Papilledema was more pronounced in the left eye than the right and there were some hemorrhages around the optic disc. Although EEG and skull films were normal the neurosurgeon suspected intracranial bleeding. Burr holes revealed a large subdural hematoma which appeared to cover the entire convexity of the left cerebral hemisphere. The hematoma was evacuated and the patient recovered uneventfully.

D.C. was up and about and feeling normal within two days following the surgery. He was examined neuropsychologically on the third postoperative day (about three weeks after the injury).

Neuropsychological Examination

D.C. was an advanced graduate student who had almost completed his doctoral studies when this accident occurred. He earned a Verbal IQ (115) in the upper part of the High Average range (exceeding about 84% of his age peers) and a Performance IQ (122) seven points higher, in the lower part of the Superior range (exceeding 93%). Based on the distribution of subtest scores it would not be possible to infer that he had experienced any significant impairment of either Verbal or Performance intelligence.

A question might be raised about the Picture Arrangement score (11) because it was clearly lower than the general level D.C. had established on the Performance subtests, but all subtest scores ranged between 11 and 14 and any inference regarding impairment would be argued against by the consistency of performances.

The patient also performed very well generally on brain-sensitive tests. He earned an Impairment Index of 0.0 (none of the tests had scores in the

THE HALSTEAD-REITAN
NEUROPSYCHOLOGICAL TEST BATTERY

Patient _____ **D.C.** _____ Age __**25**__ Sex __**M**__ Education __**20**__ Handedness __**R**__

WECHSLER-BELLEVUE SCALE

VIQ	**115**
PIQ	**122**
FS IQ	**120**
Information	**11**
Comprehension	**14**
Digit Span	**11**
Arithmetic	**13**
Similarities	**11**
Vocabulary	**13**
Picture Arrangement	**11**
Picture Completion	**14**
Block Design	**14**
Object Assembly	**14**
Digit Symbol	**12**

TRAIL MAKING TEST

Part A: __**28**__ seconds
Part B: __**62**__ seconds

STRENGTH OF GRIP

Dominant hand: __**57.0**__ kilograms

Non-dominant hand: __**54.0**__ kilograms

REITAN-KLØVE TACTILE FORM RECOGNITION TEST

Dominant hand: __**9**__ seconds; __**0**__ errors

Non-dominant hand: __**8**__ seconds; __**0**__ errors

REITAN-KLØVE SENSORY-PERCEPTUAL EXAM — **No errors**

					Error Totals	
RH___ LH ___	Both H:	RH___ LH ___		RH___ LH ___
RH___ LF ___	Both H/F:	RH___ LF ___		RH___ LF ___
LH___ RF ___	Both H/F:	LH___ RF ___		RF___ LH ___
RE___ LE ___	Both E:	RE___ LE ___		RE___ LE ___
RV___ LV ___	Both:	RV___ LV ___		RV___ LV ___

TACTILE FINGER RECOGNITION

R 1___ 2___ 3___ 4___ 5___   R __**0**__ / **20**

L 1___ 2___ 3___ 4___ 5___   L __**0**__ / **20**

FINGER-TIP NUMBER WRITING

R 1___ 2___ 3___ 4___ 5___   R __**0**__ / **20**

L 1___ 2___ 3___ 4___ 5___   L __**0**__ / **20**

NO APHASIC SYMPTOMS.

HALSTEAD'S NEUROPSYCHOLOGICAL TEST BATTERY

Category Test __**14**__

Tactual Performance Test

Dominant hand:	**6.4**		
Non-dominant hand:	**2.6**		
Both hands:	**1.2**		
		Total Time	**10.2**
		Memory	**9**
		Localization	**8**

Seashore Rhythm Test

Number Correct __**28**__ __**2**__

Speech-sounds Perception Test

Number of Errors __**3**__

Finger Oscillation Test

Dominant hand: __**53**__ __**53**__

Non-dominant hand: __**44**__

Impairment Index __**0.0**__

MINNESOTA MULTIPHASIC PERSONALITY INVENTORY

		Hs	**47**
		D	**34**
?	**50**	Hy	**58**
L	**50**	Pd	**53**
F	**44**	Mf	**69**
K	**59**	Pa	**41**
		Pt	**54**
		Sc	**53**
		Ma	**68**

REITAN-KLØVE LATERAL-DOMINANCE EXAM

Show me how you:	
throw a ball	**R**
hammer a nail	**R**
cut with a knife	**R**
turn a door knob	**R**
use scissors	**R**
use an eraser	**R**
write your name	**R**

Record time used for spontaneous name-writing:

Preferred hand	**6**	seconds
Non-preferred hand	**21**	seconds

Show me how you:	
kick a football	**R**
step on a bug	**R**

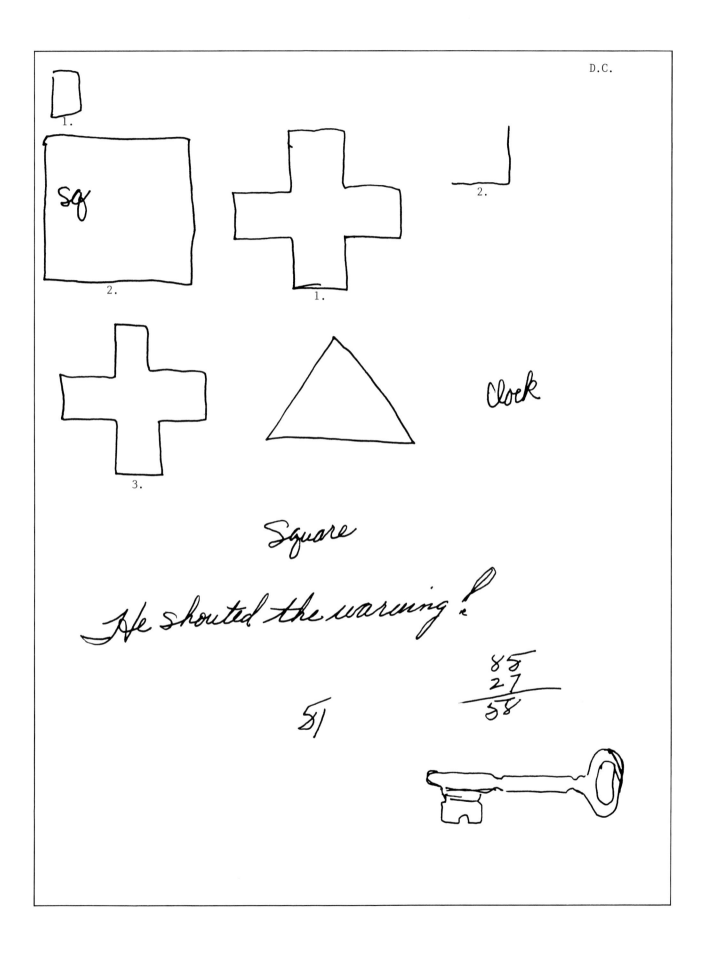

1.

2.

Sq

1.

2.

3.

Clock

Square

He shouted the warning!

51

$$\begin{array}{r} 85 \\ 27 \\ \hline 58 \end{array}$$

brain-damaged range). His scores were consistently within the normal range, indicating that his abilities were well above the average. Results on the Minnesota Multiphasic Personality Inventory were also unremarkable. The test findings make it apparent that an interpretation approach concerned exclusively with level-of-performance would conclude that this patient was functioning up to his capabilities.

Although lateralizing findings also approached the normal limits, D.C. performed quite poorly with his right (dominant) hand (6.4 min) on the Tactual Performance Test compared with his left (2.6 min). Grip strength with his right upper extremity (57.0 kg) may also have been somewhat below the expected level compared with the left upper extremity (54.0 kg). These findings might be subtle indications of mild left cerebral dysfunction.

The only finding suggesting right cerebral dysfunction was a mildly slow finger tapping speed with the left hand (44) compared with the right hand (53). The patient showed no evidence of dysphasia on the Aphasia Screening Test and his drawings were within normal limits. On the Sensory-perceptual Examination he made no mistakes on any of the trials.

One might wonder whether D.C.'s Verbal IQ was as high as might be expected from an advanced doctoral student. As noted above, the distribution of Verbal subtest scores showed little variability and provided no basis for postulating impairment. In fact, students in certain doctoral programs may be able to progress quite satisfactorily with verbal intelligence abilities in this range.

One could also question whether the mild deviation from normal relationships in performances on the two sides of the body constitutes an adequate basis for concluding that this man has sustained cerebral damage. The performance with the right hand (first trial) on the Tactual Performance Test definitely stood out as the most deviant score. It is not likely that we would have concluded that

these mild deviations were indicative of brain damage without having seen the neurosurgical report of a left subdural hematoma. In light of this medical information we could postulate that the poor performance with the right hand was a mild residual manifestation of left cerebral damage. It would appear likely that D.C. will recover completely and experience no adverse effects in the future from the very mild impairment that may presently exist. (Although we did not have an opportunity to perform follow-up examinations, we do know that D.C. later had high-level achievements.)

We included this case to demonstrate that a person may sustain a significant lesion as a result of head trauma and still escape serious neuropsychological impairment. We would presume from the test findings that the closed head injury alone was not sufficient to cause serious brain damage. Nevertheless, such an injury can tear a vessel and cause bleeding into the subdural space. The reader should be aware that persons with subdural hematomas have variable indications of neuropsychological impairment. Obviously, many patients with significant neuropsychological deficits have not had any subdural bleeding; serious damage to the brain tissue and resulting neuropsychological impairment can occur with or without a subdural hematoma.

The point illustrated by this case is that a subdural hematoma may occur with apparently negligible damage to the underlying cerebral cortex and correspondingly minimal neuropsychological deficit. However, when we became aware of D.C.'s history and neurosurgical findings we strongly advised him to discontinue playing football or engaging in any other activities that increased the risk of future head injuries. This accident probably caused very mild residual neuropsychological deficit (demonstrated particularly on the Tactual Performance Test). Clinical observation has suggested that under such circumstances a second head injury may result in impairment that is disproportionate to the severity of the blow; therefore, we would consider this man to be at risk for more significant neuropsychological impairment if he were to subsequently sustain another head blow comparable to his initial injury.

CASE #9

Name: S.G.

Age: 17

Education: 10

Sex: Female

Handedness: Right

Occupation: Student

Background Information

S.G. had recovered without complications from the usual childhood illnesses and had apparently been developing cognitive functions normally until the time of this head injury. Three days before her 17th birthday she was involved in a moving vehicle accident and was thrown through the windshield of the car in which she was a passenger. She was unconscious for 20–30 minutes after the accident. Upon regaining consciousness she began vomiting and was noted to have an enlarged left pupil. She was taken directly to a major medical center and was hospitalized within four hours after the accident occurred.

Neurological Examination

At the time of admission to the hospital the patient was slightly drowsy but coherent, cooperative, and easily arousable to verbal stimuli. She had a contusion over the top of her head and swelling and tenderness in the left frontal-temporal area. An abrasion was present over the left zygoma and around the left eye. There was dried blood in both nostrils but no evidence of leakage of cerebral spinal fluid. The left pupil was 1 mm–2 mm larger than the right but both pupils reacted to light and accommodation normally. A transitory nystagmus was noted on lateral gaze. No other aspects of the neurological examination showed any abnormalities.

A few hours after admission to the hospital the patient began to complain of diplopia. An ophthalmologist examined S.G. and found a paresis of the left medial and inferior rectus muscles and ecchymosis and subconjunctival hemorrhage (extravasation of blood below the delicate membrane that covers the front of the eyeball) of the left eye. S.G. improved quickly and within a few days seemed to be entirely normal except for the above-noted neurological findings. Results of additional examinations, however, strongly suggested that the patient had developed an intracerebral hematoma in the left frontal-parietal area.

Electroencephalography done two days after admission to the hospital showed dysrhythmia, Grade I (generalized) and Delta waves, Grade I in the left frontal-parietal area. This finding was more suggestive of either intracerebral hemorrhage or cerebral contusion than subdural or epidural hematoma. An EEG repeated 10 days later showed the same findings and plain skull films revealed a linear fracture on the left side. A pneumoencephalogram done 15 days after admission demonstrated a shift of the lateral and third ventricles to the right, suggesting a mass in the left parietal area. Left carotid angiography done 19 days after the injury indicated that the left middle cerebral artery was depressed and the left anterior cerebral artery was displaced slightly to the right. These results suggested an intracerebral hematoma in the frontal-parietal area just above the Sylvian fissure. Because the patient was making excellent progress and showed no clinical evidence of a focal brain lesion it was decided that surgical intervention might potentially be more harmful than beneficial.

S.G. was discharged from the hospital three weeks after admission and neuropsychological examination was done just before she left the hospital. The patient was followed on an out-patient basis and neuropsychological evaluation was repeated six months after the initial examination. At the time of the second testing the neurological examination was within normal limits except for slight nystagmus on lateral gaze in either direction and diplopia when looking upward and to the right, indicating a mild residual extraocular muscle paresis.

As noted above, the initial neuropsychological examination was done three weeks after the accident. At that time the neurological findings suggested that S. G. may have experienced a left frontal-parietal intracerebral hematoma, although the lesion had not been directly observed and the extent of cerebral cortical damage was not well defined. The Cornell Medical Index Health Questionnaire revealed essentially no complaints except that the patient said that her work falls to pieces when a superior is watching.

Neuropsychological Examination

S.G. earned a Verbal IQ (103) just above the Average level (exceeding about 58% of her age peers) and a Performance IQ (85) that was 18 points lower, in the middle part of the Low Average range (exceeding about 16%). These values yielded a Full Scale IQ (94) in the lower part of the Average range (exceeding 34%). Considering the fact that some variability among subtest scores is to be expected, the Verbal subtest scores do not indicate that the patient has experienced any significant impairment. Results on the Performance subtests (especially the Digit Symbol score of 7) may raise a question of cognitive deficit, but it would be difficult to confidently state that the Wechsler results reflected any loss of previously acquired abilities.

S.G. also did relatively well on Halstead's tests, earning an Impairment Index of 0.3; only the score on the Category Test (51) was in the range characteristic of brain damage. The patient performed extremely well on the Speech-sounds Perception Test, making only one error. On the Seashore Rhythm Test (28 correct) she demonstrated an above-average capability to pay attention to specific stimulus material. Thus, the general indicators suggested that this young woman had excellent abilities in focusing her attention and maintaining her concentration on well-specified tasks and had developed intelligence levels that generally were within the Low Average to Average range.

At this point we should note that S.G. performed much better on tests that were well-defined and when she knew exactly what she was supposed to do (Speech-sounds Perception Test and Seashore Rhythm Test) than on tasks that required her to define the nature of the problem before proceeding with a solution (Category Test) or a test that was fairly difficult and required her to adapt in a novel manner, deprived of the use of vision (Tactual Performance Test). Nevertheless, she did not perform particularly poorly on any of these measures.

There were essentially no signs of involvement of the left cerebral hemisphere. The patient showed no evidence of aphasia and the excellent score on the Speech-sounds Perception Test would support the hypothesis of relatively intact left cerebral functions. S.G. was a little slow in finger tapping speed with each hand (RH-40; LH-37) but the difference between the hands was almost within the normal range.

However, note that the test findings were definite in suggesting mild dysfunction of the right cerebral hemisphere. S.G. showed no improvement on the second trial (left hand) on the Tactual Performance Test although her potential for improvement (as demonstrated on the third trial) was substantial. Results on the measure of grip strength indicated that she might have been a little

THE HALSTEAD-REITAN
NEUROPSYCHOLOGICAL TEST BATTERY

Patient ___S.G.(I)___ Age __17__ Sex __F__ Education __10__ Handedness __R__

WECHSLER-BELLEVUE SCALE

VIQ	103
PIQ	85
FS IQ	94

Information	10
Comprehension	10
Digit Span	10
Arithmetic	9
Similarities	10
Vocabulary	8

Picture Arrangement	8
Picture Completion	8
Block Design	11
Object Assembly	7
Digit Symbol	7

TRAIL MAKING TEST

Part A: __24__ seconds
Part B: __76__ seconds

STRENGTH OF GRIP

Dominant hand: __16.0__ kilograms

Non-dominant hand: __13.0__ kilograms

REITAN-KLØVE TACTILE FORM RECOGNITION TEST

Dominant hand: __9__ seconds; __0__ errors

Non-dominant hand: __8__ seconds; __0__ errors

REITAN-KLØVE SENSORY-PERCEPTUAL EXAM — No errors

			Error Totals
RH___LH___	Both H: RH___LH___	RH___LH___	
RH___LF___	Both H/F: RH___LF___	RH___LF___	
LH___RF___	Both H/F: LH___RF___	RF___LH___	
RE___LE___	Both E: RE___LE___	RE___LE___	
RV___LV___	Both: RV___LV___	RV___LV___	
___ ___	___ ___		
___ ___	___ ___		

TACTILE FINGER RECOGNITION

R 1___2___3___4___5___ R __0__ / __20__

L 1___2___3___4___5___ L __0__ / __20__

FINGER-TIP NUMBER WRITING

R 1___2___3___4___5___ R __0__ / __20__

L 1___2___3___4___5___ L __0__ / __20__

NO APHASIC SYMPTOMS

HALSTEAD'S NEUROPSYCHOLOGICAL TEST BATTERY

Category Test		51

Tactual Performance Test

Dominant hand:	5.3	
Non-dominant hand:	5.3	
Both hands:	2.2	

Total Time	12.8
Memory	10
Localization	6

Seashore Rhythm Test

Number Correct	28	2

Speech-sounds Perception Test

Number of Errors	1

Finger Oscillation Test

Dominant hand:	40	40
Non-dominant hand:	37	

Impairment Index __0.3__

MINNESOTA MULTIPHASIC PERSONALITY INVENTORY

		Hs	46
		D	47
?	50	Hy	52
L	53	Pd	55
F	46	Mf	51
K	62	Pa	47
		Pt	48
		Sc	52
		Ma	35

REITAN-KLØVE LATERAL-DOMINANCE EXAM

Show me how you:

throw a ball	R
hammer a nail	R
cut with a knife	R
turn a door knob	R
use scissors	R
use an eraser	R
write your name	R

Record time used for spontaneous name-writing:

Preferred hand	9	seconds
Non-preferred hand	19	seconds

Show me how you:

kick a football	R
step on a bug	R

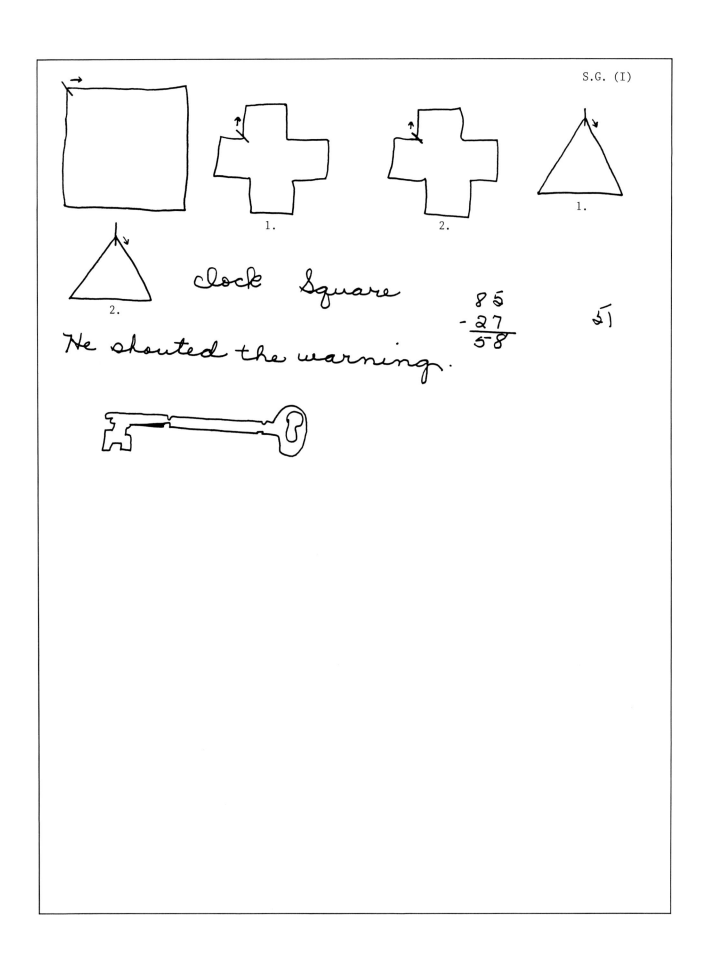

clock   Square

$$\begin{array}{r} 8\,5 \\ -\,2\,7 \\ \hline 5\text{-}8 \end{array}$$

He shouted the warning.

weak with her left upper extremity (13 kg) compared with her right (16 kg).

Finally, the patient's figure drawings were perhaps mildly deviant. The upper and lower extremities of the cross were not in the same plane in either drawing and the left extremity, when compared with the right, was somewhat out of balance in each drawing. In the drawing of the key the disparity of the upper and lower attachments of the handle to the stem must be considered somewhat unusual for a normal subject, but the general configuration is within normal limits. Thus, mild deviations from expectation were shown on certain tests related to right cerebral functioning and these results might be significant with respect to the substantial difference between Performance and Verbal IQ values.

A number of other performances were within normal limits, including the results of the Sensory-perceptual Examination. In a clinical sense one would be somewhat reluctant to place any special significance on the findings implicating mild right cerebral dysfunction, since the general indicators provided hardly any basis for inferring brain damage. From the mild indications of deficit one would postulate that this young woman experienced some impairment as a result of the head injury, but the test results yielded no findings that correlated specifically with the evidence of a left frontal-parietal intracerebral hematoma.

After being discharged from the hospital S.G. returned to school and successfully completed her third year of high school. She had no specific complaints but did feel that she was "not quite as bright" as she had been previously. The Cornell Medical Index Health Questionnaire was readministered six months after the accident and the patient's only complaints were that her eyes continually blinked or watered and were often red or inflamed, that she usually had difficulty falling or staying asleep, and she became nervous and shaky

when approached by a superior. We did not readminister the Minnesota Multiphasic Personality Inventory.

We will now compare the two sets of neuropsychological test results. Considered independently, the findings of the second testing do not provide a basis for concluding that any significant brain damage or dysfunction had occurred even though the Arithmetic score (6) on the Wechsler Scale was somewhat low. Additional findings that might be considered to deviate from normal expectancy were a slow finger tapping speed with the left hand (32), a mild reduction in grip strength with the left upper extremity (18 kg), possibly some slowness with the left hand (2.3 min) compared with the right (3.0 min) on the Tactual Performance Test, and a mildly suspicious drawing of the key (even though the general configuration was acceptable). Although these results suggested dysfunction of the right cerebral hemisphere (the mild deficits consistently involved the left upper extremity and the drawings were mildly deviant) the excellent results on many of the other tests would make it difficult to conclude that the patient had sustained any significant cerebral damage.

Comparison of the two sets of test results certainly suggested that the patient was more significantly impaired three weeks after the accident (first neuropsychological testing) than it was possible to infer confidently from the test findings. S.G. earned exactly the same Verbal IQ values (103) on both examinations, but her Performance IQ rose 26 points (from 85 to 111) on the second testing.

It is always necessary to consider the effects of practice when a test is readministered but there can be little doubt that the change in Performance IQ represents spontaneous recovery. In fact, S.G. also performed better on most of the other tests that were administered. The reduction in errors on the Category Test (from 51 to 27) and the improvement in Total Time on the Tactual Performance Test (from 12.8 min to 6.7 min) definitely

THE HALSTEAD-REITAN
NEUROPSYCHOLOGICAL TEST BATTERY

Patient ___S.G. (II)___ Age __17__ Sex __F__ Education __11__ Handedness __R__

WECHSLER-BELLEVUE SCALE

VIQ	103
PIQ	111
FS IQ	108

Information	10
Comprehension	9
Digit Span	10
Arithmetic	6
Similarities	14
Vocabulary	8

Picture Arrangement	11
Picture Completion	10
Block Design	15
Object Assembly	12
Digit Symbol	11

TRAIL MAKING TEST

Part A: __25__ seconds
Part B: __45__ seconds

STRENGTH OF GRIP

Dominant hand: __23.0__ kilograms
Non-dominant hand: __18.0__ kilograms

REITAN-KLØVE TACTILE FORM RECOGNITION TEST

Dominant hand: __8__ seconds; __0__ errors
Non-dominant hand: __8__ seconds; __0__ errors

REITAN-KLØVE SENSORY-PERCEPTUAL EXAM — No errors

					Error Totals	
RH___ LH___	Both H:	RH___ LH___		RH___ LH___		
RH___ LF___	Both H/F:	RH___ LF___		RH___ LF___		
LH___ RF___	Both H/F:	LH___ RF___		RF___ LH___		
RE___ LE___	Both E:	RE___ LE___		RE___ LE___		
RV___ LV___	Both:	RV___ LV___		RV___ LV___		
___ ___		___ ___				
___ ___		___ ___				

TACTILE FINGER RECOGNITION

R 1___ 2___ 3___ 4___ 5___ R __0__ / __20__
L 1___ 2___ 3___ 4___ 5___ L __0__ / __20__

FINGER-TIP NUMBER WRITING

R 1___ 2___ 3___ 4___ 5___ R __0__ / __20__
L 1___ 2___ 3___ 4___ 5___ L __0__ / __20__

NO APHASIC SYMPTOMS

HALSTEAD'S NEUROPSYCHOLOGICAL TEST BATTERY

Category Test		27

Tactual Performance Test

Dominant hand:	3.0	
Non-dominant hand:	2.3	
Both hands:	1.4	

Total Time	6.7
Memory	9
Localization	9

Seashore Rhythm Test

Number Correct	26	5

Speech-sounds Perception Test

Number of Errors	6

Finger Oscillation Test

Dominant hand:	45	45
Non-dominant hand:	32	

Impairment Index ___0.1___

REITAN-KLØVE
LATERAL-DOMINANCE EXAM

Show me how you:

throw a ball	R
hammer a nail	R
cut with a knife	R
turn a door knob	R
use scissors	R
use an eraser	R
write your name	R

Record time used for spontaneous name-writing:

Preferred hand	10 seconds
Non-preferred hand	17 seconds

Show me how you:

kick a football	R
step on a bug	R

1.

2.

1.

2.

clock

square

He shouted the warning.

```
  85
  27
-----
  58
```

51

exceeds the improvement expected to occur from practice effects. S.G. also performed significantly better on Part B of the Trail Making Test on the second examination (45 sec). Her grip strength was increased with both upper extremities, but the results on the initial testing probably reflected her physical inactivity while she was hospitalized for three weeks preceding the initial neuropsychological examination. The patient made no errors on the Sensory-perceptual Examination on either the first or second testing.

On the second examination the patient performed worse in finger tapping speed with her left hand than she had initially (37 vs. 32); finger tapping speed with the right hand was somewhat faster on the second testing (40 vs. 45). This finding stands independently as a possible significant indicator of deterioration of right cerebral functioning and, in the context of her excellent improvement on a number of other tests, probably is attributable to chance variation (even though such distinct changes in finger tapping speed do not occur often). S.G. also performed somewhat worse on the Speech-sounds Perception Test and the Seashore Rhythm Test. It would be difficult to propose an explanation of these changes except in terms of a gratuitous hypothesis, such as saying that the patient was not making as much of an effort on those particular tests. Finally, remembering only nine of the figures on the Memory component of the Tactual Performance Test (as contrasted with all 10 figures on the first examination) does not represent a significant change.

There is no doubt that the patient demonstrated a very substantial overall improvement on the second testing that goes well beyond practice-effect expectations. Probably the greatest improvements were on the Performance IQ and Part B of the Trail Making Test, although the improvement on the Category Test and Total Time of the Tactual Performance Test were also substantial. Even though we would interpret the results of the second testing as suggesting the presence of very mild residual dysfunction of the right cerebral hemisphere, they would also certainly indicate that the patient is presently capable of considerably more efficient and confident performances in everyday life than she had been at the time of her discharge from the hospital five months earlier. (Note that the test findings still do not demonstrate any evidence of neuropsychological impairment corresponding with the medical indications of a left intracerebral hematoma.)

Finally, a comparison of the two sets of test results for this young woman indicates the difficulty that may occur in inferring the degree of deficits when only a single examination has been given. In this case the second examination indicated quite definitely that the patient had had significant impairment of Performance intelligence at the time of the first examination. The results on the Category Test, Part B of the Trail Making Test, and the Localization component and the Total Time of the Tactual Performance Test were all significantly impaired, even though they did not appear to be particularly deficient when compared with normative data. This case clearly reinforces the value of serial testings on patients who demonstrate borderline or better values on the initial testing that may be inaccurately interpreted as reflecting normal neuropsychological functioning.

CASE #10

Name: W.B.

Age: 15

Education: 9

Sex: Male

Handedness: Right

Occupation: Student

Background Information

When W.B. was 14 years, 11 months old he was hit by a bus and sustained a fracture of his left elbow and a severe head injury. X-rays taken at a local hospital showed a large depressed fracture in the right parietal area. Three days following the injury the patient was transferred to a major medical center for further diagnostic evaluation and surgical treatment.

As a student in the latter part of his first year of high school, W.B. had been making average progress before the accident. He had not been a particularly good student but had not failed any grades. Family circumstances and other aspects of his adjustment seemed to be unremarkable.

Neurological Examination

Carotid angiograms done upon admission to the medical center showed no abnormality except for depression of the brain under the area of the skull fracture. Skull films also revealed the right parietal defect. Lumbar puncture, which indicated that the cerebral spinal fluid was under normal pressure, suggested that the fluid had previously been bloody and was clearing.

W.B. underwent surgery on the day of admission and a 6 cm x 4 cm depressed fracture in the right parietal area was elevated. The patient also had an epidural hematoma which depressed the brain about 2 cm. Exploration and needling in the

right parietal area showed edema and definite contusion but no obvious hemorrhage or laceration.

During the first two post-operative weeks W.B. was confused, completely disoriented, and combative; gradually he began to show steady improvement and by the third post-operative week (three and one-half weeks after the injury) he was lucid, rational, and cooperative. He did, however, still have complete amnesia for the accident. He also had definite left hemiparesis and hemihypesthesia in addition to some impairment in the use of his left upper extremity because of the bone fracture.

Initially after the injury W.B. did not respond even to painful stimuli on the left side of his body but withdrew his extremities when the stimulus was delivered on the right side. Babinski signs were present bilaterally and the patient showed a central facial paralysis. Physical therapy, together with spontaneous recovery, produced some improvement but a degree of motor disability remained even four weeks post-injury. W.B. also had a disturbed position and proprioceptive sense involving both left extremities. The final medical diagnoses were (1) a compound, depressed fracture in the right parietal area; (2) an epidural hematoma in the right parietal area; and (3) a contusion of the right parietal lobe.

Although the patient was completely disoriented and confused during the first two post-operative weeks, he improved rapidly and we felt that it was possible to administer neuropsychological testing about two and one-half weeks after surgery. It was necessary to make certain adaptations in the testing procedure because the patient's left arm was in a cast due to the bone fracture (e.g., he used his right upper extremity for all three trials of the Tactual Performance Test). We were not able to administer the tests of hand preference (although the patient indicated that he had always been right-handed) and the instructions for the last two items of the Aphasia Screening Test were changed so that the subject was asked to move his right hand instead of his left. It was possible to do the Sensory-perceptual Examination without any modification of the standard procedure.

Neuropsychological Examination

The patient earned a Verbal IQ (87) in the Low Average range (exceeding about 19% of his age peers), a Performance IQ (65) in the range of Mental Retardation (exceeding less than 2%), and a Full Scale IQ (74) in the range of Borderline Intelligence (exceeding 4%). W.B. showed little variability on the individual Verbal subtests and there would be no basis to infer cerebral impairment from these scores.

The Performance subtest scores tended to be somewhat lower than the Verbal scores and it appeared that W.B. may have experienced some deficit in this area, particularly on Picture Arrangement (4) and Digit Symbol (3). In addition, the 22-point disparity between Verbal and Performance IQ values suggests fairly definitely that the Performance subtest scores were somewhat reduced. However, without independent evidence of brain damage, it would be difficult to conclude definitely that this pattern of Wechsler scores reflected brain damage.

The four most sensitive indicators in the HRNTB all had scores clearly in the range of impaired brain functions. It must be remembered that there is a significant correlation between IQ values and results on these four measures (Reitan, 1956) and research has shown that the Impairment Index must be given a more liberal interpretation for persons with relatively low IQ values (Reitan, 1985). W.B.'s scores on these four variables, especially Part B of the Trail Making Test (172 sec), are strikingly deficient. Therefore, we can say that these results suggest that (1) cerebral damage has occurred and (2) the Performance IQ is affected. Considering these hypotheses, one might then raise a question of right cerebral damage.

As noted, we could not evaluate certain measures of lateralized function because the patient's left arm was in a cast; it was necessary to have the subject perform all three trials of the Tactual Performance Test with his right hand and it was not possible to measure finger tapping speed in his left hand. Nevertheless, the patient was willing to test his grip strength in the left upper extremity (despite the cast) and we were also able to perform the Sensory-perceptual Examination.

The patient showed a striking diminution of grip strength with the left upper extremity which may have been due, at least partially, to the peripheral injury and the cast. In addition, he had considerably more difficulty in tactile finger localization with his left hand (8 errors) than his right (2 errors). W.B. also showed tendencies toward a failure to perceive a tactile stimulus to the left hand when given simultaneously with the right hand and not perceive an auditory stimulus to the left ear when bilateral simultaneous stimulation was administered. The patient had only two more errors in finger-tip number writing perception with his left hand (10) than his right (8), but the examiner noted that more pressure was required on the left hand, indicating a left hypesthesia. Thus, this test contributed lateralizing evidence and suggested that the right cerebral hemisphere (parietal area) was more dysfunctional than the left.

W.B. wanted to draw large figures and therefore was permitted to use a separate sheet for each drawing. Note that the drawings of the cross and key were particularly suggestive of right cerebral

THE HALSTEAD-REITAN
NEUROPSYCHOLOGICAL TEST BATTERY

Patient __W.B. (I)__ Age __15__ Sex __M__ Education __8__ Handedness __R__

WECHSLER-BELLEVUE SCALE

VIQ	87
PIQ	65
FS IQ	74

Information	8
Comprehension	8
Digit Span	6
Arithmetic	6
Similarities	8
Vocabulary	7

Picture Arrangement	4
Picture Completion	6
Block Design	5
Object Assembly	8
Digit Symbol	3

TRAIL MAKING TEST

Part A: __56__ seconds
Part B: __172__ seconds

STRENGTH OF GRIP

Dominant hand: __38.5__ kilograms

Non-dominant hand: __14.5__ kilograms

REITAN-KLØVE TACTILE FORM RECOGNITION TEST

Dominant hand: __3__ errors

Non-dominant hand: __0__ errors

REITAN-KLØVE SENSORY-PERCEPTUAL EXAM

				Error Totals	
RH___LH___	Both H: RH___LH _2_			RH___LH _2_	
RH___LF___	Both H/F: RH___LF___			RH___LF___	
LH___RF___	Both H/F: LH___RF___			RF___LH___	
RE___LE___	Both E: RE___LE _1_			RE___LE _1_	
RV___LV___	Both: RV___LV___			RV___LV___	

TACTILE FINGER RECOGNITION

R 1___ 2 _1_ 3___ 4 _1_ 5___   R **2** / **20**

L 1___ 2 _1_ 3 _2_ 4 _3_ 5 _2_   L **8** / **20**

FINGER-TIP NUMBER WRITING

R 1 _2_ 2 _1_ 3 _1_ 4 _2_ 5 _2_   R **8** / **20**

L 1 _4_ 2 _1_ 3 _1_ 4 _2_ 5 _2_   L **10** / **20**

(MORE PRESSURE REQUIRED ON LEFT SIDE.)

HALSTEAD'S NEUROPSYCHOLOGICAL TEST BATTERY

Category Test	82

Tactual Performance Test

Right hand:	10.9
Right hand:	9.8
Right hand:	10.3

(LEFT ARM IN CAST)

Total Time	31.0
Memory	6
Localization	2

Seashore Rhythm Test

Number Correct	15	10

Speech-sounds Perception Test

Number of Errors	17

Finger Oscillation Test

Dominant hand:	41	41
Non-dominant hand:	NOT TESTED	

Impairment Index   0.9

REITAN-KLØVE
LATERAL-DOMINANCE EXAM*

Show me how you:
throw a ball	_____
hammer a nail	_____
cut with a knife	_____
turn a door knob	_____
use scissors	_____
use an eraser	_____
write your name	_____

Record time used for spontaneous name-writing:
Preferred hand	___ seconds
Non-preferred hand	___ seconds

Show me how you:
kick a football	___
step on a bug	___

*NOT GIVEN, BUT PATIENT HAD ALWAYS BEEN RIGHT-HANDED.

REITAN-INDIANA APHASIA SCREENING TEST

Form for Adults and Older Children

Name: _____ W. B. (I) _____ Age: __15__

Copy SQUARE	Repeat TRIANGLE
Name SQUARE	Repeat MASSACHUSETTS
Spell SQUARE	Repeat METHODIST EPISCOPAL " Methdis Epis "
Copy CROSS	Write SQUARE
Name CROSS	Read SEVEN
Spell CROSS	Repeat SEVEN
Copy TRIANGLE	Repeat/Explain HE SHOUTED THE WARNING.
Name TRIANGLE	Write HE SHOUTED THE WARNING.
Spell TRIANGLE	Compute 85 – 27 =
Name BABY	Compute 17 X 3 =
Write CLOCK	Name KEY
Name FORK	Demonstrate use of KEY
Read 7 SIX 2	Draw KEY
Read MGW	Read PLACE LEFT HAND TO RIGHT EAR.
Reading I	Place LEFT HAND TO RIGHT EAR Changed to RIGHT HAND TO LEFT EAR. OK.
Reading II "Here is a friendly ..."	Place LEFT HAND TO LEFT ELBOW Changed to RIGHT HAND TO RIGHT ELBOW. OK.

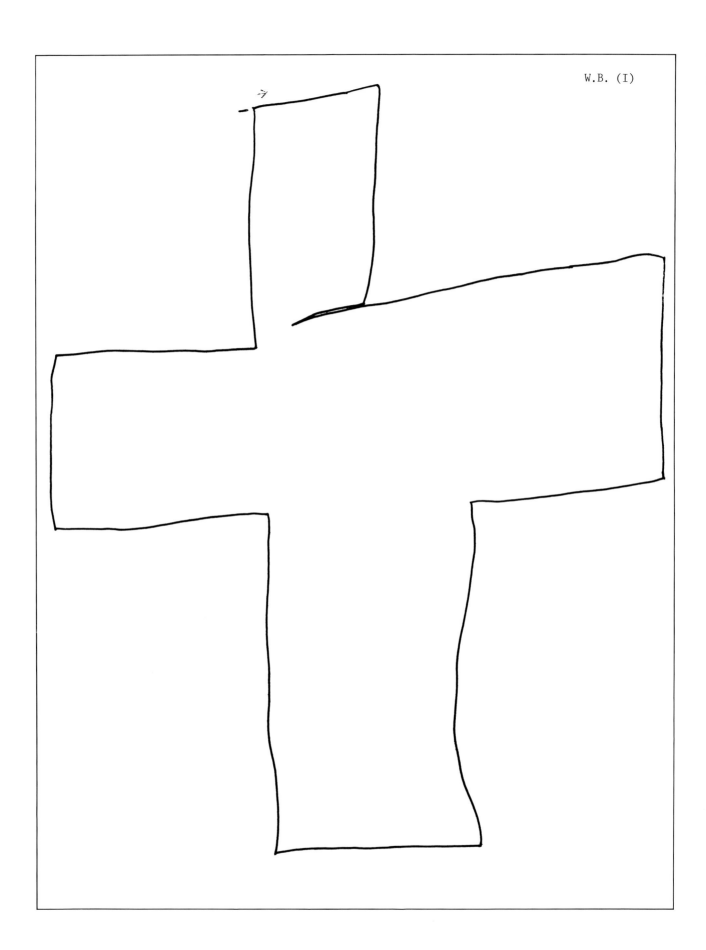

W.B. (I)

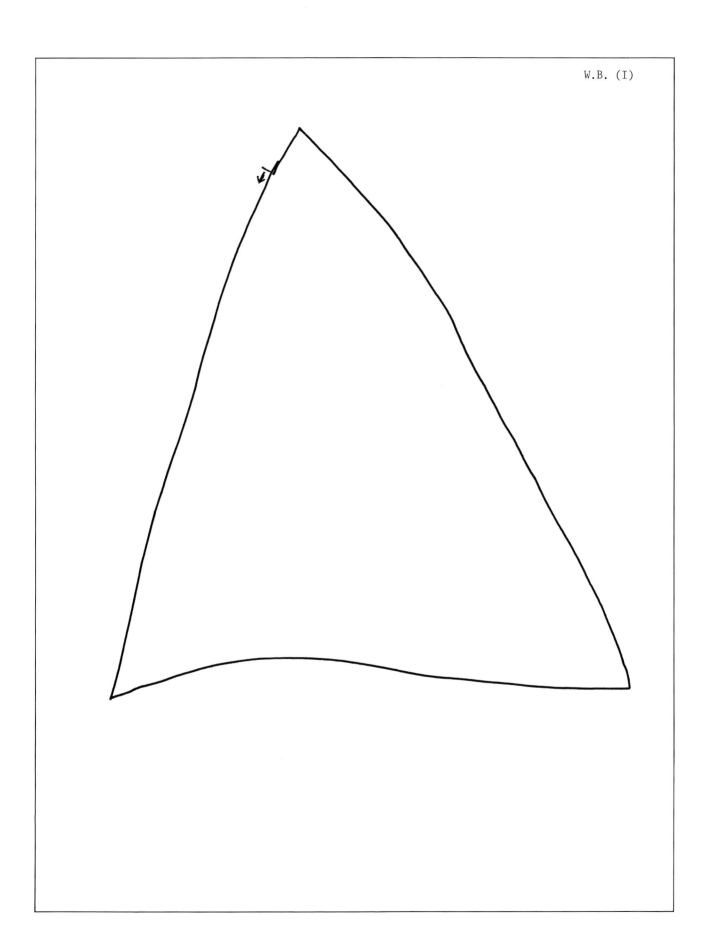

51

$\frac{85}{27}$
$\frac{}{58}$

Square

Clock

he shouted the warning

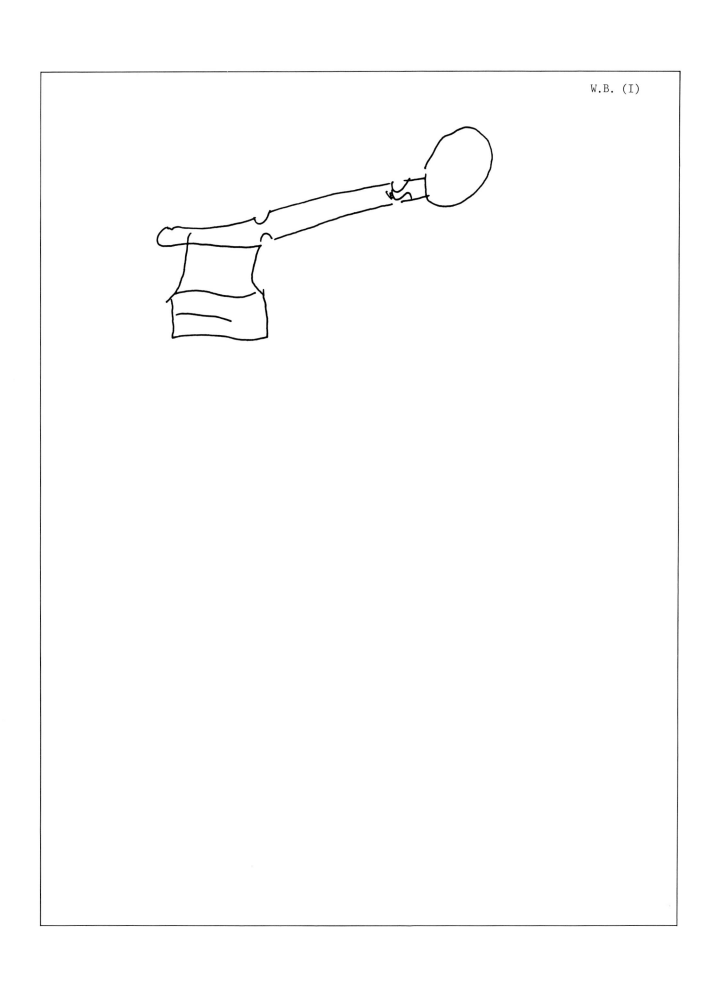

dysfunction. In his attempt to draw the cross the patient actually drew the line in the wrong direction in one instance and had to correct himself. In addition, the opposing extremities are clearly asymmetrical.

W.B. forgot to include notches on the stem of the key near the handle and attempted to put them in afterwards, but it is obvious that he was not able to draw them in an "opposing" fashion. The rest of the key was not drawn with sufficient detail to allow us to make any inferences regarding right cerebral damage. Even without the results of the Tactual Performance Test and the Finger Oscillation Test we can see that the test findings were quite convincing of right cerebral damage.

The patient also made a few mistakes that suggested left cerebral hemisphere dysfunction. On the second reading item of the Aphasia Screening Test he read the first word as "Here" instead of "HE," an unusual error that may indicate some mild difficulty in reading.

W.B.'s performance on the Tactile Form Recognition Test provided more convincing evidence of left cerebral damage. Although we did not time his responses, the patient made three mistakes in eight trials with his right hand and no mistakes with his left hand. One might attribute the single reading error to the patient's relatively low Verbal IQ, but the three errors in Tactile Form Recognition with the right hand cannot be ignored or attributed to lack of education.

W.B. also demonstrated some impairment on general indicators of brain-related functions. His Total Time on the Tactual Performance Test (31.0 min) exceeded the average time for brain-damaged subjects by a considerable margin and he performed very poorly on the Seashore Rhythm Test (15 errors). The score on the Speech-sounds Perception Test (17) was a little worse than the average score for brain-damaged subjects; considering his Verbal IQ, 17 is not a particularly bad score for this patient if we were to consider him to be a brain-damaged subject.

Including both general and lateralizing indicators, the overall neuropsychological pattern is unequivocal in its significance for impaired brain functions. The right cerebral indicators focus particularly on motor and tactile-perceptual deficits and include some difficulty on the tests for bilateral auditory perception and the drawings of the cross and key. All of these findings could be explained by postulating a lesion in the middle part of the right cerebral hemisphere.

The relatively severe deficits shown by the general indicators lead us to postulate two possibilities: either the lesion has occurred rather recently or it is progressive in nature. A progressive lesion is usually lateralized and focal, and W.B. had definite indications of both left and right cerebral damage. Looking at the overall picture, then, the test results are more typical of cerebral trauma than a focal lesion developing within the brain. In fact, the findings are almost perfectly compatible with the history information and neurosurgical findings of definite contusion of brain tissue underlying the depressed skull fracture over the middle part of the right cerebral hemisphere.

Considering the force of the blow and the mechanisms of head injury it is somewhat unusual that the patient did not show more evidence of left cerebral damage. Some investigators have suggested, though, that a depressed skull fracture may actually absorb some of the impact of the blow and therefore limit the transmission of shock waves through the rest of the brain and the shearing effects that often occur with closed head injuries.

W.B. was admitted to the hospital for a cranioplasty about four months after we first tested him and we were able to re-examine him at that time. His behavior was reportedly normal; he had returned to school and had been promoted to the next grade. Neurological examination revealed no apparent motor disability in practical aspects of behavior, but the patient did have slightly increased deep tendon reflexes (especially of the left lower extremity) and mild difficulty hopping on his left leg. The EEG was within normal limits.

The Cornell Medical Index Health Questionnaire revealed very few complaints, although the patient did indicate that at times he has had bad nosebleeds, sweats a great deal even in cold weather, is often troubled with boils, has constant numbness or tingling in parts of his body, is frequently ill and confined to bed, and often has small accidents and injuries. He denied having any other problems of either a somatic or emotional nature.

The reader is probably aware that positive practice-effect may be prominent when such a short time has elapsed between testings; however, the first four months following the injury should also represent a time when the patient experiences a substantial degree of spontaneous recovery. Taking both of these factors into account, we would expect W.B. to perform considerably better on a number of the tests than he had initially. First, we will analyze the test results for evidence of residual impairment.

W.B. earned a Verbal IQ (99) almost exactly at the Average level (exceeding 47% of his age peers) and a Performance IQ 17 points higher, in the High Average range (exceeding 86%). These values yielded a Full Scale IQ (108) in the upper part of the Average range (exceeding 70%).

The Verbal subtests did not show any significant variability to suggest cerebral damage. Although the Performance subtests were generally well done, the lowest score (10 on Digit Symbol) possibly represented mild impairment. On the basis of the Wechsler scores alone one certainly could not conclude that the patient had experienced any brain damage.

Note, however, that the four most sensitive tests yielded strong evidence of mild brain impairment, particularly considering W.B.'s adequate IQ values. Although W.B. earned an Impairment Index of 0.6, three of the four tests that had scores in the brain-damaged range — Category Test (53), Seashore Rhythm Test (25 correct), and Finger

Oscillation Test (49) — were near the cut-off point. W.B.'s only grossly deficient performance occurred on the Total Time (21.9 min) of the Tactual Performance Test, but even that score was well below the average of 25 minutes required by brain-damaged persons in general. Therefore, the analysis of the test results on which the Impairment Index is based indicates that the patient had only mild impairment. We should also note that W.B.'s score on Part B of the Trail Making Test (86 sec) must also be considered to be a sign of mild impairment, even though it was just within the normal range.

Lateralizing indicators implicated the right cerebral hemisphere to a greater extent than the left. On the initial examination it had not been possible to administer the Tactual Performance Test in the usual sequence or the Finger Oscillation Test because the patient had a cast on his left arm. On the second examination these tests were important for the interpretation; both scores indicated definite impairment of the left upper extremity. Also, the patient was probably slightly weaker than would normally be expected with his left upper extremity (42 kg) compared with his right (48 kg).

W.B. showed no evidence of aphasia but had mild difficulties copying the cross and key. The first cross was probably within normal limits but the second attempt showed a definite disparity of the vertical as well as lateral extremities. The general configuration of the drawing of the key was adequate but the patient had some difficulty with the notches near the handle and failed to draw the handle properly. This is a rather unusual type of difficulty but probably reflects very mild impairment (stemming from right hemisphere damage) in dealing with simple spatial configurations.

Finally, besides the motor and higher-level deficits involving the right cerebral hemisphere, W.B. had definite difficulty localizing fingers on his left hand (6 errors) compared with his right (1 error). He also made several mistakes reporting bilateral

THE HALSTEAD-REITAN
NEUROPSYCHOLOGICAL TEST BATTERY

Patient __W.B. (II)__ Age __15__ Sex __M__ Education __9__ Handedness __R__

WECHSLER-BELLEVUE SCALE

VIQ	99
PIQ	116
FS IQ	108

Information	10
Comprehension	9
Digit Span	7
Arithmetic	9
Similarities	10
Vocabulary	8

Picture Arrangement	15
Picture Completion	12
Block Design	11
Object Assembly	12
Digit Symbol	10

TRAIL MAKING TEST

Part A: __23__ seconds
Part B: __86__ seconds

STRENGTH OF GRIP

Dominant hand: __48__ kilograms
Non-dominant hand: __42__ kilograms

REITAN-KLØVE TACTILE FORM RECOGNITION TEST

Dominant hand: __1__ errors
Non-dominant hand: __0__ errors

REITAN-KLØVE SENSORY-PERCEPTUAL EXAM

			Error Totals	
RH___LH___	Both H:	RH___LH_1_	RH___LH_1_	
RH___LF___	Both H/F:	RH_1_LF___	RH_1_LF___	
LH___RF___	Both H/F:	LH___RF___	RF___LH___	
RE___LE___	Both E:	RE___LE___	RE___LE___	
RV___LV___	Both:	RV___LV___	RV_1_LV_1_	
			_1_ _1_	

TACTILE FINGER RECOGNITION

R 1___ 2___ 3 _1_ 4___ 5___   R _1_ / 20
L 1 _1_ 2 _1_ 3___ 4 _2_ 5 _2_   L _6_ / 20

FINGER-TIP NUMBER WRITING

R 1 _1_ 2 _1_ 3 _1_ 4___ 5 _1_   R _4_ / 20
L 1 _1_ 2___ 3___ 4 _1_ 5___   L _2_ / 20

HALSTEAD'S NEUROPSYCHOLOGICAL TEST BATTERY

Category Test __53__

Tactual Performance Test

Dominant hand:	7.3	
Non-dominant hand:	11.4	
Both hands:	3.2	

Total Time	21.9
Memory	8
Localization	5

Seashore Rhythm Test

Number Correct __25__ __6__

Speech-sounds Perception Test

Number of Errors __5__

Finger Oscillation Test

Dominant hand:	49	49
Non-dominant hand:	39	

Impairment Index __0.6__

REITAN-KLØVE
LATERAL-DOMINANCE EXAM

Show me how you:
throw a ball	R
hammer a nail	R
cut with a knife	R
turn a door knob	R
use scissors	R
use an eraser	R
write your name	R

Record time used for spontaneous name-writing:
Preferred hand	__4__ seconds
Non-preferred hand	__14__ seconds

Show me how you:
kick a football	R
step on a bug	R

REITAN-INDIANA APHASIA SCREENING TEST

Form for Adults and Older Children

Name: _____ W. B. (II) _____ Age: _15_

Copy SQUARE	Repeat TRIANGLE
Name SQUARE	Repeat MASSACHUSETTS
Spell SQUARE	Repeat METHODIST EPISCOPAL "Mesodis Episcobal"
Copy CROSS	Write SQUARE
Name CROSS	Read SEVEN
Spell CROSS	Repeat SEVEN
Copy TRIANGLE	Repeat/Explain HE SHOUTED THE WARNING.
Name TRIANGLE	Write HE SHOUTED THE WARNING.
Spell TRIANGLE	Compute 85 – 27 =
Name BABY	Compute 17 X 3 =
Write CLOCK	Name KEY
Name FORK	Demonstrate use of KEY
Read 7 SIX 2	Draw KEY
Read MGW	Read PLACE LEFT HAND TO RIGHT EAR.
Reading I	Place LEFT HAND TO RIGHT EAR
Reading II	Place LEFT HAND TO LEFT ELBOW

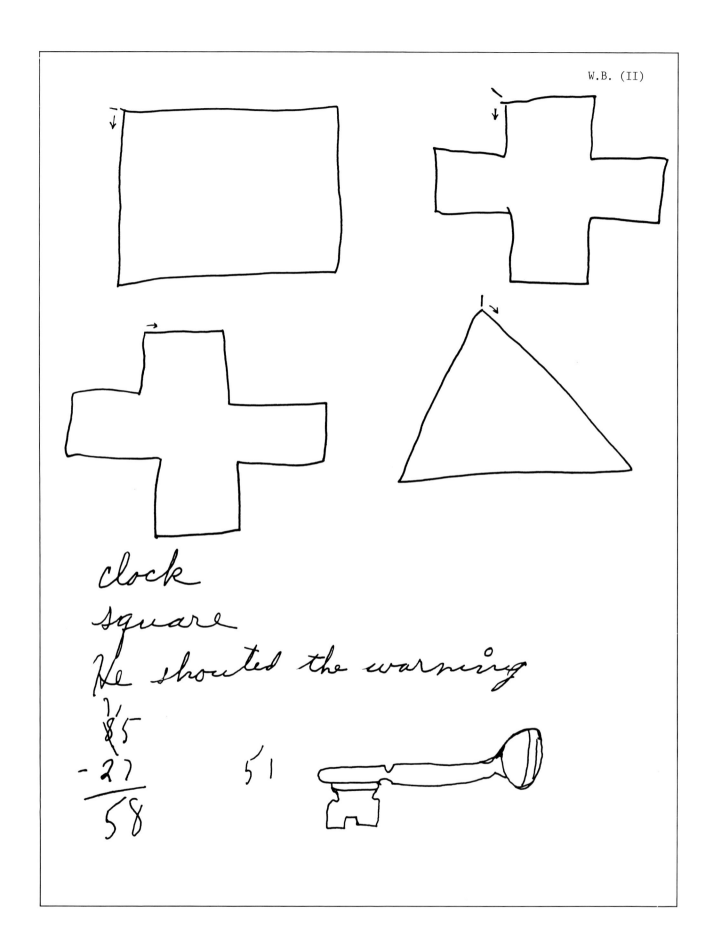

clock

square

He shouted the warning

85
− 27
‾‾‾‾
58

51

tactile and visual stimuli, but these errors were equally distributed on the two sides. However, the fact that mistakes occurred is probably a valid indication of impaired brain functions; errors of this kind are rarely seen in normal subjects.

The only demonstrations of left cerebral damage included one mistake with the right hand in Tactile Form Recognition and slightly more difficulty on the right hand (4 errors) than the left (2 errors) in finger-tip number writing perception.

It is clear from these results than the patient's right cerebral hemisphere is more impaired than his left. The lateralizing findings reinforce the hypothesis of mild cerebral damage suggested by the general indicators. These findings, like the results of the first examination, could be explained by postulating traumatic damage to the middle part of the right cerebral hemisphere resulting in both mild generalized deficits and indications of left cerebral dysfunction.

The results of the second examination validate the deficits demonstrated during the first examination done four months earlier. Even considering positive practice-effect, the patient undoubtedly made a significant and genuine improvement. His Verbal IQ was 12 points higher and his Performance IQ had risen 51 points (from 65 to 116). His Impairment Index had decreased from 0.9 to 0.6. He still showed mild impairment on the Category Test but the improvement in his score (from 82 to 53) was substantially greater than would be expected from practice-effect.

A great improvement was made on Part B of the Trail Making Test, reducing the time required from 172 to 86 seconds. The Total Time score on the Tactual Performance Test was also strikingly reduced; except for the poor score obtained with the left hand (11.4 min), the performance approached the normal range. Grip strength was better, especially in the left arm. On the Seashore Rhythm Test (25 correct) and Speech-sounds Perception Test (5) his scores improved considerably.

The patient continued to show mild impairment in his ability to copy simple figures and also demonstrated mild difficulties on the Sensory-perceptual Examination. The results of the second examination increases one's awareness of the severity of the deficits shown by this young man at the time of the first examination. With such pronounced improvement occurring over a period of less than four months we would postulate that the patient was still on a recovery course and had the potential for additional spontaneous improvement, even though the rate of improvement will probably be diminished in ensuing months.

CASE #11

Name: B.B.

Age: 24

Education: 12

Sex: Female

Handedness: Right

Occupation: Telephone Operator

Background Information

This 24-year-old woman had completed high school with approximately average grades and was working as a long-distance telephone operator. Her cognitive development had apparently been normal and she was leading a relatively routine life.

One evening, while sitting in her home, B.B. was shot from behind with a .22 caliber hand gun. Her heavy wig gave her some protection but the bullet penetrated the right posterior parietal area of her brain. Her assailant escaped but B.B. managed to call the police and summon an ambulance. During this time she was fully conscious, alert, oriented and cooperative.

In the hospital E.R. a small bullet wound with very little associated bleeding or general damage was obvious in the right posterior parietal area. The patient's pupils were equal and reacted to light and there was no paralysis of the extraocular muscles. However, she did have a dense left homonymous hemianopia, left facial weakness, and a left hemiparesis that was more profound in her arm than her leg. Deep tendon reflexes were normal on both sides. Plain skull films showed that the bullet had penetrated the skull slightly to the right of the midline in the posterior parietal area and had lodged in the suprasellar area. Metallic bullet fragments and depressed bone fragments were evident near the site of the penetration. The dorsum sella was also fractured.

B.B. was taken to surgery and a right frontal craniotomy was performed to remove the bullet which had lodged just posterior to the right optic chiasm near the right optic tract. A small craniectomy was performed at the site of penetration to remove any foreign matter and debride the wound.

Neurological Evaluation

Post-operatively the patient did very well. The left hemiparesis and left facial weakness gradually resolved; the left homonymous hemianopia, however, remained essentially unchanged. B.B. was somewhat confused shortly after the surgery but her mental status improved during the post-operative course. Electroencephalography done nine days after the injury showed diffuse abnormalities over the right cerebral hemisphere.

Neuropsychological Evaluation

Neuropsychological examination was done 15 days after the injury. In giving the Tactual Performance Test to this patient it was necessary to deviate from standard testing procedure. B.B. experienced considerable stiffness of her left upper extremity, particularly in the shoulder area. Because it was painful for her to use her left upper extremity for this test we gave three trials using only her right hand. In other respects standard aspects of administration were followed.

This woman showed evidence of significant neuropsychological impairment. Her deficits principally indicated right cerebral hemisphere dysfunction although some of the specific results also suggested left cerebral damage.

The patient earned a Verbal IQ (93) in the lower part of the Average range (exceeding about 32% of her age peers). Her Performance IQ (59) was 34 points lower, in the range of Mild Mental Retardation and exceeding less than 1%. Although an average of these values can be obtained and referred to as a Full Scale IQ there would appear to be little point in averaging the scores of a relatively normal and a severely impaired performance.

Except for Digit Span (6) and Similarities (6), the Verbal subtest scores were at approximately the Average level. Our experience has indicated that a low Digit Span score is characteristic of many neurological patients and probably has no specific significance regarding neuropsychological functioning. However, it is possible that the patient has suffered some impairment on the Similarities subtest (a finding that would be supported by the evidence of aphasia to be described later).

Except for Object Assembly (8) the patient was significantly impaired on all of the Performance subtests. We suspect that she may have earned points on this test as a result of chance success (note the extreme impairment she demonstrates in her drawings of simple spatial configurations). Although the marked disparity between Verbal and Performance IQ values certainly would suggest that B.B. may have experienced right cerebral damage, the remainder of the neuropsychological evaluation again indicates the limitations of the Wechsler Scale for general neuropsychological assessment.

B.B. performed very poorly on each of the four most sensitive measures in the HRNTB. The Category Test score (118) indicates that she has great difficulty in abstraction, reasoning, and analyzing the nature of complex situations, despite her relatively average scores on certain Verbal subtests.

We would judge that she is severely impaired in her ability to draw reasonable conclusions on the basis of her observations.

As noted above, it was painful for B.B. to use her left upper extremity and we administered the Tactual Performance Test by asking her to do it three times using her right hand alone. She had a great deal of difficulty on the first two trials but finally grasped the essential nature of the problem and was able to complete the task on the third trial. From this data one can conclude that the patient has significant impairment in her ability to analyze and solve complex problems and that she will need very careful instruction in determining the essential elements of procedure if she is to have any success in analyzing the type of complex situations that occur in everyday life. B.B. was able to remember five of the shapes on the Tactual Performance Test but was significantly impaired in her ability to localize them.

Her deficits in analyzing complex situations, being flexible in thought processes, and keeping more than one aspect of a situation in mind at the same time were also clearly demonstrated by her performance on Part B of the Trail Making Test (405 sec). It is apparent from the poor score on Part A (160 sec), however, that part of her difficulty involved the spatial nature of the task; the poor performance on Part A almost certainly reflected a problem in being able to scan the page and find the spatial location of the next number. Poor scores on both Part A and Part B are fairly characteristic of persons with severe damage of the right cerebral hemisphere.

Despite evidence of very severe impairment of higher-level brain functions, B.B. did have the basic capability to pay relatively close attention to specific stimulus material. Her score on the Speech-sounds Perception Test (11) was not grossly impaired and indicated that she was able to attend to the test stimuli and correlate them with the correct responses on her answer sheet. She did not do as well on the Seashore Rhythm

THE HALSTEAD-REITAN
NEUROPSYCHOLOGICAL TEST BATTERY

Patient _____ **B.B.** _____ Age __ **24** __ Sex __ **F** __ Education __ **12** __ Handedness __ **R** __

WECHSLER-BELLEVUE SCALE

VIQ	**93**
PIQ	**59**
FS IQ	**74**
Information	**10**
Comprehension	**10**
Digit Span	**6**
Arithmetic	**9**
Similarities	**6**
Vocabulary	**10**
Picture Arrangement	**4**
Picture Completion	**3**
Block Design	**3**
Object Assembly	**8**
Digit Symbol	**3**

TRAIL MAKING TEST

Part A: __ **160** __ seconds
Part B: __ **405** __ seconds

STRENGTH OF GRIP

Dominant hand: __ **23.5** __ kilograms
Non-dominant hand: __ **11.0** __ kilograms

REITAN-KLØVE SENSORY-PERCEPTUAL EXAM

						Error Totals		
RH ___	LH ___	Both H:	RH ___	LH **4**		RH ___	LH **4**	
RH ___	LF ___	Both H/F:	RH **1**	LF **1**		RH **1**	LF **1**	
LH ___	RF ___	Both H/F:	LH **3**	RF ___		RF ___	LH **3**	
RE ___	LE ___	Both E:	RE **1**	LE **2**		RE **1**	LE **2**	
RV ___	LV ___	Both:	RV ___	LV ___		LEFT		
___	___		___	___		VISUAL		
___	___		___	___		FIELD DEFECT		

TACTILE FINGER RECOGNITION

R 1 ___ 2 **1** 3 **2** 4 3 5 ___   R **6** / **20**

L 1 **2** 2 **2** 3 **2** 4 **2** 5 **1**   L **9** / **20**

FINGER-TIP NUMBER WRITING

R 1 **4** 2 **3** 3 **1** 4 **3** 5 **3**   R **14** / **20**

L 1 **3** 2 **4** 3 **2** 4 **3** 5 **2**   L **14** / **20**

VISUAL FIELD EXAMINATION: LEFT HOMONYMOUS HEMIANOPSIA.

HALSTEAD'S NEUROPSYCHOLOGICAL TEST BATTERY

Category Test	**118**

Tactual Performance Test

Right hand:	**15.0 (3 blocks in)**
Right hand:	**15.0 (2 blocks in)**
Right hand:	**11.1**

Total Time	**41.1 (15 blocks in)**
Memory	**5**
Localization	**1**

Seashore Rhythm Test

Number Correct __ **19** __   **10**

Speech-sounds Perception Test

Number of Errors   **11**

Finger Oscillation Test

Dominant hand:	**34**	**34**
Non-dominant hand:	**27**	

Impairment Index __ **1.0** __

REITAN-KLØVE LATERAL-DOMINANCE EXAM

Show me how you:

throw a ball	**R**
hammer a nail	**R**
cut with a knife	**R**
turn a door knob	**R**
use scissors	**R**
use an eraser	**R**
write your name	**R**

Record time used for spontaneous name-writing:

Preferred hand	**7** seconds
Non-preferred hand	**25** seconds

Show me how you:

kick a football	**R**
step on a bug	**R**

REITAN-INDIANA APHASIA SCREENING TEST

Form for Adults and Older Children

Name: _____B. B._____ Age: __24__

Copy SQUARE	Repeat TRIANGLE

Name SQUARE
       "Triangle"
	Repeat MASSACHUSETTS
	       "Massatoosess"

Spell SQUARE	Repeat METHODIST EPISCOPAL "Methodist Epistical"
Copy CROSS	Write SQUARE

Name CROSS
       "Red Cross emblem"
	Read SEVEN
	       "oven"

Spell CROSS	Repeat SEVEN
Copy TRIANGLE	Repeat/Explain HE SHOUTED THE WARNING.
Name TRIANGLE "Pyramid"	Write HE SHOUTED THE WARNING.
Spell TRIANGLE Wrote and spelled simultaneously. "T-R-A-N-I-A-A-G-L-E"	Compute 85 – 27 =
Name BABY	Compute 17 X 3 = Done quickly and correctly.
Write CLOCK	Name KEY
Name FORK "Sp -- a fork."	Demonstrate use of KEY

Read 7 SIX 2
       "Times 2 -- 2 times, six, X's
       2 -- X's 2."
	Draw KEY

Read MGW
       "G - W"
	Read PLACE LEFT HAND TO RIGHT EAR.
	       "Ace hand right ear."

Reading I Hesitatingly but OK.	Place LEFT HAND TO RIGHT EAR
Reading II "Friendly famous dog shows."	Place LEFT HAND TO LEFT ELBOW Right to left; then left to right; finally tried left to left - said, "I don't think so."

B.B.

Clock

II.

1. SQUARE

2. Square

Truiiaagle

I.

"He Shouled the
Warxing!"

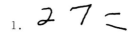

1. 27 =

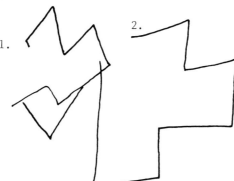

1.

2.

2. 5 – 27 = 22

51

85 (Examiner wrote
problem.)
– 27
─────
68

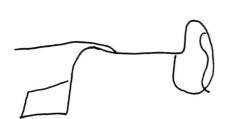

Test, but the poor score (19 correct) was probably related to the content of the procedure rather than her ability to pay attention to the stimuli.

Lateralizing indications were prominent in this patient's test results. Findings suggesting right cerebral damage included a mild deficit in finger tapping speed with the left hand compared with the right (although both hands were extremely slow) and a very pronounced loss in grip strength of the left upper extremity (11 kg).

As might be expected from a patient with a bullet wound entering the right parietal area, sensory-perceptual deficits were more prominent than indications of motor impairment. B.B. had a left homonymous hemianopia, probably caused by the path of the bullet through the geniculostriate tract.

She also had a distinct tendency to fail to perceive tactile stimuli on the left side of the body when given simultaneously with stimuli on the right side. Even though she made more mistakes on the left side, the patient made one mistake on the right side in both tactile and auditory bilateral simultaneous stimulation. Considered independently, it would be difficult to use these findings as evidence of left cerebral damage. A patient with severe generalized impairment is sometimes not quite as alert and accurate in responding as would be desired. Thus, these right-sided errors could have been either failures in reporting by the patient, chance errors, indications of left cerebral damage, or any combination of these factors.

On tactile finger recognition the patient had more difficulty on her left hand than her right, implicating the right cerebral hemisphere but in this case the number of errors on the right hand certainly suggests the possibility of left cerebral damage as well. In finger-tip number writing perception the large number of errors on each hand may be a result of the patient's general confusion or may represent bilateral cerebral damage.

The patient's performances on the Aphasia Screening Test contributed evidence of both left

and right cerebral damage. B.B. had a pronounced tendency to fail to perceive the left side of stimulus configurations, a finding characteristic of patients with acutely destructive lesions of the right cerebral hemisphere. When asked to read MGW she omitted the "M." When reading HE IS A FRIENDLY ANIMAL, A FAMOUS WINNER OF DOG SHOWS the patient read only the words on the right side of the configuration. She read SEVEN as "oven" and read the first word as "ace" when reading PLACE LEFT HAND TO RIGHT EAR. She also omitted "TO" (the first word on the left side of the line) in reading this sentence, a deficit more commonly observed in persons with right than left cerebral damage.

The types of difficulty shown by this woman in her attempts to solve the problem $85 - 27 =$ are quite characteristic of persons with severe right cerebral damage. The examiner instructed B.B. to write the problem on the sheet of paper and try to solve it. At first the patient ignored the left side of the stimulus ($85 - 27 =$) and wrote only "$27 =$"; she did not know how to proceed further. The examiner again instructed her to write the problem; this time B.B. was able to write "$5 - 27 = 22$." Once more she had omitted the left side of the stimulus configuration but realized that the problem involved subtraction and apparently subtracted the 5 from 27. Finally, the examiner wrote the problem on the paper for the patient, using a minus sign and placing the 27 below the 85. B.B. originally made a mistake in solving the problem, obtaining "68" as the answer, but was able to correct the answer herself. It was clear that she had great difficulties solving this simple arithmetic problem, stemming largely from not being able to visually perceive the spatial configuration of the stimulus material correctly. When asked to mentally compute 17×3 she had no difficulty and quickly and correctly wrote down the answer.

In examining B.B.'s drawings we see that she also showed significant deficits in the ability to copy simple spatial configurations. She was able to draw the general shape of the square and triangle but became completely confused when attempting to draw the cross. She also had severe difficulty drawing the key.

It is interesting to observe B.B.'s printing and writing after seeing the problems she had in dealing with simple spatial configurations. She was able to print and write quickly, spontaneously, and without difficulty, even though the spatial configurations represented by this type of communication certainly appear to be much more complex than those represented by a Greek cross. These seemingly contradictory findings can be explained quite simply: The spatial nature of writing and printing have been absorbed by the brain into the framework of language and verbal communication and are presented by the *left,* not the right, cerebral hemisphere (Wheeler & Reitan, 1962).

As stated earlier, the Aphasia Screening Test yielded unequivocal evidence of damage of the left as well as the right cerebral hemisphere. None of the information available from neurological diagnostic techniques or neurosurgery implicated the left cerebral hemisphere. Nevertheless, as we have previously noted in the review of mechanisms of head injury, *it is not at all uncommon to see the neuropsychological test results reflect widespread and bilateral damage even when the principal lesion involves only one cerebral hemisphere.*

This patient showed distinct naming difficulties and such problems clearly implicate the left cerebral hemisphere (Wheeler & Reitan, 1962). B.B. named the SQUARE as "triangle," the TRIANGLE as "pyramid," and began to name the FORK as "spoon" before correcting herself. One could question whether the first of these mistakes was only a temporary lapse and, because a few control subjects also give this response, there is some question whether "pyramid" is a valid indication of dysnomia in response to naming the TRIANGLE. However, beginning to name the FORK as a "spoon" is quite characteristic of persons with left cerebral damage.

The patient also had a number of other problems. Her confusion in spelling TRIANGLE is a rather distinct manifestation of left cerebral dysfunction. Her problem reading 7 SIX 2 probably relates to right cerebral damage (a tendency to ignore the left side of the spatial configuration) but also seems to suggest some difficulty understanding the symbolic significance of the material. We would not consider the patient's mild problem in enunciating MASSACHUSETTS and METHODIST EPISCOPAL indicative of a significant brain-related deficit. However, her right-left confusion, demonstrated when she was asked to PLACE LEFT HAND TO LEFT ELBOW, is quite characteristic of patients with left cerebral damage (Wheeler & Reitan, 1962).

Thus, the overall results are definite in indicating severe impairment of adaptive abilities dependent upon brain functions and the right cerebral hemisphere appears to be more seriously damaged than the left. Right cerebral indicators included (1) severe impairment of Performance IQ; (2) a tendency to ignore the left side of spatial configurations; (3) severe constructional dyspraxia; and (4) both motor and sensory-perceptual deficits that were more pronounced on the left side of the body than the right.

Left cerebral manifestations included (1) dysphasic symptoms (dysnomia, spelling dyspraxia, and possible dyslexia); and (2) right-left confusion. The relatively good score on the Speech-sounds Perception Test (although in the impaired range) suggests that the left cerebral damage was relatively discrete and probably not represented by extensive structural damage. The general indicators, which included the four most sensitive measures, represented the overall severity of impairment experienced by this woman.

Therefore, because of the nature of her disabilities, the task in rehabilitating B.B. would involve much more than attention to specific types of deficits; she needs not only retraining of her specific cognitive losses but also (and probably more significantly) extensive remediation in abstraction, reasoning, and logical analysis skills, the ability to draw conclusions from observations, and the ability to simultaneously consider several elements of complex situations.

CASE #12

Name: H.C.

Age: 53

Education: 18

Sex: Male

Handedness: Right

Occupation: Veterinarian

Background Information

This 53-year-old veterinarian was in good health until he slipped on icy steps as he left a college football stadium, fell, and hit the left side of his head on the corner of a cement step. Friends who were with him said that he initially indicated that he was alright but he quickly lapsed into a coma and was taken to the university hospital where medical examination revealed a depressed skull fracture over the left ear. During surgical repair of this injury an epidural hematoma was found and evacuated.

H.C. was unconscious for a total of approximately 24 hours following the injury. After regaining consciousness he had a right hemiparesis and some speech difficulties, a partial third nerve paralysis, and a significant left otorrhea (discharge from the auditory canal). Except for the residual left-sided hearing loss, ptosis of the left eye, and lateral deviation of the left eye (due to paresis of the medial rectus muscle), H.C. showed rapid improvement and it appeared that he had made a complete recovery by the time he was discharged from the hospital.

Six weeks after the injury H.C. sought evaluation by another neurosurgeon because he had encountered a number of problems. Because of his apparently good physical recovery he had expected to be able to return to work and function normally; instead he found it difficult to even read the newspaper. He tired very easily, was unable to concentrate well enough to read his professional journals,

and was not able to get anything accomplished in his work as a veterinarian. Although he had tried to resume his usual activities, he realized that he had been essentially inactive and had been able to accomplish very little productive activity.

Neurological Examination

Neurological examination indicated a left parietal skull defect, a complete hearing loss on the left side, ptosis of the left eyelid and lateral deviation of the eye, and a slightly enlarged left pupil that did not respond to light as well as the right pupil. Visual acuity was retained on the left side. The neurosurgeon could find no evidence of speech deficits and, except for the above findings, H.C.'s general physical and neurological examinations were within normal limits.

It did not seem that the patient's deficits were sufficiently severe to account for his ineffectiveness and the physician believed that H.C. was experiencing a stress reaction to the injury, hospitalization, and surgery. The neurosurgeon and the patient discussed this matter in detail and decided that the best plan would be for H.C. to take an extended winter vacation for several months, especially since he was not working very effectively anyway. At that point the patient was referred for neuropsychological examination to determine whether there were any significant aspects of brain-behavior relationships that were not apparent to the neurosurgeon.

Neuropsychological Evaluation

When asked about his problems H.C. reviewed the residual deficits involving his left eye and ear and also indicated that he seemed to be having some type of memory failure. On the Cornell Medical Index Health Questionnaire the patient indicated a number of somatic complaints but no emotional problems of adjustment. He said that his nose continually felt stuffed up, he had a hearing loss on the left side since his injury, he often had difficulty breathing, and he suffered from frequent severe headaches and pressure or pain in his head since the accident. At this time six weeks had elapsed since the injury.

The Wechsler Scale yielded IQ values in the High Average range, with the Verbal IQ (111) six points lower than the Performance IQ (117). The Verbal IQ exceeded about 77% of H.C.'s age peers and the Performance IQ exceeded about 87%. The Verbal subtest scores showed little variability.

The Performance scores also were within a rather restricted range, but scores on Picture Arrangement (8) and Digit Symbol (8) were lower than results on any of the other subtests. It certainly would not be possible to draw a conclusion of cerebral damage on the basis of the distribution of the Performance subtest scores, but it is possible that the Picture Arrangement and Digit Symbol scores reflected a mild degree of impairment.

The four most sensitive indicators in the Halstead-Reitan Battery were much more definitive in their significance. H.C. earned an Impairment Index of 1.0, performed worse than the average brain-damaged subject on the Category Test (69), was quite slow on Part B of the Trail Making Test (142 sec) and was not able to localize any of the figures in his drawing of the Tactual Performance Test board. The scores on which the Impairment Index is based suggested that this man had moderately severe impairment of abilities generally; however, it must be remembered that the Impairment Index reflects *consistency* of deficit rather than *severity* of deficit.

H.C. did slightly better than the average brain-damaged subject on some tests but, in general, performed somewhat worse than average despite pre-morbid intellectual functions (as well as current IQ values) that were above average. Thus, there would be little doubt from these findings that the patient had experienced some generalized impairment of adaptive abilities. On this basis alone one would predict that he would probably not be able to perform at a level that matched his pre-morbid capabilities, either in his professional work or routine activities of daily living.

Results on the Minnesota Multiphasic Personality Inventory were essentially within normal limits, so neither the MMPI nor the Cornell Medical Index indicated that the patient was experiencing any significant or serious emotional stress. The existing circumstances, however, were exactly the type likely to bring about significant emotional problems in time. That is, neurological evaluation failed to reveal any deficits sufficiently severe to impair the patient's performances; nevertheless, he was clearly impaired, to the point of being unable to read his professional journals or even a newspaper satisfactorily. In addition, his efficiency of performance in his work as a veterinarian appeared to be seriously compromised. Facing problems of this kind without any adequate explanation or understanding tends to induce a great deal of emotional distress in many patients and often produces generalized anxiety, depressive reactions, feelings of guilt, etc.

Evaluation of lateralizing findings yielded additional significant evidence of cerebral dysfunction. Although the relationships between performances of the two hands were within normal limits in finger tapping speed and grip strength, the patient was severely impaired in use of his right upper extremity for complex, adaptive performances (Tactual Performance Test). It is not uncommon

THE HALSTEAD-REITAN
NEUROPSYCHOLOGICAL TEST BATTERY

Patient __H.C.__ Age __53__ Sex __M__ Education __18__ Handedness __R__

WECHSLER-BELLEVUE SCALE

VIQ	111
PIQ	117
FS IQ	114

Information	11
Comprehension	11
Digit Span	10
Arithmetic	10
Similarities	11
Vocabulary	10

Picture Arrangement	8
Picture Completion	10
Block Design	10
Object Assembly	12
Digit Symbol	8

TRAIL MAKING TEST

Part A: __105__ seconds
Part B: __142__ seconds

STRENGTH OF GRIP

Dominant hand: __41.0__ kilograms
Non-dominant hand: __37.5__ kilograms

REITAN-KLØVE TACTILE FORM RECOGNITION TEST

Dominant hand: __17__ seconds; __0__ errors
Non-dominant hand: __9__ seconds; __0__ errors

REITAN-KLØVE SENSORY-PERCEPTUAL EXAM

				Error Totals	
RH ___ LH ___	Both H:	RH ___ LH ___		RH ___ LH ___	
RH ___ LF ___	Both H/F:	RH ___ LF ___		RH ___ LF ___	
LH ___ RF ___	Both H/F:	LH ___ RF __1__		RF __1__ LH ___	
RE __1__ LE ___	Both E:	RE ___ LE ___		RE ___ LE ___	
RV ___ LV ___	Both V:	RV ___ LV ___		RV ___ LV ___	
___ ___		___ ___	} Not		
___ ___		___ ___	} Done		

TACTILE FINGER RECOGNITION

R 1___ 2___ 3___ 4___ 5___   R __0__ / __20__
L 1___ 2___ 3___ 4___ 5___   L __0__ / __20__

FINGER-TIP NUMBER WRITING

R 1__2__ 2___ 3___ 4___ 5__1__   R __3__ / __20__
L 1__2__ 2___ 3___ 4___ 5___   L __2__ / __20__

HALSTEAD'S NEUROPSYCHOLOGICAL TEST BATTERY

Category Test __69__

Tactual Performance Test
Dominant hand: __10.0 (1 block in)__
Non-dominant hand: __5.2__
Both hands: __7.6__

Total Time	22.8 (21 blocks in)
Memory	2
Localization	0

Seashore Rhythm Test
Number Correct __25__   __6__

Speech-sounds Perception Test
Number of Errors   __13__

Finger Oscillation Test
Dominant hand: __46__   __46__
Non-dominant hand: __42__

Impairment Index __1.0__

MINNESOTA MULTIPHASIC PERSONALITY INVENTORY

		Hs	49
		D	63
?	50	Hy	62
L	43	Pd	53
F	50	Mf	41
K	51	Pa	50
		Pt	58
		Sc	59
		Ma	40

REITAN-KLØVE LATERAL-DOMINANCE EXAM

Show me how you:
throw a ball	R
hammer a nail	R
cut with a knife	R
turn a door knob	R
use scissors	R
use an eraser	R
write your name	R

Record time used for spontaneous name-writing:
Preferred hand	__7__ seconds
Non-preferred hand	__14__ seconds

Show me how you:
kick a football	R
step on a bug	L

REITAN-INDIANA APHASIA SCREENING TEST

Form for Adults and Older Children

Name: _____ H. C. _____ Age: __53__

Copy SQUARE	Repeat TRIANGLE
Name SQUARE	Repeat MASSACHUSETTS "Massachuchetts"
Spell SQUARE	Repeat METHODIST EPISCOPAL
Copy CROSS	Write SQUARE

Name CROSS
   "It's not a cross. I don't know the
   name of it."
	Read SEVEN

Spell CROSS	Repeat SEVEN
Copy TRIANGLE	Repeat/Explain HE SHOUTED THE WARNING.
Name TRIANGLE "Pyramid"	Write HE SHOUTED THE WARNING.
Spell TRIANGLE	Compute 85 − 27 =

Name BABY
    "Nude baby − no, it has diapers
    on."
	Compute 17 X 3 =

Write CLOCK	Name KEY
Name FORK	Demonstrate use of KEY
Read 7 SIX 2	Draw KEY
Read MGW	Read PLACE LEFT HAND TO RIGHT EAR.
Reading I	Place LEFT HAND TO RIGHT EAR
Reading II	Place LEFT HAND TO LEFT ELBOW

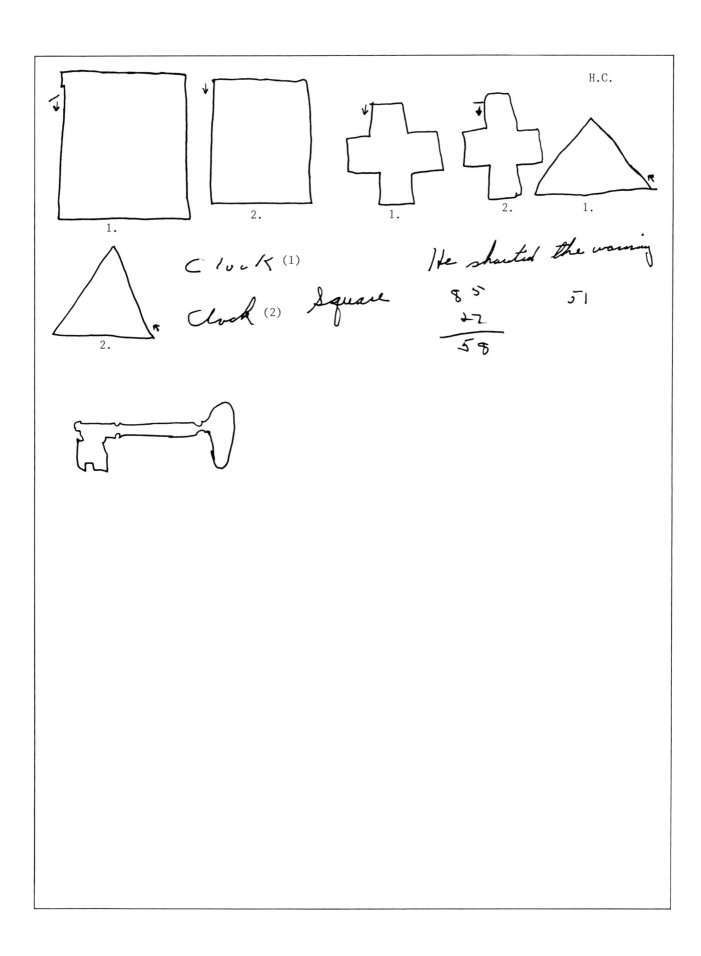

1.

2.

1.

2.

1.

2.

Clock (1)

Clock (2)   Square

He shouted the warning

8 5
2 2
---
5 8

5 1

to discover primary motor impairment in the neurological examination, but psychomotor deficit (impairment of motor problem-solving capabilities) is frequently overlooked on medical evaluation. In this instance there was a striking disparity between primary motor functions and adaptive problem-solving skills of a motoric nature.

The patient also had impairment of tactile form recognition abilities with his right hand as compared with his left and made one error perceiving a tactile stimulus to the right face. Although this finding fits the general pattern of results, a single mistake is not necessarily significant. The ptosis of the left eye precluded the test of bilateral simultaneous stimulation. Even though H.C. had a hearing loss involving the left ear, he had no difficulty perceiving bilateral simultaneous auditory stimulation.

The Aphasia Screening Test contributed additional valuable information, but we would not conclude from these mild deficits that the patient had definite dysphasia. When asked to name the CROSS, the patient responded, "It's not a cross. I don't know the name of it." It is likely that this response is not due to a visual form dysgnosia because the patient was able to recognize many other visual configurations without any particular difficulty. Even though he in effect named the figure by negating the name, the response probably represents a mild degree of impairment or uncertainty concerning the name of the figure.

When asked to name TRIANGLE, the patient said "pyramid." This response, which occasionally occurs among non-brain-damaged subjects and generally does not have pathognomonic significance, probably also indicates a mild tendency toward dysnomia in this particular case. Evidence of the patient's ability in visual form perception (evidence against visual form dysgnosia) was demonstrated by his observation that the baby was wearing diapers. Finally, H.C.'s enunciation of

MASSACHUSETTS included an error that is probably suggestive of left cerebral dysfunction: he inserted the "ch" sound for the "s" sound toward the end of the word. The above findings are not strong enough to classify the patient as dysphasic, but they do represent the types of disorders seen in persons with left cerebral damage.

It is not surprising that the neurosurgeon would fail to note any evidence of organic language dysfunction in this man. Elicitation of mild language difficulties of the type manifested by persons with left cerebral damage is dependent upon use of standardized stimulus material in which comparative observations have been made with many thousands of patients. In fact, H.C.'s responses on the Aphasia Screening Test are entirely consistent with observation of more serious organic language deficits shortly after the injury and almost certainly represent abnormalities, even though mild, of language capabilities due to cerebral damage.

We would even postulate that for this man the score of 13 errors on the Speech-sounds Perception Test indicated a mild degree of deficit in dealing with language symbols. Even though the patient's score was almost identical with the average for brain-damaged subjects, it must be remembered that the Speech-sounds Perception Test score correlates closely with Verbal IQ, and this patient should have performed somewhat better, considering the fact that his Verbal IQ exceeded about 77% of his age peers.

Thus, even though the indications of left cerebral damage were mild (except for the right-handed performances on the Tactual Performance Test and the Tactile Form Recognition Test), they were quite definite. No corresponding indications were present to implicate the right cerebral hemisphere. Although the drawings of figures were mildly deviant (especially the cross), we would not be able to conclude that they had any definite pathological significance.

In summary, H.C. showed significant generalized impairment of adaptive abilities dependent upon brain functions and specific indications of left cerebral damage. Considering the neuropsychological findings, it is not at all surprising that he was having difficulty resuming his pre-morbid occupational functions as a veterinarian. Even his impairment in reading the newspaper and professional journals would be expected in light of the evidence of mild difficulty in dealing with language symbols for communicational purposes. With such definite indications of impairment in the right upper extremity one would expect that H.C.'s efficiency in bimanual problem-solving tasks would be greatly reduced. In fact, when permitted to use both hands on the third trial of the Tactual Performance Test, the patient used his left hand almost exclusively.

However, the most significant deficits concerning overall efficiency of performance of both professional and everyday activities relates to the type of impairment shown on the general indicators (e.g., the Category Test, Part B of the Trail Making Test, and the Localization component of the Tactual Performance Test). H.C.'s difficulty on these general indicators is behaviorally reflected by a significant reduction in his general problem-solving capabilities, his inability to analyze problems very effectively, and an inflexibility in his thought processes that prevents him from balancing one aspect of a situation with another. Consequently, H.C. does not know where to begin to solve complex problems and as a result appears generally inefficient.

It is highly unlikely that an extended winter vacation would provide effective treatment for these types of problems. It is probable, however, that H.C. will show additional spontaneous improvement, since the injury was sustained only six weeks prior to this testing. The more effective approach to this man's rehabilitation would be to institute selected brain retraining procedures at the time when progress would be facilitated by spontaneous recovery. Although the REHABIT program had not been developed at the time this man was examined, he would have been an excellent candidate for brain training, beginning with Track C and gradually incorporating and integrating material from Tracks B and A. During the cognitive-retraining period we would recommend that H.C. return to his professional activities, but on a basis in which he was not stressing himself or expecting his work output (either in quality or quantity) to compare with his pre-morbid level.

We realize how difficult it is to effectively accomplish such a plan and are aware that it cannot be done merely by advising the patient to follow such recommendations. Continued counseling is necessary to give the patient an opportunity to ventilate his frustrations, failures, disappointments, and other emotional responses to his neuropsychological impairment. Such counseling sessions supplement the direct brain-retraining sessions by providing the patient with some insight into the realistic neuropsychological basis of his failures. In addition, counseling also creates the opportunity to identify and develop alternative mechanisms of adaptation to recurring problems. Finally, physical therapy, emphasizing a range of adaptive movements, would probably facilitate improvement of functional use of the right upper extremity. A therapeutic plan ("to take an extended winter vacation") based on limited understanding of the patient's deficits and ensuing problems is not an adequate answer and demonstrates a gross insensitivity to the patient's problems.

CASE #13

Name: B.B.

Age: 17 (Testing I)
            18 (Testing II)

Education: 11 (Testing I)
            12 (Testing II)

Sex: Female

Handedness: Left

Occupation: Student (Testing I)
            Receptionist (Testing II)

Background Information

B.B. was 16 years old when she suffered a severe head injury in an automobile accident. She had a vague recollection of another car approaching in the wrong lane and an impending head-on crash; her next memory was having the lacerations on her chin sutured in the County Hospital several hours after the accident.

The patient said that when she regained consciousness she felt light-headed and quite weak and had blurred vision that was not helped by her glasses. She was able to be out of bed 48 hours after the injury but remained in the hospital for seven days. The neurological examination at that time was within normal limits and she was given a diagnosis of cerebral concussion.

B.B.'s medical history was not remarkable. She reportedly suffered from occasional migraine headaches prior to the injury but had not experienced any such headaches for some time. She had two younger siblings, both of whom were in good health.

The patient continued to experience light-headed episodes and blurred vision after being discharged from the hospital. Although her vision cleared within a few weeks, B.B. did not feel that she was able to read normally for approximately five months. She did not experience the type of migraine headaches that she had previously, but

did have occasional headaches which seemed to start in the occipital region and, in a generalized fashion, progressed to the frontal areas. These headaches, which usually lasted two to three days, were not accompanied by nausea, vomiting, or dizziness.

This young woman had been approximately a "B" student in high school but after the head injury her grades dropped to a "D" average; she did so poorly in algebra that she was forced to drop the course and was not able to catch up in shorthand. The patient's mother reported that her daughter did not seem to concentrate as well as she did before the accident and was not able to make decisions and follow through with activities. Her family said that after the injury B.B. had become very difficult to get along with and seemed to project her emotional distress onto others. When she became angry she would accuse her parents and siblings of various activities that had no factual basis.

About 7½ months after the injury this young woman unsuccessfully attempted to commit suicide by taking an overdose of aspirin. She became ill and was absent from school two days, then was able to return to classes. Even after the school year finished the situation seemed to be showing no improvement and approximately 10 months after the injury the patient and her parents decided to seek medical help.

Neurological Examination

The neurological and physical examinations were within normal limits. An EEG showed diffuse abnormality with bilateral slowing most evident in the temporal regions. There was no sharp or spike wave activity. A radionuclide brain scan was normal. Although the EEG abnormality may have been caused by brain damage, the neurological evaluation did not reveal any condition which could be treated medically and it was at this point that the patient was referred for neuropsychological examination.

Neuropsychological Examination

When asked about the nature of her problem this young woman reported that she had been in an automobile accident approximately 11 months earlier and was unconscious for about 45 minutes. She said that at present she was having dizzy spells, some trouble in school, and did not seem to be her usual self. On the Cornell Medical Index Health Questionnaire she indicated a number of somatic complaints, including bad spells of sneezing; a continually stuffed up nose; frequent heavy chest colds that usually kept her miserable all winter; attacks of hayfever and asthma; pains in the heart or chest area; cold hands and feet even in hot weather; frequent spells of severe dizziness; episodes of fainting; twitching of the face, head or shoulders; great difficulty in sleeping; and spells of complete exhaustion or fatigue.

She also had a number of emotional problems, including great apprehension during examinations; feeling nervous and shaky when approached by a superior; finding that her work deteriorated when she was closely observed; always getting directions and orders wrong; having to do things very slowly in order to avoid mistakes; having great difficulty making up her mind and wishing she always had someone at her side to advise her; being a touchy person whose feelings are easily hurt and who is always upset by criticism; usually being misunderstood by others and having to be on guard even with friends; doing things on sudden impulse; easily becoming upset and irritated; becoming angry whenever anyone tells her what to do; often feeling annoyed and irritated by people; flaring up in anger if not permitted to do what she wants to do right away; jumping or shaking badly with sudden noises; often becoming suddenly scared for no reason; and trembling or feeling weak when others shout at her.

These responses suggested that the patient felt apprehensive, anxious, and unsure of herself. Because we had been advised by the National Institutes of Health to refrain from giving the test to minors for research purposes we did not administer the Minnesota Multiphasic Personality Inventory. However, results on the Cornell Medical Index Health Questionnaire certainly suggest that an evaluation of her emotional status would have been advisable.

The patient earned a Verbal IQ (100) exactly at the Average level and a Performance IQ 18 points lower (82) in the Low Average range, exceeding only 11% of her age peers. The Full Scale IQ (91) was in the lower part of the Average range, exceeding 27%.

B.B. showed a considerable degree of variability among the Verbal subtest scores; Digit Span (3) was quite low and the other scores were almost at the average level or above. Although Digit Span has been shown to be the only subtest in the Wechsler Scale that does not show a significant difference between groups with and without cerebral damage (Reitan, 1959a), the particularly low score in this instance probably does have some significance. Considering the scores on the Seashore Rhythm Test (29 correct) and Speech-sounds Perception Test (4), it would hardly seem that the low score on Digit Span is attributable to an inability to attend to immediate stimulus material.

Except for Digit Symbol, the patient performed worse on the Performance subtests than the Verbal

THE HALSTEAD-REITAN
NEUROPSYCHOLOGICAL TEST BATTERY

Patient __B.B.(I)__ Age __17__ Sex __F__ Education __11__ Handedness __L__

WECHSLER-BELLEVUE SCALE

VIQ	100
PIQ	82
FS IQ	91

Information	12
Comprehension	11
Digit Span	3
Arithmetic	9
Similarities	12
Vocabulary	10

Picture Arrangement	5
Picture Completion	6
Block Design	8
Object Assembly	7
Digit Symbol	13

TRAIL MAKING TEST

Part A: __21__ seconds
Part B: __62__ seconds

STRENGTH OF GRIP

Dominant hand: __16__ kilograms

Non-dominant hand: __19__ kilograms

REITAN-KLØVE TACTILE FORM RECOGNITION TEST

Dominant hand: __9__ seconds; __0__ errors

Non-dominant hand: __8__ seconds; __0__ errors

HALSTEAD'S NEUROPSYCHOLOGICAL TEST BATTERY

Category Test		67

Tactual Performance Test

Dominant hand:	3.9	
Non-dominant hand:	2.8	
Both hands:	2.0	
	Total Time	8.7
	Memory	7
	Localization	6

Seashore Rhythm Test

Number Correct	29	1

Speech-sounds Perception Test

Number of Errors		4

Finger Oscillation Test

Dominant hand:	44	44
Non-dominant hand:	42	

Impairment Index __0.3__

REITAN-KLØVE
LATERAL-DOMINANCE EXAM

Show me how you:

throw a ball	R
hammer a nail	L
cut with a knife	L
turn a door knob	R
use scissors	L
use an eraser	L
write your name	L

Record time used for spontaneous name-writing:

Preferred hand	8 seconds
Non-preferred hand	16 seconds

Show me how you:

kick a football	L
step on a bug	L

REITAN-KLØVE SENSORY-PERCEPTUAL EXAM — **No errors**

Error Totals

RH___LH ___	Both H:	RH___LH ___	RH___LH ___
RH___LF ___	Both H/F:	RH___LF ___	RH___LF ___
LH___RF ___	Both H/F:	LH___RF ___	RF___LH ___
RE___LE ___	Both E:	RE___LE ___	RE___LE ___
RV___LV ___	Both	RV___LV ___	RV___LV ___

TACTILE FINGER RECOGNITION

R 1___ 2___ 3___ 4___ 5___ R __0__ / __20__

L 1___ 2___ 3___ 4___ 5___ L __0__ / __20__

FINGER-TIP NUMBER WRITING

R 1__1__ 2___ 3___ 4___ 5___ R __1__ / __20__

L 1___ 2___ 3___ 4___ 5___ L __0__ / __20__

REITAN-INDIANA APHASIA SCREENING TEST

Form for Adults and Older Children

Name: _____ B. B. (I) _____ Age: __17__

Copy SQUARE	Repeat TRIANGLE
Name SQUARE	Repeat MASSACHUSETTS
Spell SQUARE	Repeat METHODIST EPISCOPAL
Copy CROSS	Write SQUARE
Name CROSS	Read SEVEN
Spell CROSS	Repeat SEVEN
Copy TRIANGLE	Repeat/Explain HE SHOUTED THE WARNING.
Name TRIANGLE	Write HE SHOUTED THE WARNING.
Spell TRIANGLE	Compute 85 – 27 =
Name BABY	Compute 17 X 3 = "41." Examiner gave 12 x 5, and patient responded correctly.
Write CLOCK	Name KEY
Name FORK	Demonstrate use of KEY
Read 7 SIX 2	Draw KEY
Read MGW	Read PLACE LEFT HAND TO RIGHT EAR.
Reading I	Place LEFT HAND TO RIGHT EAR
Reading II	Place LEFT HAND TO LEFT ELBOW

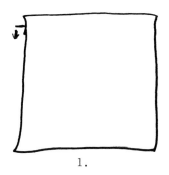

1.

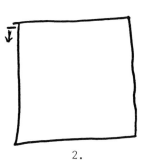

2.

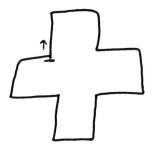

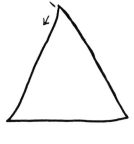

clock

square

He shouted the warning

$$\begin{array}{r} \overset{7}{8}5 \\ -27 \\ \hline 58 \end{array}$$ 41   60
         (17 x 3) (12 x 5)

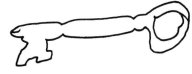

subtests. Her quickness and alertness in performing the Digit Symbol subtest is an unusual finding for a person with cerebral damage. Nevertheless, the relatively low scores on the other Performance subtests may have some significance with respect to impaired brain functions.

The four most sensitive indicators in the HRNTB yielded variable results. The Impairment Index of 0.3 was within the normal range, but it should be noted that the Category Test score (67) contributed to the Impairment Index and actually was worse than the average score for brain-damaged subjects. The other score contributing to the Impairment Index was finger tapping speed with the dominant hand (44) but we would not attribute much significance to this score. (It has been demonstrated that women tap somewhat more slowly than men.) The patient performed relatively well on Part B of the Trail Making Test (62 sec) and the Localization component of the Tactual Performance Test (6). Thus, the four most sensitive indicators clearly suggest that B.B. is neither grossly nor seriously impaired in terms of her basic adaptive abilities.

Although lateralizing indicators were not striking, certain findings were sufficient to suggest mild right cerebral damage. Since B.B. was left-handed, we would expect better performances in grip strength and finger tapping speed with the left hand than the right. She was only slightly better in finger tapping speed with the left hand (44) than the right (42), a finding suggesting a very mild deficit with the left hand. In the measure of grip strength the results were more definite. The patient should have had a greater grip strength in her left hand than her right; however, she measured 16 kg (left) compared with 19 kg (right).

It must be recognized that the Finger Oscillation Test and the Strength of Grip Measurement results relate strictly to motor functions (primary speed and strength); therefore, they can readily be affected by peripheral damage. Poor performances on these measures may (but not necessarily) indicate cerebral dysfunction.

Note, however, that this patient showed mild difficulties in drawing simple spatial configurations in addition to her poor performances on Grip Strength and Finger Tapping. Careful inspection of her drawing of the square indicates that she started on the left side, drawing a vertical line downward. She drew the second line somewhat too far to the right and was forced to continue within the framework that had been established which caused a closure problem when she was ready to complete the figure. Even though the lateral extremities were slightly out of balance, the drawing of the cross was within normal limits and on the basis of this drawing it would be difficult to conclude that the patient had sustained right cerebral damage. However, the drawing of the key provided mild but fairly definite evidence of impairment. B.B. had difficulty achieving symmetry in the teeth of the key and made an error with respect to size in her initial attempt to draw the nose. Thus, even though only very mildly deviant, her drawings appear to represent brain-related deficits.

These indications of mild right cerebral hemisphere impairment, based on specific signs as well as comparisons of performances on the two sides of the body, further validate the significance of the difference between the Verbal and Performance IQ values. In the total context of her test results we can be fairly confident in saying that this young woman has experienced a degree of impairment of Performance intelligence. In summary, the overall findings indicate impairment of right cerebral function with no comparable evidence present to implicate the left cerebral hemisphere.

The remainder of the test results essentially fall within normal limits. B.B. clearly had the ability to pay close and continuing attention to specific stimulus material (demonstrated by her scores on the Seashore Rhythm Test and Speech-sounds Perception Test) and performed very well when she understood exactly what she was supposed to do.

Conversely, her poorest score was on the Category Test, a task that required her to define the nature of the problem before she could proceed with its solution.

Persons who have good basic abilities but who tend to become confused and bewildered when trying to analyze and define complex situations frequently find that their intact abilities are relatively useless when they are faced with new or difficult situations. Understandably, circumstances of this kind tend to generate a certain degree of anxiety. The pattern of deficits shown by this woman, even though quite mild in nature, are consistent with residual effects of a closed head injury as well as the emotional problems that had been reported.

It should be recalled that this patient sustained her brain injury nearly 10 months before the present examination; therefore, it would be likely that a considerable amount of spontaneous recovery would have occurred by this time. However, in such instances it must also be remembered that residual deficits imply that considerably more serious impairment existed during the period shortly after the injury. It is probable that this woman had to fight her way back confronted with deficits that were considerably more pronounced than represented by the present test findings. Even when spontaneous recovery occurs, such deficits can cause serious problems and are quite threatening and disturbing to the patient.

Over and beyond these considerations, some individuals show a definite tendency toward exacerbation of pre-existing emotional problems after sustaining a head injury. Aita and Reitan (1948) reviewed the cases of approximately 500 brain-injured soldiers and found four who had developed "post-traumatic psychotic behavior." However, when these four cases were investigated thoroughly regarding their pre-injury psychiatric status, each patient was found to have significant and serious problems that pre-dated the head injury and were only exacerbated (rather than caused) by the cerebral trauma. There appears to be a basic mechanism, which operates more definitely in some cases than others, that elicits pre-existing tendencies toward emotional abnormalities as a result of cranio-cerebral trauma.

Returning to the present case, B.B. went on to finish high school and found a job as a receptionist-typist at a small local college. She performed this work satisfactorily for a period of nearly one and one-half years, although she admitted that she had "emotional problems" and was taking a "nerve pill" every four hours.

One day B.B. had a sudden onset of numbness on the left side of her body that lasted for several minutes. She gradually regained a normal feeling, but felt that her perception was not quite the same as it had been. Within about an hour she noticed a similar but somewhat milder sensation of numbness involving her right side. These episodes frightened her and she went to see her physician who in turn referred her to a medical center for an evaluation.

About three weeks elapsed before B.B. arranged an appointment at the medical center; the episodes of numbness occurred just before Christmas and she was reluctant to interrupt the holiday season. Her physician at the medical center reported that the neurological examination was entirely within normal limits and B.B. was referred for neuropsychological evaluation to determine whether any evidence of progressive cerebral damage was present.

Considering that (1) B.B.'s initial neuropsychological deficits were a result of head trauma; (2) most patients show some progressive degree of recovery in time; and (3) the initial set of test results (obtained nearly 18 months earlier) had reflected a relatively chronic, static condition of the brain, one would not expect this woman to show any very striking improvement. In fact, some patients who have sustained head injury show neuropsychological regression in certain respects, possibly correlated with such factors as the development of epileptic foci. In this case the patient may have experienced some type of sensory fit, although it is also possible that her behavioral manifestation was related to her emotional stresses.

This time on the Cornell Medical Index Health Questionnaire B.B. indicated that she suffers from hayfever and asthma; gets out of breath long before anyone else; has cold hands and feet even in hot weather; suffers from frequent cramps in her legs; has a poor appetite; gulps her food and usually feels bloated after eating; has hot or cold spells; has spells of severe dizziness; frequently feels faint; has numbness or tingling in her body as well as twitching of the face, head and shoulders; usually gets up tired and exhausted in the morning; and often gets spells of complete exhaustion or fatigue.

The patient again answered positively to many questions that related to emotional aspects of adjustment, with essentially identical responses to those given initially. However, at the present time she also indicated that she must constantly attempt to control herself in order to avoid going to pieces.

Neuropsychological Evaluation

Upon re-administration of the Wechsler-Bellevue Scale B.B. earned a Verbal IQ (110) in the lower limit of the High Average range (exceeding about 75% of her age peers), a Performance IQ (87) that was 23 points lower, in the Low Average range (exceeding 19%), and a Full Scale IQ (99) nearly exactly at the Average level (exceeding 47%).

The distribution of Verbal subtest scores showed that the patient performed above the average level on most of the subtests, with relatively poor scores occurring only on Digit Span (7) and Arithmetic (6). It is apparent from these values that in the past B.B. had an opportunity to develop normal intellectual capabilities.

Except for Digit Symbol (11) the Performance subtests were consistently below the average level. Although some individuals normally show a disparity of this magnitude between Verbal and Performance scores, in this case one could readily

raise a hypothesis of some impairment of Performance intelligence.

The patient performed relatively well on the four indicators most sensitive to brain damage; only the Category score (53) was in the impaired range. Thus, it would appear that her general level of ability is fairly adequate.

Some of the lateralizing scores suggested impairment of the right cerebral hemisphere. Taking into account that this woman was left-handed, she performed quite poorly with her left hand (10.4 min) compared with her right (2.7 min) on the Tactual Performance Test, was scarcely any faster with her left hand (46) than her right (45) in finger tapping speed, had less grip strength in her left upper extremity (17.0 kg) than her right (20.5 kg), and made three mistakes in finger-tip number writing perception on her left hand but no mistakes on her right hand.

The consistency and magnitude of these findings are sufficient to postulate some impairment of the right cerebral hemisphere. The nature of the findings focuses particularly on motor and tactile-perceptual deficits. B.B.'s excellent scores when using her right hand (2.7 min) and both hands (1.3 min) on the Tactual Performance Test demonstrate that she is not generally impaired in the higher-level requirements of the test. The poor score with the left hand (10.4 min) on the TPT, as well as the deficient performances on finger tapping, grip strength, and finger-tip number writing perception, are probably reflections of primary motor and/or tactile-perceptual dysfunction. The overall results would therefore suggest a focal lesion in the right posterior frontal and parietal areas which is chronic and static in nature, not causing serious generalized disruption of cerebral functions (judging from the good scores on most of the tests), and possibly epileptogenic.

The patient's drawings were not grossly defective, although one could question the first drawing

THE HALSTEAD-REITAN
NEUROPSYCHOLOGICAL TEST BATTERY

Patient **B.B. (II)** Age **18** Sex **F** Education **12** Handedness **L**

WECHSLER-BELLEVUE SCALE

VIQ	110
PIQ	87
FS IQ	99
Information	12
Comprehension	14
Digit Span	7
Arithmetic	6
Similarities	16
Vocabulary	11
Picture Arrangement	7
Picture Completion	8
Block Design	9
Object Assembly	7
Digit Symbol	11

TRAIL MAKING TEST

Part A: **24** seconds
Part B: **65** seconds

STRENGTH OF GRIP

Dominant hand: **17.0** kilograms
Non-dominant hand: **20.5** kilograms

REITAN-KLØVE TACTILE FORM RECOGNITION TEST

Dominant hand: **12** seconds; **0** errors
Non-dominant hand: **10** seconds; **0** errors

REITAN-KLØVE SENSORY-PERCEPTUAL EXAM — No errors

			Error Totals	
RH___ LH___	Both H:	RH___ LH___	RH___ LH___	
RH___ LF___	Both H/F:	RH___ LF___	RH___ LF___	
LH___ RF___	Both H/F:	LH___ RF___	RF___ LH___	
RE___ LE___	Both E:	RE___ LE___	RE___ LE___	
RV___ LV___	Both:	RV___ LV___	RV___ LV___	
___ ___		___ ___		
___ ___		___ ___		

TACTILE FINGER RECOGNITION

R 1___ 2___ 3___ 4___ 5___ R **0** / **20**
L 1___ 2___ 3___ 4___ 5___ L **0** / **20**

FINGER-TIP NUMBER WRITING

R 1___ 2___ 3___ 4___ 5___ R **0** / **20**
L 1 **2** 2 ___ 3 **1** 4 ___ 5___ L **3** / **20**

HALSTEAD'S NEUROPSYCHOLOGICAL TEST BATTERY

Category Test   53

Tactual Performance Test

Dominant hand: **10.4**
Non-dominant hand: **2.7**
Both hands: **1.3**

Total Time	14.4
Memory	8
Localization	6

Seashore Rhythm Test

Number Correct **26**   5

Speech-sounds Perception Test

Number of Errors   2

Finger Oscillation Test

Dominant hand: **46**   46
Non-dominant hand: **45**

Impairment Index   0.3

MINNESOTA MULTIPHASIC PERSONALITY INVENTORY

		Hs	58
		D	46
?	50	Hy	64
L	43	Pd	81
F	60	Mf	38
K	48	Pa	70
		Pt	55
		Sc	61
		Ma	73

REITAN-KLØVE LATERAL-DOMINANCE EXAM

Show me how you:

throw a ball	R
hammer a nail	L
cut with a knife	L
turn a door knob	R
use scissors	L
use an eraser	L
write your name	L

Record time used for spontaneous name-writing:

Preferred hand	**8** seconds
Non-preferred hand	**16** seconds

Show me how you:

kick a football	L
step on a bug	L

REITAN-INDIANA APHASIA SCREENING TEST

Form for Adults and Older Children

Name: _____ B. B. (II) _____ Age: __18__

Copy SQUARE	Repeat TRIANGLE
Name SQUARE	Repeat MASSACHUSETTS
Spell SQUARE	Repeat METHODIST EPISCOPAL
Copy CROSS	Write SQUARE
Name CROSS	Read SEVEN
Spell CROSS	Repeat SEVEN
Copy TRIANGLE	Repeat/Explain HE SHOUTED THE WARNING.
Name TRIANGLE	Write HE SHOUTED THE WARNING.
Spell TRIANGLE	Compute 85 – 27 =
Name BABY	Compute 17 X 3 = "41"; self corrected.
Write CLOCK	Name KEY
Name FORK	Demonstrate use of KEY
Read 7 SIX 2	Draw KEY
Read MGW	Read PLACE LEFT HAND TO RIGHT EAR.
Reading I	Place LEFT HAND TO RIGHT EAR
Reading II	Place LEFT HAND TO LEFT ELBOW

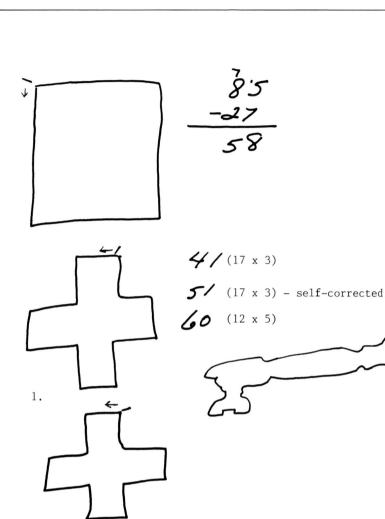

$$\begin{array}{r} \overset{7}{8}5 \\ -27 \\ \hline 58 \end{array}$$

41 (17 x 3)

51 (17 x 3) – self-corrected

60 (12 x 5)

1.

2.

1.

2.

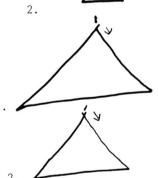

grandfather clock

square

We shouted the warning

of the cross (because of disparity of the lateral extremities) and the generally disproportional drawing of the key. However, it would be difficult to be confident that these drawings are a specific reflection of right cerebral damage.

The results on the Minnesota Multiphasic Personality Inventory show a pattern of deviant scores suggesting significant difficulties in relationships with others as well as in behavior more generally. The most common MMPI pattern among brain-damaged subjects is elevation of the first three clinical scales (Hypochondriasis, Depression, and Hysteria) and this patient does not show this particular pattern. It is likely that B.B. believes that she has been treated unfairly, has some feelings of hostility, and may demonstrate impulsive tendencies. Considering the relatively mild indications of impairment of her cognitive ability structure, it would be difficult to say that her emotional problems are directly related to the brain injury.

Comparison of the patient's performances on the two neuropsychological examinations indicates that she gained ten points in Verbal IQ and five points in Performance IQ values. The same general pattern of results on the Wechsler Scale was present initially, although on the second examination the scores for individual subtests were generally a little higher. Obviously, part of this improvement may be due to positive practice-effect but it is also likely that the patient has shown some genuine improvement as well. She also performed a little better on the Category Test, but it is not uncommon to see a substantial degree of positive practice-effect on this test and we could not be confident that the improved score represents a genuine improvement. Many of the other test results show very minimal gains, but the general patterns of relationships, both among various tests and in terms of lateralized deviations, were maintained.

Note, though that the performance with the left hand (first trial) on the Tactual Performance Test was much worse on the second examination.

The patient also had significant difficulty in fingertip number writing perception with the left hand compared with the right, a finding that was not present on the initial testing. These two factors, combined with the continuing pattern of left-sided impairment in finger tapping speed and grip strength, created a more striking set of indications pointing toward focal involvement in the middle part of the right cerebral hemisphere.

It would seem possible that the patient may have developed an epileptogenic lesion by the time of the second examination and her clinical complaints had some validity in this regard. The practical implications of the second set of findings would relate to recommending that additional effort be made to determine the presence of a developing epilepsy as well as appropriate treatment. Because the initial set of neuropsychological findings suggested that the patient's condition was relatively stabilized (consistent with history information that the injury had occurred nearly 10 months before testing) we did not expect to see any substantial improvement in level of performance on the second examination and this hypothesis was essentially confirmed by the neuropsychological test results.

CASE #14

Name: R.H.

Age: 38

Education: 9

Sex: Male

Handedness: Right

Occupation: Fireman

Background Information

R.H. sustained a severe concussion at the age of 23 (15 years before the present neuropsychological examination). During military combat the blast of an artillery shell threw him across a road 30 feet wide; he remained unconscious for several hours and was stunned and confused upon awakening. Medical examination at that time showed no objective evidence of neurological deficits. From this accident R.H. also sustained a bullet wound of his right arm that caused both nerve and muscle damage and residual weakness and numbness. Aside from these injuries the patient had no history of illnesses or events likely to have caused nervous system damage.

R.H. was discharged from military service less than one year following the artillery blast. Within a few months he began to have episodes in which he would become nauseated and dizzy and have diplopia and blurred vision in the right eye. These episodes, which lasted about 30 seconds, occurred every three to four months. Although R.H. had a "strange" feeling, these episodes lasted only a short time and he was able to ignore them.

Over the years these attacks increased in frequency, occurring four to five times a day, and seemed to be growing more severe. At this time the patient sought medical attention and was admitted to a major medical center for a complete neurological evaluation.

Neurological Examination

Physical and neurological examinations documented obvious damage and mild deformation of the right arm as a result of the earlier bullet wound and an area of hypesthesia and hypalgesia in the distribution of the ulnar nerve. Two electroencephalograms were done; one was within normal limits and the other showed definite dysrhythmia in the right temporal area, suggesting an epileptogenic focus. A pneumoencephalogram and bilateral cerebral angiograms were within normal limits. R.H. was placed on antiepileptic medications and the attacks (now classified as complex partial epilepsy) were less severe and reduced in frequency to about one per day. Neuropsychological examination was done during this hospitalization.

About seven months after he was discharged from the hospital the patient decided to go on a regimen of vitamins and dietary supplementation. His seizures promptly increased to five to six per day and on one occasion the patient experienced a partial motor seizure which spread to involve adjacent muscles (Jacksonian epilepsy). The seizure began in the patient's left upper extremity and rendered him unconscious for about 15 to 20 minutes. Following this episode R.H. returned for neurological consultation. He was again placed on antiepileptic medications and his seizures quickly decreased to about one mild, brief episode a day.

This sequence of events strongly suggested that the blast concussion sustained 15 years ago had caused the development of complex partial epilepsy with particular involvement of the right cerebral hemisphere. Kløve and Matthews (1969) have shown that patients with complex partial epilepsy generally show milder neuropsychological deficits than persons with other categories of epilepsy.

As noted, neurological examination at the time of admission revealed a mild degree of bilateral hearing loss, weakness of the right biceps femoris that was particularly expressed in the fourth and fifth fingers of the right hand, and hypesthesia and hypalgesia of the medial and dorsal aspects of the right arm. The findings involving the right upper extremity were almost certainly related to the bullet wound sustained 15 years before the current examination.

Neuropsychological Examination

Despite the fact that he had been working quite satisfactorily as a city fireman for several years, R.H.'s history strongly suggested that he would demonstrate some generalized impairment of neuropsychological functions. Some findings implicating the right cerebral hemisphere might be expected, considering the evidence for an epileptogenic focus in the right cerebral hemisphere (and especially the occurrence of a Jacksonian seizure that began in the left upper extremity).

However, it should be remembered that the types of brain disorders which cause epilepsy are basically electrophysiologic and neuropsychological findings correlate more closely with structural damage than electrical abnormalities. Thus, although it would not be possible to predict confidently that specific evidence of right cerebral damage would emerge in the neuropsychological data, the test results should reflect some weakness in the right upper extremity associated with the bullet wound sustained 15 years earlier. The hypesthesia and hypalgesia might also produce tactile-perceptual deficits of the right hand.

Since the initial injury occurred approximately 15 years before neuropsychological testing we certainly would not expect to find evidence of an acutely destructive or rapidly progressive focal lesion of either cerebral hemisphere. In summary, we would predict (1) mild generalized impairment; (2) possible indicators of right cerebral hemisphere dysfunction; and (3) some deficits involving the right upper extremity caused by peripheral damage.

The patient had very few complaints on the Cornell Medical Index Health Questionnaire. He indicated that pressure or pain in his head often makes life miserable, he has hot or cold spells, and experiences constant numbness or tingling in parts of his body. He denied any other problems. However, results on the Minnesota Multiphasic Personality Inventory were distinctly elevated on the Hypochondriasis and Hysteria scales, yielding a definite Conversion V configuration.

The patient earned a Verbal IQ (107) in the upper part of the Average range (exceeding about 68% of his age peers) and a Performance IQ (112) a few points higher, in the lower part of the High Average range (exceeding about 79%). R.H. had a very low score (4) on Digit Span, but this is not uncommon in hospitalized patients. The low score (5) on Digit Symbol, however, would certainly raise a question about impairment of brain functions (unless motor impairment of the right upper extremity were responsible). One might also be concerned about a score of 9 on Picture Arrangement in the context of the other Performance subtest scores; it might suggest right temporal lobe dysfunction.

Results on the four most sensitive indicators in the HRNTB yielded evidence of generalized neuropsychological deficit. The patient earned an Impairment Index of 0.7, with only the scores on the Speech-sounds Perception Test (7) and the Memory component of the Tactual Performance Test (7) being in the normal range. The score on the Category Test (75) was considerably worse than

THE HALSTEAD-REITAN
NEUROPSYCHOLOGICAL TEST BATTERY

Patient **R.H.** Age **38** Sex **M** Education **9** Handedness **R**

WECHSLER-BELLEVUE SCALE

VIQ	107
PIQ	112
FS IQ	110

Information	11
Comprehension	14
Digit Span	4
Arithmetic	12
Similarities	11
Vocabulary	11

Picture Arrangement	9
Picture Completion	14
Block Design	11
Object Assembly	13
Digit Symbol	5

TRAIL MAKING TEST

Part A: **30** seconds
Part B: **87** seconds

STRENGTH OF GRIP

Dominant hand: **38.0** kilograms
Non-dominant hand: **46.5** kilograms

REITAN-KLØVE TACTILE FORM RECOGNITION TEST

Dominant hand: **10** seconds; **0** errors
Non-dominant hand: **8** seconds; **0** errors

REITAN-KLØVE SENSORY-PERCEPTUAL EXAM — No errors

			Error Totals	
RH ___ LH ___	Both H:	RH ___ LH ___	RH ___ LH ___	
RH ___ LH ___	Both H:	RH ___ LH ___	RH ___ LH ___	
LH ___ LH ___	Both H:	RH ___ LH ___	RH ___ LH ___	
RE ___ LH ___	Both H:	RH ___ LH ___	RH ___ LH ___	
RV ___ LV ___	Both:	RV ___ LV ___	RV ___ LV ___	

TACTILE FINGER RECOGNITION

R 1___ 2___ 3___ 4___ 5___   R **0** / 20

L 1___ 2___ 3___ 4___ 5___   L **0** / 20

FINGER-TIP NUMBER WRITING

R 1 **1** 2___ 3___ 4___ 5___   R **1** / 20

L 1___ 2___ 3___ 4___ 5___   L **0** / 20

HALSTEAD'S NEUROPSYCHOLOGICAL TEST BATTERY

Category Test 75

Tactual Performance Test

Dominant hand:	**6.4**	
Non-dominant hand:	**9.0**	
Both hands:	**4.8**	

Total Time	20.2
Memory	7
Localization	3

Seashore Rhythm Test

Number Correct **22** 10

Speech-sounds Perception Test

Number of Errors 7

Finger Oscillation Test

Dominant hand:	49	49
Non-dominant hand:	45	

Impairment Index 0.7

MINNESOTA MULTIPHASIC PERSONALITY INVENTORY

		Hs	77
		D	53
?	50	Hy	71
L	66	Pd	62
F	50	Mf	49
K	70	Pa	50
		Pt	52
		Sc	59
		Ma	50

REITAN-KLØVE LATERAL-DOMINANCE EXAM

Show me how you:

throw a ball	**R**
hammer a nail	**R**
cut with a knife	**R**
turn a door knob	**R**
use scissors	**R**
use an eraser	**R**
write your name	**R**

Record time used for spontaneous name-writing:

Preferred hand	**10** seconds
Non-preferred hand	**29** seconds

Show me how you:

kick a football	**R**
step on a bug	**R**

REITAN-INDIANA APHASIA SCREENING TEST

Form for Adults and Older Children

Name: _____ R. H. _____ Age: __38__

Copy SQUARE	Repeat TRIANGLE
Name SQUARE	Repeat MASSACHUSETTS
Spell SQUARE "S–Q–U–A–R"	Repeat METHODIST EPISCOPAL
Copy CROSS	Write SQUARE
Name CROSS	Read SEVEN
Spell CROSS	Repeat SEVEN
Copy TRIANGLE	Repeat/Explain HE SHOUTED THE WARNING.
Name TRIANGLE	Write HE SHOUTED THE WARNING.
Spell TRIANGLE "T–R–Y–A–N–G–L–E"	Compute 85 – 27 =
Name BABY	Compute 17 X 3 =
Write CLOCK	Name KEY
Name FORK	Demonstrate use of KEY
Read 7 SIX 2	Draw KEY
Read MGW	Read PLACE LEFT HAND TO RIGHT EAR.
Reading I	Place LEFT HAND TO RIGHT EAR
Reading II	Place LEFT HAND TO LEFT ELBOW

R.H.

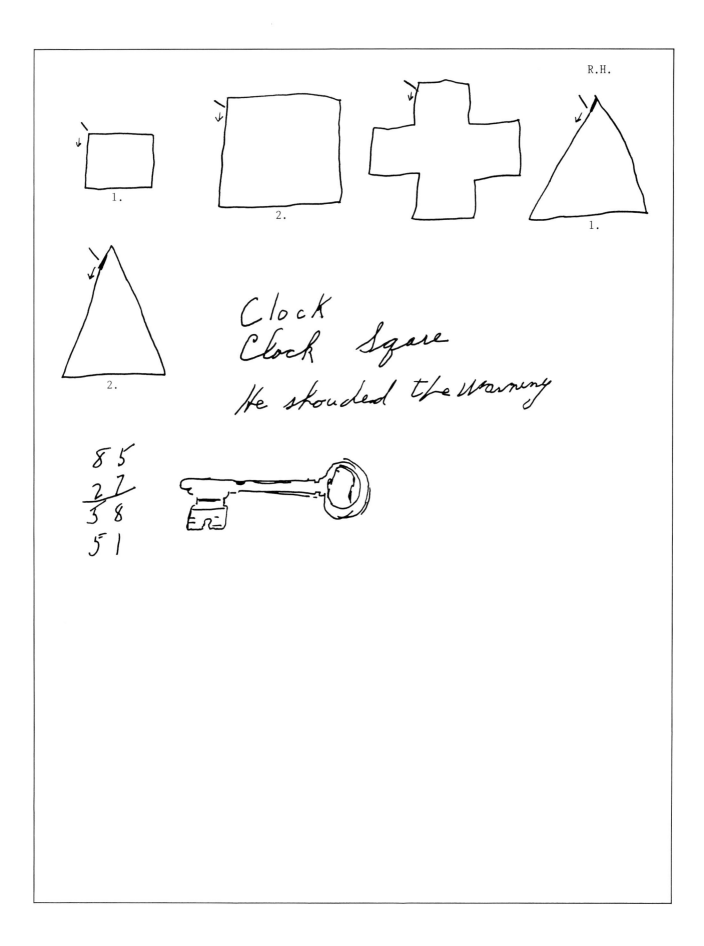

1.

2.

1.

2.

Clock
Clock Sqare

He shouded the Worning

8 5
2 7
3 8
5 1

that of the average brain-damaged patient. R.H. was within the normal range on Part B of the Trail Making Test (87 sec) but, in light of the IQ values, even this score must be considered suggestive of mild cerebral dysfunction. Thus, based on the scores on brain-sensitive tests, there is little doubt that this man had at least mild impairment of adaptive abilities and this impression was reinforced by his relatively good IQ values (Reitan, 1985).

Lateralizing signs were not pronounced. The patient showed no imperception of bilateral simultaneous sensory stimuli and was able to do the tests for tactile finger localization and finger-tip number writing perception almost entirely without error. The examiner noted that more pressure was required on the fingers on the right hand (corresponding with the neurological findings of hypalgesia and hypesthesia), but when sufficient pressure was used so that the patient could feel the stimulus being applied, he showed no signs of cerebral cortical difficulties. In other words, the test results clearly indicate peripheral tactile impairment but the cortical requirement of the tasks, relating to differential judgments of the stimulus material, was unimpaired.

R.H. did, however, have a distinctly reduced grip strength in his right upper extremity (38.0 kg) compared with his left (46.5 kg). The Tactual Performance Test demonstrated distinct impairment of the left upper extremity compared with the right. The patient's right-handed performance (first trial) was essentially within the normal range (6.4 min); however, R.H. required significantly more time (9.0 min) on the second trial (left hand). In all probability this was a valid reflection of the

right cerebral hemisphere being more impaired than the left, even though there were no additional specific indicators. The patient's drawings were within normal limits.

Impaired grip strength with the right upper extremity was the only indicator of left cerebral damage. (Note that the Speech-sounds Perception Test score [7] was quite adequate.) The Aphasia Test demonstrated some spelling deficiencies, but they were quite typical for persons with relatively inadequate educational backgrounds. The patient omitted the "E" in spelling SQUARE, and used a "Y" instead of an "I" in spelling TRIANGLE, and a "D" instead of a "T" in writing SHOUTED.

The above-mentioned errors are not sufficient by themselves to implicate the left cerebral hemisphere but a somewhat more suspicious result occurred when the patient attempted to write SQUARE while looking at the printed stimulus. He omitted the "U," and even among poorly educated people this mistake is unusual when the printed letters are immediately available as an illustration. This latter finding could be a valid indication of impaired ability to deal with language symbols, but it would be difficult to draw such a conclusion confidently from this minimal evidence alone.

In summary, the findings were essentially in line with expectation considering the nature of the injury, the evidence of complex partial epilepsy, and the duration of time that had elapsed since the injury. It should be noted that even if the MMPI's suggestion of conversion tendencies is correct, it certainly is not a basis for ruling out mild impairment of brain functions in this man.

CASE #15

Name: C.L.

Age: 33

Education: 20

Sex: Male

Handedness: Right

Occupation: University Professor

Background Information

C.L. had earned a Ph.D. and currently was an associate professor of economics at a major university. He had been discharged from the Navy because of high blood pressure. In the past he had experienced migraine headaches but had had no headaches for the last few years and his blood pressure was in the normal range without medication. Three months before C.L. sustained the current head injury he had undergone an anterior cervical fusion. He had no prior medical symptoms or findings that suggested the presence of cerebral disease or damage.

C.L. had been involved in a moving vehicle accident three weeks before the current neuropsychological examination. He was immediately rendered unconscious by the collision and recalled nothing about the accident or even the events occurring a short time before the injury. A large laceration on his forehead was sutured in the hospital E.R.

The patient was probably unconscious for about 10 hours before he gradually began to regain consciousness in his hospital room. He demonstrated varying degrees of alertness; generally he was quite lethargic but at times appeared to be very restless and confused. He also had severe headaches and during the first several days of hospitalization he vomited several times. When he tried to get up and walk he had a dizzy, lightheaded sensation. These symptoms, together with his general state of lethargy and confusion, concerned his physicians and raised the possibility of a subdural accumulation of blood or fluid.

Neurological Examination

Except for C.L.'s extreme lethargy, neurological examination was within normal limits; although his responses were slow, he was oriented to time, place and person. Cranial nerve functions were intact. Inspection of the eye grounds suggested papilledema of the left optic disc and it was not possible to discern any venous pulsations. Although the right optic disc was not elevated, no venous pulsations were seen. There was no muscle weakness and muscle stretch reflexes were normal and equal on both sides. C.L. did have some difficulty with the finger-to-nose test and seemed to be somewhat slow in performing rapid tapping with each hand, especially the left.

Because of the patient's continued lethargy, impaired alertness, and dizzy spells when he tried to walk, a more intensive neurological investigation was performed. An echoencephalogram revealed no shift of midline brain structures.

Because the patient had shown no particular improvement during the first week after his injury and examination of the eye grounds was even more suggestive of early papilledema, bilateral carotid angiography was done and the results were essentially within normal limits. However, an EEG showed slow wave activity bilaterally, more prominent on the right side.

Eleven days after the injury the papilledema had progressed to the point that some extravasation of blood was present around the optic disc on the left side. A second echoencephalogram again showed no shift of midline structures but did suggest that the third ventricle was somewhat increased in width. This finding, together with the progressive papilledema, suggested a posterior fossa lesion. A suboccipital craniectomy was performed and revealed an extensive amount of subdural fluid in the posterior fossa. After this fluid was evacuated burr holes were placed bilaterally over the convexity where more subdural fluid was found on both sides and aspirated.

The patient improved slowly following surgery; within five days the extravasation of blood around the optic disc had partially cleared and it was possible to discern pulsation of the veins in the retina. C.L. continued to improve, gradually became more active, had no further severe headaches, and was discharged from the hospital three weeks following the injury.

At this point one would wonder about the possibility of significant residual cerebral damage. The presence of a subdural hygroma certainly suggests that the patient had experienced a significant head injury. The most likely mechanism would be tearing of the arachnoid tissue as a result of the head blow and cerebral spinal fluid escaping into the subdural space. The fact that the hygroma was present in the posterior fossa as well as over each cerebral hemisphere suggested that the effects of the head injury were fairly extensive.

A subdural hygroma acts in essentially the same manner as a subdural hematoma; in some cases the lesion does not cause any significant damage to the underlying brain tissue and in other instances the brain damage is extensive and severe, resulting from pressure waves and shearing forces (which may occur with or without the subdural

hygroma). C.L. was given a neuropsychological examination at the time of discharge from the hospital in order to evaluate the behavioral consequences of his head injury.

Neuropsychological Evaluation

At the time of neuropsychological examination the testing technician asked the patient why he was hospitalized. C.L. reported in a very matter-of-fact manner that he had been in an automobile accident three weeks earlier, bumped his head, and underwent surgery to relieve pressure on his brain. On the Cornell Medical Index Health Questionnaire he had absolutely no complaints at all.

The reader should be aware that it is not uncommon for persons who have experienced significant head injury, hospitalization, and even brain surgery to have no complaints, especially if they have come through the procedures well, are feeling better, are ready to be discharged from the hospital, and have not yet had a chance to check out the consequences of any brain damage that may have been sustained. It is not particularly surprising then, that C.L.'s results on the Minnesota Multiphasic Personality Inventory were also generally within the normal range. Occasionally patients deny any problems on direct questioning (such as the Cornell Medical Index Health Questionnaire) but show evidence of definite underlying anxiety and emotional distress on the MMPI.

As would be expected from a faculty member in economics at a major university, the Wechsler results indicate that C.L. had developed intellectual functions quite normally. His Verbal IQ (129), which was in the Superior range, exceeded about 97% of the normative sample. The patient performed a little poorly on Digit Span (11), but this is not at all uncommon for hospitalized patients. Considering the variability among the Verbal subtests, there would be no reason to postulate that

THE HALSTEAD-REITAN
NEUROPSYCHOLOGICAL TEST BATTERY

Patient ___C.L. (I)___ Age __33__ Sex __M__ Education __20__ Handedness __R__

WECHSLER-BELLEVUE SCALE
VIQ	129
PIQ	110
FS IQ	121

Information	12
Comprehension	17
Digit Span	11
Arithmetic	17
Similarities	14
Vocabulary	14

Picture Arrangement	10
Picture Completion	13
Block Design	11
Object Assembly	10
Digit Symbol	9

TRAIL MAKING TEST
Part A: __38__ seconds
Part B: __98__ seconds

STRENGTH OF GRIP
Dominant hand: __49.0__ kilograms
Non-dominant hand: __43.5__ kilograms

REITAN-KLØVE TACTILE FORM RECOGNITION TEST
Dominant hand: __8__ seconds; __0__ errors
Non-dominant hand: __9__ seconds; __0__ errors

REITAN-KLØVE SENSORY-PERCEPTUAL EXAM – No errors

			Error Totals	
RH___ LH___	Both H: RH___ LH___	RH___ LH___		
RH___ LF___	Both H/F: RH___ LF___	RH___ LF___		
LH___ RF___	Both H/F: LH___ RF___	RF___ LH___		
RE___ LE___	Both E: RE___ LE___	RE___ LE___		
RV___ LV___	Both: RV___ LV___	RV___ LV___		

TACTILE FINGER RECOGNITION
R 1___ 2___ 3___ 4___ 5___ R __0__ / __20__
L 1___ 2___ 3___ 4___ 5___ L __0__ / __20__

FINGER-TIP NUMBER WRITING
R 1___ 2___ 3___ 4___ 5___ R __0__ / __20__
L 1__1__ 2___ 3___ 4___ 5___ L __1__ / __20__

HALSTEAD'S NEUROPSYCHOLOGICAL TEST BATTERY

Category Test __46__

Tactual Performance Test
Dominant hand: __7.4__
Non-dominant hand: __9.5__
Both hands: __4.1__

Total Time __21.0__
Memory __5__
Localization __1__

Seashore Rhythm Test
Number Correct __22__ __10__

Speech-sounds Perception Test
Number of Errors __6__

Finger Oscillation Test
Dominant hand: __46__ __46__
Non-dominant hand: __40__

Impairment Index __0.7__

MINNESOTA MULTIPHASIC PERSONALITY INVENTORY

		Hs	49	
		D	44	
?	50	Hy	55	
L	46	Pd	50	
F	44	Mf	65	
K	64	Pa	53	
		Pt	52	
		Sc	48	
		Ma	45	

REITAN-KLØVE LATERAL-DOMINANCE EXAM

Show me how you:
throw a ball	R
hammer a nail	R
cut with a knife	R
turn a door knob	R
use scissors	R
use an eraser	R
write your name	R

Record time used for spontaneous name-writing:
Preferred hand	__6__ seconds
Non-preferred hand	__23__ seconds

Show me how you:
kick a football	R
step on a bug	R

REITAN-INDIANA APHASIA SCREENING TEST

Form for Adults and Older Children

Name: _____C. L. (I)_____ Age: _33___

Copy SQUARE	Repeat TRIANGLE
Name SQUARE	Repeat MASSACHUSETTS
Spell SQUARE	Repeat METHODIST EPISCOPAL
Copy CROSS	Write SQUARE
Name CROSS	Read SEVEN
Spell CROSS	Repeat SEVEN
Copy TRIANGLE	Repeat/Explain HE SHOUTED THE WARNING.
Name TRIANGLE	Write HE SHOUTED THE WARNING.
Spell TRIANGLE	Compute 85 – 27 =
Name BABY	Compute 17 X 3 =
Write CLOCK	Name KEY
Name FORK	Demonstrate use of KEY
Read 7 SIX 2	Draw KEY Patient had omitted the hole in the handle. Examiner asked if he wished to add anything. Patient then completed the drawing.
Read MGW	Read PLACE LEFT HAND TO RIGHT EAR.
Reading I	Place LEFT HAND TO RIGHT EAR
Reading II	Place LEFT HAND TO LEFT ELBOW

1.

2.

clock

square

He shouted the warning.

85
27
___
58

51

C.L. had experienced any significant cognitive impairment.

However, C.L.'s Performance IQ (110) fell at the lower limits of the High Average range (exceeding about 75%). Scores for individual Performance subtests were consistently at the Average level (except for Picture Completion [13], which often tends to deviate in the direction of the Verbal subtests when there is some impairment of Performance intelligence). Thus, with this distribution of scores, one could raise a question about possible generalized impairment of Performance intelligence. Since it is not unusual for academic personnel to have higher Verbal than Performance IQ values, one would wonder whether these IQ values actually reflected an impairment of Performance intelligence.

Results on the four most sensitive measures in the Halstead-Reitan Battery strongly suggest at least a mild degree of impairment. The worst of these scores occurred on the Localization component of the Tactual Performance Test (1). The Impairment Index (0.7) was definitely in the impaired range and the patient performed poorly on Part B of the Trail Making Test (98 sec). Although the cut-off point on the Category Test is 50 errors (based on Halstead's data), our studies have indicated that using 45 errors as the cut-off point would reduce the number of misclassifications (false negatives).

The Impairment Index (as well as the other tests in this group) have correlations with IQ values of approximately 0.5 to 0.6. Therefore, from a person with a doctorate degree and relatively high IQ values one would expect a performance that is better — rather than worse — than the average person. Even though C.L. was not grossly impaired compared with many other individuals, in light of his background, education and general intelligence it would appear quite definitely that he had suffered significant impairment of higher-level brain functions.

The scores on the lateralizing indicators suggested right hemisphere dysfunction but no specific signs of left cerebral damage were found. C.L., who was distinctly right-handed, performed poorly with his left hand (9.5 min) compared with his right (7.4 min) on the Tactual Performance Test and had more difficulty than would be expected drawing the key.

Although one could question the disparity in placement of the extremities of the cross, we would classify the drawings of the square, cross and triangle within normal limits. However, the teeth of the key were definitely not symmetrical and it was only as an afterthought that C.L. attempted to place notches on the stem. The patient did not complete drawing the handle of the key and inserted the center part only after prompting by the examiner. Thus, these results suggest that C.L. does have some mild difficulty dealing with spatial configurations and supports the hypothesis of right cerebral dysfunction formulated on the performance with the left hand on the Tactual Performance Test and the decreased Performance IQ score.

In summary, C.L. had generalized impairment of his higher-level adaptive abilities and showed few specific deficits of a pathognomonic nature. The absence of errors on the Sensory-perceptual Examination is not unusual for persons with generalized (rather than focal) traumatic brain damage. We would interpret the test results as suggesting that (1) the patient did not have focal involvement of the cerebral cortex; (2) the accumulation of cerebral spinal fluid in the subdural space was probably due to a tear of the arachnoid tissue with no associated specific damage to underlying cerebral cortex; and (3) the impairment shown on neuropsychological testing was due to diffuse damage rather than an effect of the subdural hygromas.

C.L. returned for a follow-up examination about five and one-half months after the initial testing. Often a comparison of results obtained after the brain has had a chance for spontaneous recovery is helpful in assessing the deficits that were present initially. Our studies have indicated that spontaneous recovery is usually most pronounced in the areas of initial deficit. (Dikmen & Reitan, 1976). *In other words, the recovery process does not have a beneficial effect on functions that were not originally impaired; instead, recovery manifests itself on the measures that were initially performed poorly.*

In this instance we would expect (1) some improvement of Performance intelligence compared with Verbal intelligence; (2) distinctly better scores on the Category Test, the Trail Making Test and the Tactual Performance Test (particularly in terms of Total Time, the left-hand performance, and the Localization component); (4) improved drawings on the Aphasia Screening Test; and (5) possibly faster finger tapping speed. Clinical observations have shown that most patients continue to demonstrate some residual deficits after head injury and do not achieve a perfectly consistent recovery on all of the measures that were initially performed poorly. As expected in individual cases, and as shown below, these predictions of recovery were only partially confirmed.

Although there was some variability in the scores on particular subtests, the patient's Verbal IQ (130) showed essentially no change from the initial examination. However, except for Picture Arrangement (9), the Performance subtests consistently demonstrated some improvement. Rather than representing only practice-effect, it is likely that the improvement is definite and genuine on Digit Symbol (14). The general improvement in Full Scale IQ (from 121 to 128) also probably represents genuine improvement and not practice-effect alone.

As noted previously, the patient did not perform as well on Picture Arrangement as he had initially. This test is often depressed in persons with specific right anterior temporal lobectomies

for intractable epilepsy (Meier & French, 1966). Thus, it is possible that C.L.'s score on Picture Arrangement represents a mild degree of permanent residual impairment.

The patient showed definite improvement on the Category Test (from 46 to 23 errors) but only minor change on the Impairment Index (from 0.7 to 0.6). Because it is a generally sensitive measure reflecting *consistency* of impairment rather than *severity* of impairment, the Impairment Index often does not show any very striking change when there are residual deficits following a head injury. Therefore, it is always important to evaluate the results on the individual tests that make up the Impairment Index.

C.L. showed remarkable improvement on the Total Time of the Tactual Performance Test (from 21.0 min to 9.2 min), exceeding any improvement expected from practice-effect. The greatest improvement on the Tactual Performance Test occurred with the left hand (from 9.5 min to 2.8 min), which represented the worst performance in the three trials on the initial examination.

The patient showed only minimal improvement in the Trail Making Test and actually performed a little worse than initially on the Memory and Localization components of the Tactual Performance Test. Finger tapping speed was slightly improved with each hand and grip strength improved significantly with the right hand. (Grip strength is often reduced in bed-ridden persons who have had little physical activity. This could be the reason for the marked improvement in grip strength with the right upper extremity but does not explain the minimal changes with the left upper extremity.)

Although the patient did not draw the key in much detail, it clearly represents a better performance than the initial effort. The square, cross and triangle were essentially within normal limits on the first examination and continued to be adequately done on the second testing. Note, however, that the current drawing of the cross shows some

THE HALSTEAD-REITAN
NEUROPSYCHOLOGICAL TEST BATTERY

Patient __C.L. (II)__ Age __33__ Sex __M__ Education __20__ Handedness __R__

WECHSLER-BELLEVUE SCALE

VIQ	130
PIQ	121
FS IQ	128

Information	11
Comprehension	14
Digit Span	13
Arithmetic	18
Similarities	16
Vocabulary	14

Picture Arrangement	9
Picture Completion	14
Block Design	13
Object Assembly	12
Digit Symbol	14

TRAIL MAKING TEST

Part A: __34__ seconds
Part B: __92__ seconds

STRENGTH OF GRIP

Dominant hand: __57.0__ kilograms
Non-dominant hand: __43.0__ kilograms

REITAN-KLØVE TACTILE FORM RECOGNITION TEST

Dominant hand: __9__ seconds; __0__ errors
Non-dominant hand: __8__ seconds; __0__ errors

REITAN-KLØVE SENSORY-PERCEPTUAL EXAM — No errors

				Error Totals	
RH___ LH___	Both H:	RH___ LH___		RH___ LH___	
RH___ LF___	Both H/F:	RH___ LF___		RH___ LF___	
LH___ RF___	Both H/F:	LH___ RF___		RF___ LH___	
RE___ LE___	Both E:	RE___ LE___		RE___ LE___	
RV___ LV___	Both:	RV___ LV___		RV___ LV___	
___ ___		___ ___			
___ ___		___ ___			

TACTILE FINGER RECOGNITION

R 1___ 2___ 3___ 4___ 5___ R __0__ / 20
L 1___ 2___ 3___ 4___ 5___ L __0__ / 20

FINGER-TIP NUMBER WRITING

R 1 _3_ 2___ 3___ 4___ 5___ R __3__ / 20
L 1___ 2___ 3___ 4___ 5___ L __0__ / 20

NO APHASIC SYMPTOMS.

HALSTEAD'S NEUROPSYCHOLOGICAL TEST BATTERY

Category Test _____ 23

Tactual Performance Test

Dominant hand:	4.3
Non-dominant hand:	2.8
Both hands:	2.1

Total Time	9.2
Memory	4
Localization	0

Seashore Rhythm Test

Number Correct __24__ _____ 8

Speech-sounds Perception Test

Number of Errors _____ 5

Finger Oscillation Test

Dominant hand:	49	49
Non-dominant hand:	42	

__Impairment Index__ __0.6__

MINNESOTA MULTIPHASIC PERSONALITY INVENTORY

		Hs	54
		D	56
?	50	Hy	69
L	43	Pd	62
F	44	Mf	57
K	70	Pa	56
		Pt	62
		Sc	59
		Ma	63

REITAN-KLØVE LATERAL-DOMINANCE EXAM

Show me how you:
throw a ball	R
hammer a nail	R
cut with a knife	R
turn a door knob	R
use scissors	R
use an eraser	R
write your name	R

Record time used for spontaneous name-writing:
Preferred hand	5 seconds
Non-preferred hand	16 seconds

Show me how you:
kick a football	R
step on a bug	R

1.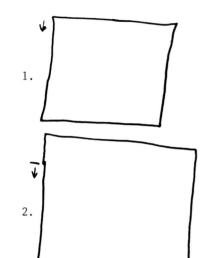

$$85 - 27 = 58$$

51

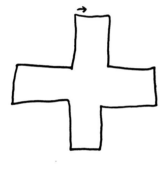

2.

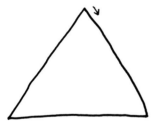

CLOCK
clock

square

He shouted the warning.

disparity in the lateral extremities that may have some significance. Also, the patient did not plan carefully in drawing the third line of the square and found it necessary to close the figure after completing the last horizontal line. Thus, even though they are generally comparable to the drawings done by control subjects, for C.L. these drawings probably reflect very mild residual difficulties.

The patient performed slightly worse with his right hand in finger-tip number writing perception (3 errors) than he did on the initial examination (0 errors). However, all of the mistakes occurred on the thumb and, unless the test is done very carefully, it is sometimes difficult to draw numbers on a person's thumb. A less-experienced examiner gave the second examination and this factor could have influenced the results. In any case, the interpretation of the test scores was not significantly affected by this single indicator of possible left cerebral dysfunction.

In summary, although results on certain measures still indicated a mild degree of residual deficit, the patient showed significant improvement on the second evaluation, principally on the tests that had demonstrated deficit on the initial examination. The improvement shown on the second examination independently validates the impairment demonstrated at the time of the first testing.

Even though they may be gradually resolving, the presence of cognitive deficits over a five-month period can have an unsettling effect on the patient. Although C.L. had no complaints on the Cornell Medical Index Health Questionnaire at the time of the first examination, at the second testing he indicated that he often gets spells of complete exhaustion or fatigue, working tires him out completely, and every little effort wears him out. Thus, it appears that C.L. may feel more strain now than during the period immediately following his brain surgery.

Results on the Minnesota Multiphasic Personality Inventory also suggest that this man is feeling more stress and general anxiety at present than he did five months ago (at the time of the first examination). Even though they may be only relatively mildly impaired, it is not uncommon for patients to show such indications of emotional stress and difficulty after a period of time has elapsed and the impairment has had an opportunity to influence the activities of everyday living. This type of emotional response does not occur in every instance of head injury, but it does indicate the importance of recognizing that neuropsychological deficits can have an unsettling and even distressing effect on emotional aspects of adjustment.

In summary, based on the results of the second examination, it would be difficult to conclude that the patient had any significant residual impairment. The deficits on the left side in finger tapping speed and grip strength stand out rather clearly and the results on finger-tip number writing perception (if valid) also deviate from normal expectancy. The poor scores on the Memory and Localization components of the Tactual performance Test and Part B of the Trail Making Test would also be unusual for this man, given his general intelligence levels and other abilities. The Picture Arrangement score was low compared to the other Performance subtests. Nevertheless, it would have been difficult to conclude confidently that, if seen independently, the second set of test results reflected significant cerebral damage.

When compared with the initial findings, however, the results of the second testing definitely suggest that the patient has some residual impairment and it is possible that this degree of deficit may be permanent. Although there have not been any careful studies of the particular tests or areas of function in which spontaneous improvement is most likely to be manifested, it is not unusual to see as much improvement as shown by this man on retesting after approximately a six-month period of spontaneous recovery.

CASE #16

Name: R.D.

Age: 26

Education: 19

Sex: Male

Handedness: Left

Occupation: Student

Background Information and Neurological Findings

Approximately one month before this examination R.D., an advanced graduate student in the final phases of completing his Ph.D. dissertation, was involved in a moving vehicle accident and sustained a very severe closed head injury. When admitted to the hospital his blood pressure was 40/0. He was deeply comatose and responded only to strong painful stimuli; it appeared that he was able to move his right extremities better than his left.

After several hours of observation the patient had hypoactive bowel sounds, his hemoglobin had dropped from 13 gm/% to 9 gm/%, and hematuria was evident. His pulse was 140 and both pupils were constricted. At this point R.D. was transferred to a major medical center.

R.D. remained hypotensive after receiving numerous blood transfusions and an exploratory laparotomy was performed because of this problem. Surgery revealed a small tear in the capsule of the spleen and a huge retroperitoneal hematoma on the right side, apparently involving the right kidney. Examination of the kidney showed that it was fractured and its pedicle was transsected. Both a spleenectomy and right nephrectomy were performed immediately.

The patient recovered uneventfully from the operative procedures but remained in a comatose state for about one week before gradually regaining consciousness. Cerebral angiograms did not show any displacement of structures or indications of a mass lesion of the brain; however, they did suggest pronounced spasm of the internal carotid arteries bilaterally. During the second week after the injury the patient was still occasionally disoriented to time, person, and place.

Neuropsychological Examination

Neuropsychological examination was done approximately one month post-injury. When R.D. was discharged from the hospital 11 days later he was able to walk, feed himself, and had partial bowel and bladder control. It was apparent, however, that his psychological functioning was seriously impaired. The neurological diagnosis was severe closed head injury with multiple diffuse contusions of the brain.

When we administered the Cornell Medical Index Health Questionnaire we saw that the patient was giving random responses and the test was discontinued. Results on the Minnesota Multiphasic Personality Inventory deviated significantly from normal, but the validity scales were also quite deviant and no attempt was made to do a specific interpretation.

This man showed evidence of serious generalized impairment of brain-related abilities. He earned a Verbal IQ (74) in the range of Borderline intelligence (exceeding only 4% of his age peers) and Performance (58) and Full Scale (64) IQ values in the range of Mild Mental Retardation (exceeding less than 2%).

Although the distribution of subtest scores indicated that the patient was generally impaired, the average scores on the Information (10) and Digit Span (10) subtests suggested that R.D. had higher IQ values in the past than he presently demonstrated. Judging from the scores alone, it would be perfectly reasonable to presume that the patient had suffered significant impairment on a number of the subtests. Of course, knowing that he had nearly completed requirements for the doctorate degree would be an obvious basis for presuming that at one time his general intelligence had been considerably higher.

Some of the low scores, particularly the 0 on the Vocabulary subtest, might be questioned. One would expect this man to be able to give the definitions of at least the simplest words; however, he had difficulty that seemed to reflect extreme impairment in abstraction ability as well as dysphasia. For example, he defined an apple as "red clothing" and donkey as "brown clothing." He probably was using colors to refer to the apple and donkey but was perseverating verbally in his repetition of "clothing."

With other words he was not able to offer relevant responses (e.g., he defined nuisance as "get away"). It is surprising that R.D. performed as well as he did on Digit Span (10), but this test (as well as Object Assembly) often yields somewhat deviant results.

There is no doubt that qualitative analysis of the responses may add additional significant information in evaluating the Wechsler subtest scores, even though our emphasis, in an effort to relate quantitative aspects of the data, has been upon the actual test scores. On the Information subtest this man was not able to name the President or the previous President but was able to earn credit for identifying the Koran as well as the author of Faust. Inconsistent responses of this kind, with respect to the difficulty level, are certainly valid indications of impairment from pre-morbid levels.

R.D. had great difficulty on many of the tests in the Halstead-Reitan Battery, performing especially poorly on tasks that were complex in nature and required him to analyze the problem or keep more than one element of the task in mind at the same time. Except for the first two subtests (which are rather simple) the patient was able to do no better than chance on the Category Test, earning a final score of 150 errors. Although he finally finished Part A of the Trail Making Test with great difficulty (240 sec) he could not complete Part B. He earned a score of 0 on the Localization component of the Tactual Performance Test, a task that was just too difficult for him to manage.

R.D. did somewhat better on the Seashore Rhythm Test (22 correct), clearly performing better than a chance level. On the Speech-sounds Perception Test his score (8 errors) was nearly within the normal range and was, in fact, much better than would have been predicted from his IQ values. It is apparent from his score on the Speech-sounds Perception Test that the first level of central processing (concerned with ability to pay attention and maintain concentration) was more intact than the highest levels, which reflect abstraction, reasoning, and logical analysis abilities (Reitan & Wolfson, 1985a).

Lateralizing indicators implicated the left cerebral hemisphere to a much greater extent than the right. Since the patient was definitely left-handed one would expect somewhat better performances in grip strength and finger tapping speed with the left hand than the right. As it turned out, the left-handed performances were far better, demonstrating definite impairment of the right upper extremity.

The Tactual Performance Test also suggested more difficulties with the right hand than the left, although the generally poor performance impairs the confidence with which this inference can be drawn. In other words, the Tactual Performance Test represented such a high level of difficulty for

THE HALSTEAD-REITAN
NEUROPSYCHOLOGICAL TEST BATTERY

Patient **R.D.** Age **26** Sex **M** Education **19** Handedness **L**

WECHSLER-BELLEVUE SCALE

VIQ	74
PIQ	58
FS IQ	64

Information	10
Comprehension	3
Digit Span	10
Arithmetic	0
Similarities	2
Vocabulary	0

Picture Arrangement	3
Picture Completion	4
Block Design	1
Object Assembly	7
Digit Symbol	2

TRAIL MAKING TEST

Part A: **240** seconds
Part B: _____ seconds
(Discontinued; 300″ at F)

STRENGTH OF GRIP

Dominant hand: **23.0** kilograms
Non-dominant hand: **9.5** kilograms

REITAN-KLØVE TACTILE FORM RECOGNITION TEST

Dominant hand: **22** seconds; **3** errors
Non-dominant hand: **36** seconds; **3** errors

REITAN-KLØVE SENSORY-PERCEPTUAL EXAM

				Error Totals	
RH___ LH___	Both H:	RH___ LH___	RH___ LH___		
RH___ LF___	Both H/F:	RH **2** LF___	RH **2** LF___		
LH___ RF___	Both H/F:	LH **4** RF___	RF___ LH **4**		
RE___ LE___	Both E:	RE **2** LE **2**	RE **2** LE **2**		
RV___ LV___	Both:	RV___ LV___	RV___ LV___		

TACTILE FINGER RECOGNITION

R 1 _1_ 2 _1_ 3 _4_ 4 _1_ 5 _1_   R _8_ / 20
L 1 ___ 2 ___ 3 _2_ 4 _1_ 5 _2_   L _5_ / 20

FINGER-TIP NUMBER WRITING

R 1 _3_ 2 _1_ 3 _2_ 4 _4_ 5 _2_   R _12_ / 20
L 1 _3_ 2 _1_ 3 _1_ 4 ___ 5 ___   L _5_ / 20

HALSTEAD'S NEUROPSYCHOLOGICAL TEST BATTERY

Category Test		**150**

Tactual Performance Test

Dominant hand:	**10.0 (2 blocks)**
Non-dominant hand:	**10.0 (0 blocks)**
Both hands:	**10.0 (3 blocks)**
Total Time	**30.0 (5 blocks)**
Memory	**1**
Localization	**0**

Seashore Rhythm Test

Number Correct **22**   **10**

Speech-sounds Perception Test

Number of Errors   **8**

Finger Oscillation Test

Dominant hand:	**42**	**42**
Non-dominant hand:	**18**	

Impairment Index   1.0

MINNESOTA MULTIPHASIC PERSONALITY INVENTORY

		Hs	82
		D	82
?	50	Hy	75
L	73	Pd	83
F	120+	Mf	69
K	51	Pa	105
		Pt	79
		Sc	120+
		Ma	81

REITAN-KLØVE LATERAL-DOMINANCE EXAM

Show me how you:
throw a ball	**L**
hammer a nail	**L**
cut with a knife	**L**
turn a door knob	**L**
use scissors	**L**
use an eraser	**L**
write your name	**L**

Record time used for spontaneous name-writing:
Preferred hand	**23** seconds
Non-preferred hand	**90** seconds

Show me how you:
kick a football	**R**
step on a bug	**L**

REITAN-INDIANA APHASIA SCREENING TEST

Form for Adults and Older Children

Name: _____R. D._____ Age: ___26___

Copy SQUARE	Repeat TRIANGLE
Name SQUARE "Triangle"	Repeat MASSACHUSETTS "Massasoosetts"
Spell SQUARE "S-Q-U-U-A-R-E"	Repeat METHODIST EPISCOPAL
Copy CROSS	Write SQUARE
Name CROSS "Triangle"	Read SEVEN
Spell CROSS	Repeat SEVEN
Copy TRIANGLE	Repeat/Explain HE SHOUTED THE WARNING.
Name TRIANGLE	Write HE SHOUTED THE WARNING.
Spell TRIANGLE	Compute 85 – 27 = Copied problem incorrectly. Given 24 – 13 and was confused (see).
Name BABY "Metamorphosis"	Compute 17 X 3 =
Write CLOCK	Name KEY
Name FORK	Demonstrate use of KEY
Read 7 SIX 2 "7 S-I-X 2."	Draw KEY
Read MGW "W-G-W – no – M-G-W."	Read PLACE LEFT HAND TO RIGHT EAR. "Please stand at rail ear."
Reading I	Place LEFT HAND TO RIGHT EAR Right hand to right ear.
Reading II "He is a free man – animal, a famous winner of dog shows."	Place LEFT HAND TO LEFT ELBOW Right hand to left elbow.

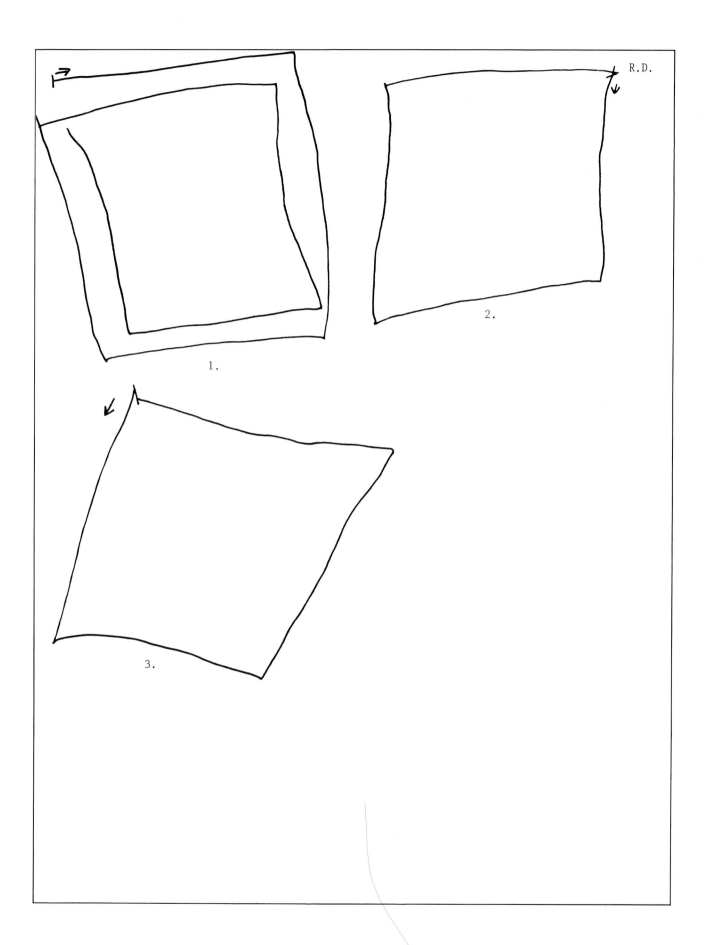

R.D.

1.

2.

3.

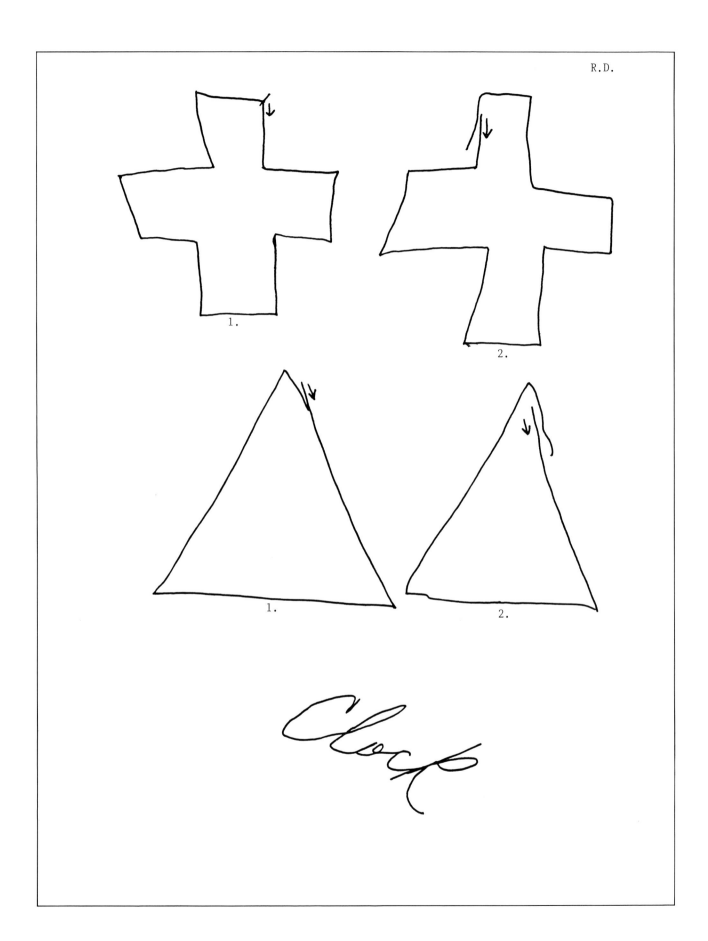

1.

2.

1.

2.

Clock

Square

He shouted the warning.

$$35 - 27 = 8$$ (85 – 27)

Examiner wrote problem.

$$\begin{array}{r} 2\ 4 \\ -\ 1\ 3 \\ \hline 5\ 7 \\ 2\ 7 \\ \hline 2\ 9\ 8 \end{array}$$

Examiner wrote problem.

$$\begin{array}{r} 8 \\ -\ 3 \\ \hline 5 \end{array}$$

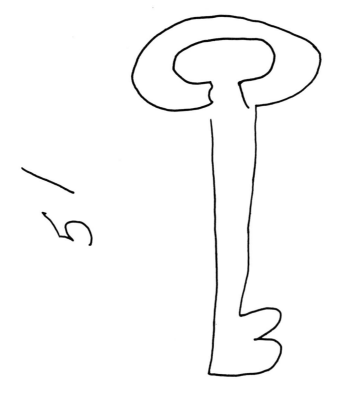

51

this man that he was not able to make much progress even using his left upper extremity and, as a result, differential performances of the left and right upper extremities were obscured.

Sensory-perceptual deficits were also prominent. R.D. had difficulty with tests of bilateral simultaneous tactile stimulation, particularly when the hand was required to compete with the face. In cases of severe generalized impairment of cerebral functions it is not uncommon to find that the patient is able to respond to the stimulus given to the face but does not perceive the stimulus given to the hand. When the cerebral damage is severe, insensitivity of the hand may be observed regardless of whether the stimulus to the face is given ipsilaterally or contralaterally. The fact that R.D. failed to perceive stimuli to the hands and reported only the stimuli to the face strongly suggests generalized impairment of brain functions. However, R.D. consistently failed to appreciate the stimulus to the left hand when it was given simultaneously with a stimulus to the right face, suggesting that the right cerebral hemisphere might be more severely damaged than the left.

With auditory stimulation the patient failed to report that both stimuli were administered simultaneously in any of the trials. This is an unusual response and is probably indicative of cerebral damage, but obviously has no lateralizing significance.

On tests of tactile finger localization and finger-tip number writing perception R.D. showed significant difficulties on both sides but clearly had more difficulty on the right hand than the left. These findings, therefore, suggest the presence of more serious damage of the left than right cerebral hemisphere.

Note that the patient also had a number of obvious dysphasic symptoms. In right-handed persons who have had the opportunity to develop brain-behavior relationships normally (without damage to the brain early in life which may have

affected the developmental organization of neuropsychological functions), dysphasia is nearly always a manifestation of left cerebral dysfunction. Left-handed persons also usually depend upon their left cerebral hemispheres for language functions (Penfield & Roberts, 1959), but a small proportion of left-handed individuals appear to have language localized in their right cerebral hemisphere. Reitan observed an unreported case of a man who had been strongly left-handed all of his life and had no apparent impairment of language functions whatsoever after a left cerebral hemispherectomy. Thus, it appears that there are instances of left-handed persons whose language functions are strongly lateralized to the right cerebral hemisphere.

In this case one might question whether the patient's aphasic difficulties stemmed from right or left cerebral damage. The fact that both motor and sensory-perceptual functions generally showed more serious impairment on the right side of the body implied that the left cerebral hemisphere was more seriously damaged than the right and might serve as a basis for presuming that the dysphasic manifestations also were a function of left cerebral damage. However, in this instance the overall picture also included definite evidence of constructional dyspraxia. With positive findings implicating each cerebral hemisphere the question of where R.D.'s language functions are located would still exist. Perhaps the greater impairment on the right side of his body (which definitely implies more serious involvement of the left hemisphere) is associated with constructional dyspraxia rather than language difficulties. It appears likely that in the case of this man the dysphasia is related to left cerebral damage, but because of the findings of generalized deficits the question probably cannot be answered unequivocally.

As the reader can see, R.D.'s aphasic symptoms were quite definite. He called the SQUARE a "triangle" and perseverated verbally by also calling the CROSS a "triangle." Confusion in spelling was manifested by the attempt to spell SQUARE. R.D. also gave a highly unusual response ("metamorphosis") in attempting to name the BABY. This response probably represents a manifestation of some type of disordered reasoning rather than dysnomia. However, giving the wrong name for the SQUARE and CROSS are almost certainly manifestations of dysnomia.

Whether one would identify this man's symptoms as spelling dyspraxia would be open to question, but repetition of the "U" in spelling SQUARE is almost certainly a manifestation of left cerebral dysfunction. (Whether or not to use specific diagnostic terminology to identify dysphasic deficits in the case of an individual subject is a matter of clinical judgement based upon the type and severity of the defective response; however, one should not let the question of terminology stand in the way of observing the patient's response and recognizing its significance for impaired brain functions.)

When R.D. read the letters individually and failed to identify the middle number in 7 SIX 2 he demonstrated a response typical of patients with impaired ability to recognize the symbolic significance of language material. Failing to read the letters MGW correctly is a response seen only in persons with quite serious impairment of language functions. Even though the patient corrected his mistake, the fact that he initially made an error indicates clearly that his ability to recognize individual letters is seriously impaired and we would classify this response as visual letter dysgnosia.

R.D. had difficulty reading several other items. He was initially confused in the first part of the second reading item, but then was able to pull his intellectual abilities together and finish the sentence correctly. When he attempted to read PLACE LEFT HAND TO RIGHT EAR he responded, "Please stand at rail ear." Obviously, in this instance, he was much more confused in attempting to understand the symbolic significance of the printed material.

The patient had some difficulty in enunciating MASSACHUSETTS and the error probably suggests the presence of mild central dysarthria. He actually substituted an "S" sound for the "CH" sound, a type of error that differs from the slurring of the sound made by some non-brain-damaged subjects. Thus, even this response is probably part of the overall picture of organic language impairment.

This man also had considerable difficulty in performing simple arithmetic problems. When asked to do $85 - 27 =$, he copied the problem incorrectly although he recorded the correct answer. However, writing "35" instead of "85" is suspicious in its own right regarding the symbolic significance of numbers. The examiner pursued this question further by writing two problems on the paper for the patient to solve. The patient demonstrated a considerable degree of arithmetical confusion on the first problem, $24 - 13$. He probably added the 4 and 3 but it is difficult to discern his reasoning for deciding upon 5 as the next number. The additional computations that he attempted at this point also seem beyond comprehension, but there is no doubt that he was significantly confused with respect to performance of simple arithmetical problems and we would identify this difficulty as dyscalculia.

Although R.D.'s writing was within normal limits, his attempts to copy simple spatial configurations demonstrated significant deficits. His first attempt to copy the square showed that he was confused about the inside and outside lines. He was trying to achieve a wide border, but obviously became confused. The examiner asked him to try the task again, ignoring the wide border and drawing only the outside line, and then the patient was able to do somewhat better. On the third attempt he again had a little difficulty achieving lines of equal length along the four sides.

The first drawing of the cross, showing imbalance of the extremities, was mildly deviant from a normal performance. In the patient's second attempt the problem was even more serious and he needed to extend the upper extremity to affect a balanced closure. The patient even had some difficulty in copying the triangle, especially in trying to attain closure.

We can see that these figures clearly indicate a moderate degree of impairment in dealing with simple spatial relationships, a problem which became even more apparent in the attempt to copy the key. The teeth of the key were drawn so simply that it is difficult to evaluate. However, R.D. became quite confused trying to reproduce the handle and demonstrated typical constructional dyspraxia.

It is interesting to note that patients with brain lesions are sometimes able to perform simple tasks quite satisfactorily and in other instances they become entirely confused. Head (1926) noticed this difficulty in successive evaluations of aphasic patients and questioned the classification of aphasic syndromes and their reliability, since a patient might not show the same deficit on a successive examinations and demonstrate other deficits that had not been present initially. Aphasic manifestations and discrepancies of this kind occur frequently among persons with cerebral damage and the inconsistency of response in its own right may be a further manifestation of impaired brain functions.

In this case, for example, R.D. became completely confused when attempting to solve a simple arithmetic problem that had been written on the paper by the examiner; however, when asked to multiply 17 × 3 mentally and write only the answer on his paper, he did so with no difficulty whatsoever. Some professionals have considered such inconsistencies in a patient's performance to represent malingering. It is the clinician's responsibility to learn to recognize the apparent inconsistencies that are demonstrated by brain-damaged persons and interpret such performances in the context of the overall set of test results.

In summary, this man showed very severe impairment of higher-level abilities, particularly in tasks that required abstraction, reasoning, logical analysis, ability to keep several elements of a task in mind at the same time, and competence in complex problem-solving situations. He manifested "flashes" of his prior abilities on certain tasks, but the severe nature of generalized impairment was obvious.

R.D. also had evidence of damage of each cerebral hemisphere, including clear demonstrations of dysphasia and constructional dyspraxia. The left cerebral hemisphere definitely seemed to be more seriously damaged than the right, but the overall results were consistent with significant generalized cerebral damage.

The patient performed relatively well on the Speech-sounds Perception Test and the reader may wonder how such a score could be achieved in the face of significant impairment of reading skill as well as other aphasic deficits. This, again, is one of the types of inconsistencies that is frequently demonstrated by brain-damaged persons and in this case the Speech-sounds Perception Test score almost certainly reflects R.D.'s pre-morbid verbal abilities. This particular disparity therefore provides additional evidence that the patient had much better abilities before his injury, but it cannot be used as a basis for discounting the significance of the positive indications of language deficit on the Aphasia Screening Test.

We included this case not only because of the teaching value of the configuration of test findings, but also to illustrate the severity of impairment that is occasionally seen in persons with head injuries. In fact, a great number of persons sustain severe head injuries and devastating impairment of higher-level brain functions, and many are so severely and obviously impaired that they are not even referred for neuropsychological examination.

Although neuropsychological testing may detect evidence of significant impairment even when other approaches yield negative results, it is a mistake to neglect neuropsychological evaluation in cases of severe head injury that have documented neurological findings. First, it is important to establish a baseline for purposes of assessing eventual improvement due to spontaneous recovery and/or brain retraining. Second, a full evaluation of the effects of brain injury is needed in every case in order to recognize the patient's problems as a basis for counseling and to develop a plan of remediation.

CASE #17

Name: C.H.

Age: 40

Education: 12

Sex: Male

Handedness: Right

Occupation: Retired Navy
             radio operator

Background Information

C.H. had spent most of his adult life in the Navy working principally as a radio operator. He was admitted to the hospital at this time because he had experienced a major motor seizure on two separate days during the preceding week. The patient lost consciousness, fell to the ground (on one occasion striking the back of his head with considerable force) and experienced tonic-clonic contractions for about five minutes. Upon regaining consciousness he reported that he felt tired and had sore muscles for several days.

These seizures began occurring suddenly without any type of aura about two years ago. Although C.H. had been taking antiepileptic medication, the seizures had not been adequately controlled.

The patient denied having had any serious illnesses or surgical procedures. He admitted that he had a rather quick temper and was chronically nervous and anxious. Two years before the epileptic attacks began C.H. was seriously injured in a moving vehicle accident. Both of his legs were broken and he had contusions and abrasions over much of his body. He sustained a head blow and had several facial fractures which required orthopedic wiring. He was unconscious for approximately 10 hours after the automobile injury.

Neurological Examination

Physical and neurological examinations yielded findings that were within normal limits. An electroencephalogram showed a relatively mild generalized dysrhythmia. Although non-specific and of no localizing significance, the tracings were definitely considered to be abnormal and were judged to be compatible with a convulsive disorder but not pathognomonic for epilepsy.

Although a pneumoencephalogram showed no displacement of structures, a slight but definite dilatation of the anterior horns of the lateral ventricles was noted on both sides. The head injury sustained four years earlier was presumably responsible for the development of the epileptic attacks. During the course of this hospitalization the patient's antiepileptic medications were monitored and adjusted.

Neuropsychological Evaluation

Neuropsychological examination was done three weeks after C.H. entered the hospital. On the Cornell Medical Index Health Questionnaire he had a number of complaints. He said that he has pains in the heart or chest area, often suffers from an upset stomach, often has spells of severe dizziness and frequently feels faint, and has great difficulty sleeping. He also felt that he was a nervous and sensitive person, that his feelings are easily hurt and he is always upset by criticism. He believed that he does things impulsively, lets little things get on his nerves and make him angry, is easily upset and irritated, and becomes angry when anyone tells him what to do. Sudden noises make him jump or shake badly and frightening thoughts keep coming back into his mind. The Minnesota Multiphasic Personality Inventory was not strikingly deviant but did suggest that the patient may resist conventional regulations and constraints and probably is somewhat impulsive.

Results of the Wechsler Scale indicated that C.H.'s general intelligence level was well above average. He earned a Verbal IQ (126) in the Superior range (exceeding about 96% of his age peers) and a Performance IQ (117) in the High Average range (exceeding 87%). These values yielded a Full Scale IQ (123) in the Superior range (exceeding 94%).

The Verbal subtest scores indicated that the patient performed consistently well on all measures except Digit Span (7). As we have frequently noted, a low score on Digit Span is not unusual in hospitalized persons, even those who have no past or present evidence of cerebral disease or damage.

Except for Object Assembly (8) and Digit Symbol (8) the Performance subtests were also generally above average. Object Assembly tends to be rather variable and the low score may reflect an inability to grasp one of the problems. The low Digit Symbol score may be an indication of brain damage, but it would be difficult to draw this conclusion from the Wechsler scores alone.

The four most sensitive indicators in the Halstead-Reitan Battery were generally done poorly. C.H. earned an Impairment Index of 0.7 (70% of the tests had scores in the brain-damaged range), performed worse than the average brain-damaged subject on the Category Test (70) despite his high IQ values, and did poorly on the Localization component of the Tactual Performance Test (3). On the other hand, C.H. performed remarkably well on Part B of the Trail Making Test (39 sec), indicating that he is quick, alert, and able to keep both alphabetical and numerical series in mind at

the same time while searching for the location of the appropriate symbol.

Under such circumstances, many psychologists are tempted to average the scores, apparently presuming that the patient was lucky on the Trail Making Test and unlucky on the other measures. A more appropriate approach to interpreting the Halstead-Reitan Battery is to accept every score as representative of an aspect of the patient's brain functions (recognizing that all of the measures are necessary to adequately reflect brain functions in an overall sense and that some tests may be performed better than others, even with a damaged brain).

The three measures that reflected deficient performances all correlate fairly well with IQ scores and C.H.'s high IQ values suggest that he should have performed better, rather than worse, than the average subject. Reitan (1985) has shown that the Impairment Index should be considered with relation to IQ values and that a poor Impairment Index takes on additional significance for brain damage when the subject's IQ values are relatively intact. Although it has not yet been formally demonstrated, the same generalization is almost certainly true for the Category Test.

In the context of the other poor scores, the good score on the Trail Making Test argues strongly against the presence of an acutely destructive or rapidly progressive lesion of either cerebral hemisphere. Other tests in the Battery were done well and can be interpreted the same way. It is clear from the results that even though C.H.'s brain may have sustained damaged, it is relatively stabilized in a biological sense.

Lateralizing signs were present to implicate both cerebral hemispheres, but the right cerebral hemisphere was definitely more involved. The relatively mild indications of left cerebral damage include some difficulty in finger-tip number writing perception with the right hand (2 errors) but no mistakes at all with the left hand. The patient also

THE HALSTEAD-REITAN
NEUROPSYCHOLOGICAL TEST BATTERY

Patient __C.H.__ Age __40__ Sex __M__ Education __12__ Handedness __R__

WECHSLER-BELLEVUE SCALE

VIQ	126
PIQ	117
FS IQ	123

Information	14
Comprehension	15
Digit Span	7
Arithmetic	16
Similarities	16
Vocabulary	14

Picture Arrangement	11
Picture Completion	14
Block Design	13
Object Assembly	8
Digit Symbol	8

TRAIL MAKING TEST

Part A: __30__ seconds
Part B: __39__ seconds

STRENGTH OF GRIP

Dominant hand: __40.0__ kilograms

Non-dominant hand: __33.5__ kilograms

REITAN-KLØVE TACTILE FORM RECOGNITION TEST

Dominant hand: __8__ seconds; __0__ errors

Non-dominant hand: __12__ seconds; __0__ errors

REITAN-KLØVE SENSORY-PERCEPTUAL EXAM — No errors

Error Totals

RH ___ LH ___	Both H:	RH ___ LH ___	RH ___ LH ___	
RH ___ LF ___	Both H/F:	RH ___ LF ___	RH ___ LF ___	
LH ___ RF ___	Both H/F:	LH ___ RF ___	RF ___ LH ___	
RE ___ LE ___	Both E:	RE ___ LE ___	RE ___ LE ___	
RV ___ LV ___	Both	RV ___ LV ___	RV ___ LV ___	
___ ___		___ ___		
___ ___		___ ___		

TACTILE FINGER RECOGNITION

R 1___ 2___ 3___ 4___ 5 **1**   R **1** / 20

L 1___ 2 **2** 3 **2** 4___ 5___   L **4** / 20

FINGER-TIP NUMBER WRITING

R 1 **1** 2___ 3 **1** 4___ 5___   R **2** / 20

L 1___ 2___ 3___ 4___ 5___   L **0** / 20

HALSTEAD'S NEUROPSYCHOLOGICAL TEST BATTERY

Category Test __70__

Tactual Performance Test

Dominant hand: __3.6__
Non-dominant hand: __6.8__
Both hands: __3.2__

Total Time	13.6
Memory	9
Localization	3

Seashore Rhythm Test

Number Correct __25__   __6__

Speech-sounds Perception Test

Number of Errors   __9__

Finger Oscillation Test

Dominant hand: __46__   46
Non-dominant hand: __41__

Impairment Index __0.7__

MINNESOTA MULTIPHASIC PERSONALITY INVENTORY

		Hs	44
		D	60
?	50	Hy	55
L	36	Pd	71
F	66	Mf	59
K	42	Pa	47
		Pt	64
		Sc	63
		Ma	78

REITAN-KLØVE LATERAL-DOMINANCE EXAM

Show me how you:
throw a ball	R
hammer a nail	R
cut with a knife	R
turn a door knob	R
use scissors	R
use an eraser	R
write your name	R

Record time used for spontaneous name-writing:
Preferred hand	10 seconds
Non-preferred hand	20 seconds

Show me how you:
kick a football	R
step on a bug	R

REITAN-INDIANA APHASIA SCREENING TEST

Form for Adults and Older Children

Name: _____ C. H. _____ Age: __40__

Copy SQUARE	Repeat TRIANGLE
Name SQUARE	Repeat MASSACHUSETTS
Spell SQUARE	Repeat METHODIST EPISCOPAL "Methodist Episcocopal"
Copy CROSS	Write SQUARE
Name CROSS	Read SEVEN
Spell CROSS	Repeat SEVEN
Copy TRIANGLE	Repeat/Explain HE SHOUTED THE WARNING.
Name TRIANGLE	Write HE SHOUTED THE WARNING.
Spell TRIANGLE	Compute 85 – 27 =
Name BABY	Compute 17 X 3 =
Write CLOCK	Name KEY
Name FORK	Demonstrate use of KEY
Read 7 SIX 2	Draw KEY
Read MGW	Read PLACE LEFT HAND TO RIGHT EAR.
Reading I	Place LEFT HAND TO RIGHT EAR
Reading II	Place LEFT HAND TO LEFT ELBOW

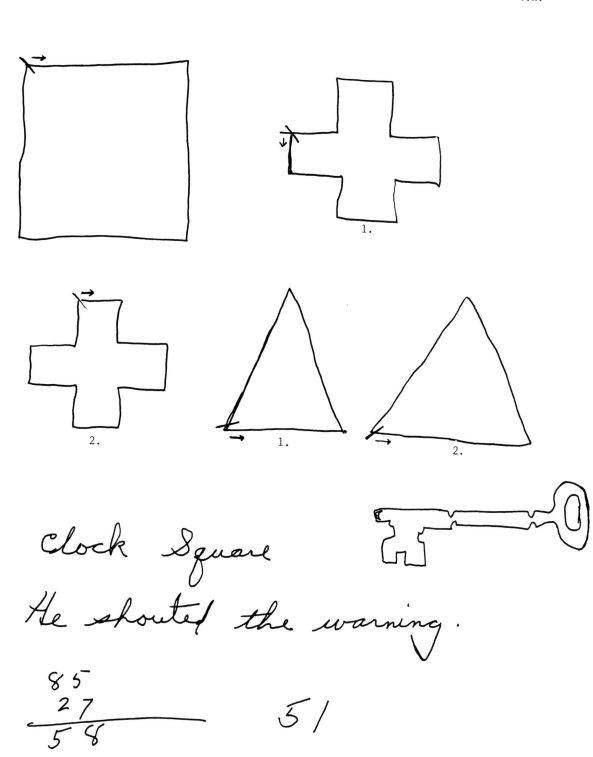

Clock Square

He shouted the warning.

$$
\begin{array}{r}
8\,5 \\
2\,7 \\
\hline
5\,8
\end{array}
$$

51

made an error in enunciating EPISCOPAL, represented by repetition (addition) of a syllable. This type of error occurs much more frequently in persons with left rather than right cerebral damage and, together with the very mild difficulty in finger-tip number writing perception, could be considered sufficient to suggest correspondingly mild left cerebral damage. The excellent Verbal IQ, the relatively good score on the Speech-sounds Perception Test (9), and the complete absence of any other indicators of aphasia certainly support the hypothesis that the left cerebral hemisphere is not seriously damaged.

Indications of right cerebral damage were shown most prominently on the Tactual Performance Test. The patient performed quite well on the first trial with his right hand (3.6 min), but required nearly double that amount of time on the second trial when using his left hand (6.8 min). His grip strength with his left extremity was also mildly reduced.

Note that the deficits involving the left upper extremity were not limited to motor manifestations; C.H. was a little slow in tactile form recognition with his left hand and made significantly more errors in finger localization with his left hand (4) than his right (1). He may also have been somewhat slow in finger tapping speed with his left hand (41) compared with his right (46), but the relationship was basically within normal limits. The deficits on the left side of the body focus rather specifically on motor and tactile-perceptual abilities.

Also note that C.H.'s drawings were within normal limits. One could postulate that the Performance IQ (which was nine points lower than the Verbal IQ) represented another indication of right cerebral damage, but the patient's performances on Picture Arrangement and Block Design (the most reliable indicators of right cerebral dysfunction in the Wechsler Scale) were not strikingly reduced. Therefore, the right cerebral indicators could be viewed as representing an area of rather focal static involvement in the middle part of the right cerebral hemisphere. Even though the EEG tracings did not show any type of focal disturbance in this area, it is not uncommon to observe neuropsychological results of this kind in patients with epilepsy.

Considering the evidence of left-sided motor and tactile-perceptual deficits, we would postulate that C.H. has a focal chronic-static lesion in the middle part of the right cerebral hemisphere, probably caused by the head injury sustained four years earlier. He also has demonstrated generalized deficits and some very mild indicators of left cerebral damage.

It is clear that C.H. is not grossly or severely impaired. Nevertheless, his adaptive abilities are compromised and he is likely to have particular difficulty in performing bimanual tasks that require the coordinated use of both hands. His impulsive tendencies (suggested in his own evaluation as well as the MMPI) may constitute a special problem for this man; he is generally quick and alert but does not have the critical judgement and analytic capabilities (shown by his score on the Category Test) that would normally have a rational modulating influence.

Finally, despite his excellent IQ values, very good scores on certain measures, and the absence of any severe impairment, C.H.'s test results definitely and distinctly deviate beyond normal limits. The findings implicating the right cerebral hemisphere, which could scarcely have occurred on a chance basis, present a typical picture of chronic-static cerebral dysfunction. In fact, it would be unlikely that an experienced neuropsychologist, familiar with interpretation of the Halstead-Reitan Battery, would be inclined to consider any possibility other than a long-standing head injury to account for these test results.

CASE #18

Name: A.B.

Age: 26

Education: 3

Sex: Male

Handedness: Right

Occupation: Unemployed

Background Information

This 26-year-old man apparently had limited ability, at least in an academic sense, all of his life. School was quite difficult for A.B. and he quit in the fourth grade; therefore, he completed only three grades satisfactorily.

A.B. had been unemployed in a variety of jobs, principally as a helper on the farm and a factory worker. He had been working as a logger for about three years when he was injured while topping a tree. A limb fell, hit him on the head, and knocked him to the ground where he lay unconscious for about four hours. Upon being found he was taken to the local hospital. He was unconscious for a total of about eight hours.

Since being discharged from the hospital A.B. had severe headaches and many dizzy spells. He reported that he has a headache all of the time and that aspirin helps very little. The headache becomes particularly severe whenever he attempts to exert himself, such as chopping wood, moving furniture, etc. Because the only work he is able to do involves manual labor, this combination of factors has rendered him unemployed since the time of the injury. A.B. also said that since the accident his memory has been significantly impaired.

It is entirely possible that this man sustained significant brain injury, but on the other hand it is also possible that his complaints (including his inability to work) represent an emotional reaction to the overall situation. Therefore, in evaluating this patient it is important to differentiate between deficits related to brain injury and problems stemming from emotional difficulties or perhaps even more significantly, the patient's limited premorbid intellectual and academic background.

We were not able to administer the Cornell Medical Index Health Questionnaire or the Minnesota Multiphasic Personality Inventory because A.B. was not able to read. The Wide Range Achievement Test was given to obtain information regarding his level of academic achievement and he earned the following grade-equivalents: Reading, 2.1; Spelling, 2.1; and Arithmetic, 2.7. It was apparent from these results that A.B. had only the most primitive academic skills.

Neurological Examination

When we examined A.B. his neurological examination and EEG were within normal limits. Therefore, the findings on these examinations have to viewed as non-contributory; the patient may have sustained significant brain damage which was not detected by these evaluations. A review of A.B.'s history revealed no evidence that he had ever sustained any significant head injuries or illnesses prior to the logging accident that might have affected his brain functions. During the neuropsychological examination the patient was pleasant, cooperative and easy-going. It appeared that he made a serious effort to do his best and we believe that valid results were obtained.

Neuropsychological Evaluation

The test results indicate that A.B. has general intelligence levels far below average, shows impairment on brain-sensitive tests as well, and has extremely limited academic abilities. At the present time it is probable that he would have great difficulty performing even a very simple type of competitive occupational job.

The patient earned a Verbal IQ (78) in the upper part of the Borderline range (exceeding about 7% of his age peers) and a Performance IQ (88) in the upper part of the Low Average range (exceeding 21%). These values yielded a Full Scale IQ (81) in the lower part of the Low Average range (exceeding about 10%).

A.B. showed a considerable degree of variability on the individual subtests. He performed particularly poorly on Information (5) and Vocabulary (3), subtests that relate to stored information and verbal abilities. We would doubt that this man ever had very high intelligence levels and it is likely that he was always somewhat below the average. It is also possible, however, that he has experienced some degree of impairment of certain aspects of general intelligence.

A.B. also performed quite poorly on the brain-sensitive tests, earning an Impairment Index of 0.7 (about 70% of the tests had scores in the brain-damaged range). His only performances in the normal range were on two measures of memory functions: the Memory (9) and Localization (7) components of the Tactual Performance Test.

The patient showed serious impairment on the Category Test, a task that required abstraction, concept formation, and reasoning abilities. He was quite limited in his capability to use logical analysis and understand cause-and-effect relationships. From his score of 116, we would postulate that A.B. is not able to reason his way through situations and probably is confused much of the time.

A.B. also had great difficulty on tasks that required flexibility and alertness in thinking. Except

for definite impairment with his right (preferred) extremity when attempting to solve complex tasks (Tactual Performance Test), his basic motor functions were relatively adequate. Conversely, he was somewhat slow in finger tapping speed with his left hand (42) compared with his right (50). Therefore, we have evidence that a number of the major areas of brain functions were definitely impaired.

A.B. also had great difficulty with tasks that involved verbal and language skills. On the Aphasia Screening Test it was apparent that his academic abilities were quite limited. He was scarcely able to spell at all, had minimal reading ability, could write only very simple material (such as his name) and even misnamed common objects. It is probable that some of his limited academic skills relate to impairment of the left cerebral hemisphere resulting from specific damage, but we would also postulate that this man has never had adequate brain training in developing verbal abilities. His very limited education was not sufficient to allow much development of spelling, reading, and writing skills.

A.B. had somewhat more ability in arithmetical functions than dealing with language symbols, but even in this area he was not particularly proficient. One cannot necessarily presume that his basic operational skills in arithmetic were adequate on the basis of the Arithmetic subtest score (9) on the Wechsler Scale, and it is not uncommon to find disparities between achievement tests of arithmetical skills.

As noted, the Wide Range Achievement Test was administered to obtain specific information about A.B.'s academic competence and we learned that his abilities ranged from the beginning to the latter part of the second grade. Academic abilities at this level are not sufficient to provide a normal adjustment in terms of the requirements of everyday living and occupational situations.

We would postulate that this man's brain has never been properly trained and many of the deficiencies that he shows are probably a result of

THE HALSTEAD-REITAN
NEUROPSYCHOLOGICAL TEST BATTERY

Patient _____**A.B.**_____ Age __**26**__ Sex __**M**__ Education __**3**__ Handedness __**R**__

WECHSLER-BELLEVUE SCALE

VIQ	78
PIQ	88
FS IQ	81

Information	5
Comprehension	9
Digit Span	6
Arithmetic	9
Similarities	7
Vocabulary	3

Picture Arrangement	6
Picture Completion	6
Block Design	11
Object Assembly	9
Digit Symbol	8

TRAIL MAKING TEST

Part A: __**52**__ seconds
Part B: __**192**__ seconds

STRENGTH OF GRIP

Dominant hand: __**39.0**__ kilograms
Non-dominant hand: __**40.5**__ kilograms

REITAN-KLØVE TACTILE FORM RECOGNITION TEST

Dominant hand: __**8**__ seconds; __**0**__ errors
Non-dominant hand: __**10**__ seconds; __**0**__ errors

REITAN-KLØVE SENSORY-PERCEPTUAL EXAM

				Error Totals	
RH ___ LH ___	Both H:	RH ___ LH ___	RH ___ LH ___	
RH ___ LF ___	Both H/F:	RH **4** LF ___	RH **4** LF ___	
LH ___ RF ___	Both H/F:	LH **2** RF ___	RF ___ LH **2**	
RE ___ LE ___	Both E:	RE ___ LE ___	RE ___ LE ___	
RV ___ LV ___	Both:	RV ___ LV ___	RV ___ LV ___	

TACTILE FINGER RECOGNITION

R 1___ 2___ 3___ 4 **2** 5___   R **2** / **20**
L 1___ 2___ 3 **1** 4 **2** 5___   L **3** / **20**

FINGER-TIP NUMBER WRITING

R 1 **1** 2 **1** 3___ 4___ 5___   R **2** / **20**
L 1___ 2___ 3___ 4___ 5___   L **0** / **20**

HALSTEAD'S NEUROPSYCHOLOGICAL TEST BATTERY

Category Test _____ 116

Tactual Performance Test

Dominant hand:	15.0
Non-dominant hand:	6.2
Both hands:	2.7

Total Time	23.9
Memory	9
Localization	7

Seashore Rhythm Test

Number Correct __**18**__ ____**10**____

Speech-sounds Perception Test

Number of Errors ____**37**____

Finger Oscillation Test

Dominant hand:	50	50
Non-dominant hand:	42	

Impairment Index __**0.7**__

REITAN-KLØVE
LATERAL-DOMINANCE EXAM

Show me how you:
throw a ball	R
hammer a nail	R
cut with a knife	R
turn a door knob	R
use scissors	R
use an eraser	R
write your name	R

Record time used for spontaneous name-writing:
Preferred hand	**15** seconds
Non-preferred hand	**27** seconds

Show me how you:
kick a football	R
step on a bug	R

REITAN-INDIANA APHASIA SCREENING TEST

Form for Adults and Older Children

Name: _____A. B._____ Age: __26___

Copy SQUARE	Repeat TRIANGLE
Name SQUARE	Repeat MASSACHUSETTS "Matchachucha"

Spell SQUARE
    " H -" (Could not spell.)
	Repeat METHODIST EPISCOPAL
	    "Mescobal Piscobal"

Copy CROSS
    Wanted to draw it again to make it
    larger.
	Write SQUARE

Name CROSS	Read SEVEN Could not read.
Spell CROSS " C - O --" (Could not spell.)	Repeat SEVEN
Copy TRIANGLE	Repeat/Explain HE SHOUTED THE WARNING. "He shotted day warning." Explanation- Recognized element of danger.
Name TRIANGLE "Warning sign." Examiner questioned, but patient knew no other name.	Write HE SHOUTED THE WARNING. Did not know how to begin.
Spell TRIANGLE " W - " (Could not spell.)	Compute 85 - 27 =" 67 "
Name BABY	Compute 17 X 3 =

Write CLOCK
    Could not write - did not know how
    to begin.
	Name KEY

Name FORK "Spoon"	Demonstrate use of KEY
Read 7 SIX 2 " 7 - - - 2." Did not know letters.	Draw KEY
Read MGW	Read PLACE LEFT HAND TO RIGHT EAR. Was able to read only the word "to."
Reading I " See the ----- boy."	Place LEFT HAND TO RIGHT EAR Tried to put right hand to right elbow.

Reading II
  " He is a ---, -- a -- ---
  to --- --."
	Place LEFT HAND TO LEFT ELBOW

85
- 27
 67   51

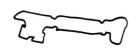

A.B.

1. S QUARE
2. square

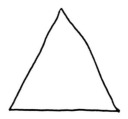

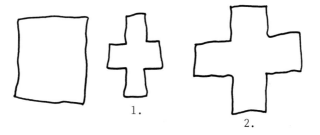

1.

2.

inadequate education. In addition, however, there are certain findings indicating the type of impairment that may be associated with craniocerebral trauma.

Measures of lateral dominance indicated that the patient was definitely right-handed. Nevertheless, his grip strength was a little weaker in his right upper extremity (39.0 kg) than his left (40.5 kg) and he performed particularly poorly on a complex manipulatory task (Tactual Performance Test) with his right hand (15.0 min).

Other findings suggested mild dysfunction of each cerebral hemisphere. A.B. had difficulty perceiving a tactile stimulus to each hand when given in competition with a stimulus to the face on the opposite side, but this was more prominent on the right hand than the left. The patient also made two errors in finger-tip number writing perception on his right hand but had no difficulty on his left hand. Considering the overall findings of this examination, the relationships of the results suggest that A.B. did experience some additional impairment of brain functions as a result of the traumatic incident that occurred about three years ago. His cognitive functions (and their behavioral correlates) had apparently not developed very well before the accident, and the effects of the craniocerebral trauma left him even less capable of functional performances. Therefore, when the accident occurred, A.B. was probably in a marginal condition and the additional impairment of brain functions was sufficient to render him incapable of normal independent occupational functioning.

In summary, the neuropsychological test results indicate that A.B. has significant dysfunction of brain-related abilities and is particularly impaired in the area of abstraction, reasoning, and logical analysis. We would predict that it is very difficult for him to understand complex situations and be able to make sense of them. He cannot be expected to analyze situations, perform in accordance with obvious needs, or engage in tasks that require serial analysis as the nature of the problem

unfolds. He does appear to have fairly good memory functions in an immediate sense, but his impairment in logical analysis and reasoning will preclude the prospect of his memory being usefully employed.

Although motor and manipulatory skills represented the patient's best abilities, he was not very proficient in this regard either. It is possible that he might be able to perform a simple manual type of job, but it is also possible that his headaches are sufficiently severe to interfere considerably with this prospect. Neuropsychological examination is not a basis for evaluating the headaches; however, we can see that this man's cognitive ability structure is quite limited and the stress that he would experience by attempting to engage in competitive employment would undoubtedly be difficult for him.

Because A.B.'s test results and history do not indicate the presence of progressive brain damage one might consider him a candidate for brain training. Given a presumably static biological condition of the brain, it is possible that some progress might be made with a vigorous program. Although we were not able to do brain retraining with A.B., we would postulate that any training efforts would have had limited success at best.

This prediction stems from our experience with patients having a similar ability structure and comparable deficits. First, it would be necessary to make up for nearly a total absence of academic training and experience in a person who has limited intelligence in addition to cerebral damage. Second, the severe impairment of reasoning and conceptual abilities (demonstrated by his score on the Category Test) would have a very limiting effect on the patient's potential for improvement.

It is possible, of course, to teach a person basic skills in abstraction, logical thinking, comprehending and postulating cause-and-effect relationships, and generally in "learning how to learn." We have found this type of deficit to be prominent in many children with learning disabilities, and the secret to teaching them academic skills is to initially concentrate on tasks that improve reasoning and abstraction abilities. However, in this case, the neuropsychological deficits are so widespread and stem from such a long history that we would predict only rather limited progress.

Some additional comments should be made regarding how it is possible to infer cerebral damage in persons with minimal educational backgrounds and limited general intelligence. The problem for many neuropsychologists is that they rely upon a level-of-performance method of inference to interpret the data. We must emphasize that level of performance (i.e., how well the patient performs on various tests) is *not* the approach to use in these types of cases. Intelligence is a variable that is normally distributed and some persons will have quite high values, others will demonstrate quite low values, and most of the sample (or population) will fall toward the center of the distribution.

Obviously, principles for inferring the presence of cerebral damage in a specific individual cannot be based solely upon the level of performance. Many bright and capable persons sustain brain damage, continue to perform better than the average on most (if not all) neuropsychological measures, and still are significantly impaired. The same consideration applies to persons with average intelligence or persons with intelligence levels below average.

From a clinical viewpoint it is necessary to use an approach to interpretation that is valid and relevant *for the individual subject*. We realized that it would be necessary to devise multiple methods of inference in order to accomplish this purpose (Reitan, 1966; Reitan, 1967b; Reitan & Wolfson, 1985a). Therefore, the Halstead-Reitan Battery was developed to measure not only the individual's level of proficiency in a broad number of areas but also evaluates (1) specific deficits that occur almost exclusively among persons with cerebral damage

(the "sign" approach); (2) patterns and relationships among test results as they reflect the differential functioning of various areas of the cerebral cortex and show deviations that go beyond normal limits; and (3) comparisons of the individual's functional efficiency on the two sides of the body.

The Halstead-Reitan Battery evaluates both motor (output) and sensory (input) skills ranging from simple to complex tasks in order to determine whether the relationships between the two sides of the body deviate from normal expectancy. Regardless of the general intelligence and educational background of the subject, comprehensive interpretation of the Halstead-Reitan Battery requires assessment using all of these methods of inference, assessing the several sub-batteries as they relate differentially to each of these approaches, and integrating the interpretation into a statement of overall brain-behavior relationships for the individual subject.

When evaluating a person with poor educational background and limited abilities, the methods of inference that depend upon interindividual comparisons are less useful than those that depend upon intraindividual evaluation. The level-of-performance approach compares the subject's scores with scores obtained by other individuals. Using this method alone, it is obvious that persons of lesser ability will compare poorly with persons having greater abilities.

The "sign" approach, an attempt to identify specific deficits that occur principally among persons with cerebral damage, is also based fundamentally on interindividual comparisons. For example, in the general population some people will draw poor geometric figures and others will do quite well. Even in performances representing limited skill, this approach often permits identification of specific deficits that tend to occur only among persons with cerebral damage. If the "sign" approach produces positive findings, the results may be helpful in identifying cerebral damage even in a person with low general abilities.

The method of inference that depends upon evaluating comparative intraindividual performances may be quite useful, but the clearest disparities of intraindividual ability structure occur in persons who initially had higher levels of ability and then sustained specific and discrete areas of deficit. This particular approach is sometimes not as helpful as it might be in persons who have always had generally low abilities or in persons who have experienced severe, widespread impairment of previously existing abilities (such as patients with Alzheimer's disease.)

The fourth inferential approach, based upon comparisons of performances on the two sides of the patient's own body, is frequently useful when evaluating persons with generally low abilities. This method is often critically significant in evaluations of children, whose abilities are in a developmental stage and are often rather variable (even among normal subjects).

A critical approach in A.B.'s case would be the evaluation of overall findings to determine whether performances on the two sides of the body deviate beyond normal expectancy. We saw that A.B.'s level of performance was generally limited. He did not do well on the Wechsler Scale and as we would expect from his general intelligence and educational limitations, performed poorly on most of the other measures.

From the pattern of test results one could not presume that A.B. had achieved abilities that even approached the normal level. On the Tactual Performance Test his relatively good scores on the third trial and the Memory and Localization components support the hypothesis of a relatively stabilized condition of the brain rather than to establish a level of performance that should have been achieved by all of the other measures in the Battery.

It is difficult to use a differential score approach effectively because A.B. demonstrated deficits on so many of the tests. It appears that he performed more poorly on difficult tasks that required a higher level of intellectual and cognitive function (such as the Category Test and Part B of the Trail Making Test) than on lower-level tests of brain functions (such as finger tapping and certain sensory-perceptual measures) but disparities of this kind cannot be used to make definite conclusions about recent craniocerebral trauma. Such findings are not uncommon, even among patients with a life-long history of mental retardation.

In this case the "sign" approach yielded some of the most valuable information about the patient's cognitive status. The Aphasia Screening Test indicated that A.B. had had limited academic skills, and results from the Wide Range Achievement Test and the patient's educational history certainly confirms this finding. Therefore, the fact that the patient had very limited reading and spelling ability could not be used as a basis to diagnose brain damage.

Note, though, that A.B. made certain mistakes more commonly seen among persons with cerebral damage than among persons with limited academic backgrounds or poor general intelligence. First, he misnamed the FORK as "spoon," a finding that tends to occur among persons with left cerebral damage. Despite his limited reading ability, he was able to read certain simple words and identify the individual letters MGW. However, when asked to read 7 SIX 2 he became entirely confused by the letters and could not read them as a word or even as individual letters. Confusion on this particular item is another type of deficit frequently manifested by persons with left cerebral damage. These two findings were strongly suggestive of damage to the left cerebral hemisphere rather than limited academic skills.

Certain other responses made by A.B. (such as his pronunciation of MASSACHUSETTS and METHODIST EPISCOPAL) would probably be considered indicative of left cerebral damage if they had been made by a subject who had more formal academic background. For A.B., mistakes of this kind (as well as a number of others, including possible right-left confusion) might possibly be attributable to poor training.

The patient's drawings were also mildly suggestive of impaired brain functions (especially the notches on the stem of the key near the handle which deviate in the same direction — a common finding in persons with right cerebral damage) but findings of this kind are also sometimes seen in persons with life-long ability limitations.

A.B.'S arithmetical skills, interpreted in the context of his other deficits, suggest that his abilities may have been better in the past than they presently appear to be. It was particularly impressive that the patient was able to write the correct answer to 17×3, again demonstrating a disparity in various manifestations of arithmetical abilities. In this case, then, the "sign" approach would definitely suggest that A.B.'s cognitive impairment was due to a recent insult of the brain rather than his life-long limitations.

By far the most convincing evidence of fairly recent craniocerebral damage was derived from comparisons of performances on the two sides of the body. Measures of lateral dominance indicated that A.B. was strongly right-handed; therefore, we would expect him to perform better on motor tasks (such as finger tapping) with his right hand. (Recall that no difference is expected in accordance with lateral dominance for sensory-perceptual tests used in the Halstead-Reitan Battery.)

A.B. showed rather convincing lateralized disparities involving the left cerebral hemisphere. We see that he (1) had less grip strength with his right hand (39.0 kg) than his left (40.5 kg); (2) performed rather poorly on the Tactual Performance Test with his right upper extremity (15.0 min)

compared with his left (6.2 min); (3) had a pronounced tendency to fail to perceive a tactile stimulus to the right hand when it was given simultaneously to the left side of the face; and (4) had some difficulty in finger-tip number writing perception on his right hand (2 errors) but made no mistakes with his left hand. These results go beyond expectation for persons with limited educational and intellectual skills and are sufficient to support a conclusion of left cerebral dysfunction.

A.B. also demonstrated both motor and tactile-receptive deficits on the left side of the body, indicating right cerebral hemisphere dysfunction. His finger tapping speed was slightly reduced with the left hand and there was a tendency to fail to perceive a tactile stimulus to the left hand when given in competition with the right side of the face. We would also consider the very mild deficits in the drawing of the key as a complementary indicator of right cerebral impairment.

An overall evaluation of the results strongly indicates that A.B. has sustained cerebral damage in addition to having low general intelligence levels and limited educational opportunities. It was possible to draw such inferences on the basis of a careful evaluation of specific deficits using the "sign" approach, and, more significantly, the disparities of performances on the two sides of the body.

The fact that the deficits involve both cerebral hemispheres (even though the left hemisphere was more involved than the right) further exemplifies a rather typical finding in cases of head injury. In fact, A.B.'s overall results are quite characteristic of a person with limited general intelligence and minimal academic competence who has sustained brain damage from a closed head injury.

CASE #19

Name: L.H.

Age: 43

Education: 8

Sex: Male

Handedness: Right

Occupation: Mechanic

Background Information

L.H. had surgery for two herniated lumbar discs about ten years before this hospital admission. Approximately three years later he had surgical repair of bilateral inguinal hernias. He was admitted to the hospital this time shortly after having been involved in a serious moving vehicle accident. While under the influence of alcohol L.H. crossed the center line on a highway and drove directly into the path of another vehicle; two people in the other car were killed. The patient, who was alone in his car, suffered multiple injuries, including a laceration of the left wrist, ecchymosis of the right knee, bruising and swelling of the left ankle, and a severe head injury with a laceration in the mid-forehead area with an underlying fracture of the left frontal bone near the midline.

Neurological Examination

L.H.'s state of consciousness was impaired at the time of admission; he was actively restless but did not verbalize. His pupils were equal and reactive to light; extraocular muscle functions and the fundi were within normal limits. Both tympanic membranes were intact but the membrane in the left external auditory canal had a slightly more bluish color. Neurological examination was within normal limits. Cranial nerve functions appeared to be intact. The patient moved all extremities with good strength and muscle stretch reflexes were equal and active. Upon admission to

the hospital L.H. experienced a small right pneumothorax followed by a complete collapse of the lung a few hours later.

The patient gradually regained consciousness and showed improvement. However, he appeared to have a short attention span and sometimes answered questions and offered comments in a rather superficial and inappropriate manner. An electroencephalogram done nine days after admission to the hospital was normal. Because L.H. appeared clinically to be impaired and inappropriate in his mentation he was kept in the hospital longer than his physical condition warranted in order to see if he would show some improvement in mental functioning. He was discharged from the hospital nearly four weeks after admission. Neuropsychological examination was done 18 days after the injury.

Neuropsychological Examination

L. H. earned Verbal (75), Performance (70), and Full Scale (70) IQ values in the range of Borderline intelligence, exceeding approximately 2%–5% of his age peers. Although he performed considerably better on Information (8) than the other ten subtests, scores on all of the subtests were well below the average level. This man had completed only eight years of school and a question might be raised regarding his pre-morbid intelligence level. There is no evidence from the Wechsler subtests to indicate that L.H. had ever had intellectual abilities that were even as high as the average level; however, the score on the Information subtest, compared with the other scores, suggests that he may have experienced some impairment on both Verbal and Performance subtests.

L.H. showed evidence of severe deficit on the four most sensitive measures in the HRNTB. The Impairment Index of 0.9 indicated that he consistently performed poorly; the only normal score on Halstead's tests was the finger tapping speed of the preferred hand (56). The patient performed very poorly on the Category Test (128). He was able to do the first and second subtests and showed a little improvement from the fifth to the sixth subtests (when the principle was repeated) but had only a chance number of correct responses on subtests three, four, five, and seven. It is apparent from these results that L.H.'s ability in reasoning and logical analysis was quite limited.

The patient demonstrated similar impairment on Part B of the Trail Making Test. He worked for 90 seconds, repeatedly made errors, and reached only the third circle. He had been able to complete the sample for Part B with constant direction and instruction from the examiner, but when he attempted to solve Part B independently he became totally confused. His drawing of the Tactual Performance Test board was very limited and inaccurate; he was able to recall four of the ten figures but could not localize any of them correctly. In fact, the patient performed poorly on every test administered except for finger tapping speed with the right hand and the tests of bilateral simultaneous sensory stimulation. He was too confused to be able to complete the Minnesota Multiphasic Personality Inventory.

An important question and one which neuropsychologists are often asked to answer might be raised at this point: Was this man always defective in his intellectual functioning or were the deficits a result of the recent brain trauma? In all probability, both of these factors contributed to his poor performances and the question cannot be answered

on the basis of general indicators and a level-of-performance inferential approach. In cases of severe generalized impairment, such as this one, identification of specific deficits and comparisons of performances on the two sides on the body contribute greatly to the identification of effects of brain damage.

This patient showed distinct and definite lateralizing signs that implicated both cerebral hemispheres. His grip strength was sharply reduced in his right upper extremity (9.0 kg) compared with his left (16.5 kg). The right-sided weakness was very probably due to left cerebral damage since there was no medical evidence to suggest any specific damage to the right upper extremity. However, considering the fact that the patient showed definite tactile-perceptual losses on the right side — as well as mild dysphasia — this inference can be drawn from the neuropsychological test results alone. Although his ability on the Tactile Form Recognition Test was at least mildly impaired on both sides, he took nearly twice as long to identify the figures with his right hand (22 sec) than his left (12 sec). L.H. had comparatively even more difficulty in tactile finger localization with the right hand (11 errors), although the four errors on the left hand also pointed toward some degree of deficit.

Interestingly, this patient was able to perform the more difficult task of finger-tip number perception with fewer errors than he made in the test for tactile finger localization. Results of this kind are somewhat unusual, but when they do occur they lend credence to the results of the finger localization test as indicators of cerebral damage. Thus, L.H. not only had evidence of impairment of motor strength on the right side but also demonstrated more serious tactile-perceptual deficits on the right side than the left. The likelihood of a cerebral lesion increases when both of these types of deficits are present.

THE HALSTEAD-REITAN
NEUROPSYCHOLOGICAL TEST BATTERY

Patient _____**L.H.**_____ Age __**43**__ Sex __**M**__ Education __**8**__ Handedness __**R**__

WECHSLER-BELLEVUE SCALE

VIQ	75
PIQ	70
FS IQ	70

Information	8
Comprehension	4
Digit Span	3
Arithmetic	4
Similarities	3
Vocabulary	4

Picture Arrangement	3
Picture Completion	3
Block Design	4
Object Assembly	0
Digit Symbol	5

TRAIL MAKING TEST

Part A: __**50**__ seconds
Part B: Discontinued at "2"; 90 seconds, 6 errors

STRENGTH OF GRIP

Dominant hand:	**9.0**	kilograms
Non-dominant hand:	**16.5**	kilograms

REITAN-KLØVE TACTILE FORM RECOGNITION TEST

Dominant hand:	**22**	seconds;	**1**	errors
Non-dominant hand:	**12**	seconds;	**1**	errors

REITAN-KLØVE SENSORY-PERCEPTUAL EXAM — No errors

				Error Totals	
RH ___ LH ___	Both H:	RH ___ LH ___		RH ___ LH ___	
RH ___ LF ___	Both H/F:	RH ___ LF ___		RH ___ LF ___	
LH ___ RF ___	Both H/F:	LH ___ RF ___		RF ___ LH ___	
RE ___ LE ___	Both E:	RE ___ LE ___		RE ___ LE ___	
RV ___ LV ___	Both:	RV ___ LV ___		RV ___ LV ___	

TACTILE FINGER RECOGNITION

R 1___ 2 **2** 3 **2** 4 **4** 5 **3**   R **11** / **20**

L 1___ 2___ 3___ 4 **2** 5 **2**   L **4** / **20**

FINGER-TIP NUMBER WRITING

R 1 **2** 2 **1** 3 **1** 4 **1** 5 ___   R **5** / **20**

L 1___ 2___ 3___ 4___ 5 **2**   L **2** / **20**

HALSTEAD'S NEUROPSYCHOLOGICAL TEST BATTERY

Category Test	128

Tactual Performance Test

Dominant hand:	**15.0 (6 blocks)**
Non-dominant hand:	**15.0 (5 blocks)**
Both hands:	**11.0**

Total Time	**41.0 (21 blocks)**
Memory	4
Localization	0

Seashore Rhythm Test

Number Correct	**18**	10

Speech-sounds Perception Test

Number of Errors	28

Finger Oscillation Test

Dominant hand:	**56**	56
Non-dominant hand:	**41**	

Impairment Index	0.9

REITAN-KLØVE
LATERAL-DOMINANCE EXAM

Show me how you:

throw a ball	R
hammer a nail	R
cut with a knife	R
turn a door knob	R
use scissors	R
use an eraser	R
write your name	R

Record time used for spontaneous name-writing:

Preferred hand	**12**	seconds
Non-preferred hand	**23**	seconds

Show me how you:

kick a football	R
step on a bug	R

REITAN-INDIANA APHASIA SCREENING TEST

Form for Adults and Older Children

Name: _____L. H._____ Age: __43___

Copy SQUARE	Repeat TRIANGLE

Name SQUARE
          "Rectangular"
	Repeat MASSACHUSETTS
	          "Massatussus"

Spell SQUARE "S-Q-U-A-I-R." Examiner asked him to try it again. "S-Q-U-I-R-E."	Repeat METHODIST EPISCOPAL "Methodist Depiscopol"
Copy CROSS	Write SQUARE
Name CROSS "Square"	Read SEVEN
Spell CROSS	Repeat SEVEN
Copy TRIANGLE	Repeat/Explain HE SHOUTED THE WARNING.
Name TRIANGLE	Write HE SHOUTED THE WARNING.
Spell TRIANGLE	Compute 85 – 27 = Confused. (See text)
Name BABY	Compute 17 X 3 = Confused. (See text)
Write CLOCK	Name KEY
Name FORK	Demonstrate use of KEY
Read 7 SIX 2	Draw KEY
Read MGW	Read PLACE LEFT HAND TO RIGHT EAR.
Reading I "S-E-E," examiner asked him to read words rather than letters. Then OK.	Place LEFT HAND TO RIGHT EAR
Reading II	Place LEFT HAND TO LEFT ELBOW Right hand to right ear. Examiner questioned. Then right hand to right elbow.

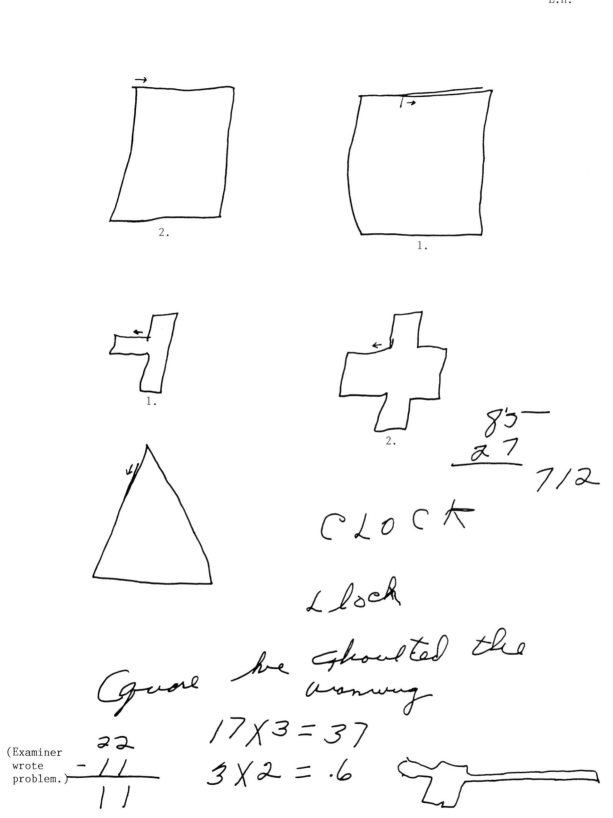

2.

1.

1.

2.

8'5
27
——
712

CLOCK

Llock

Cquore he Cshourted the uranung

17 X 3 = 37

3 X 2 = .6

(Examiner wrote problem.)

22
- 11
——
11

The patient did not show any gross evidence of aphasia and casual clinical neurological examination had not revealed any such deficits. This case provides an excellent example of the advantage of using a standardized procedure such as the Aphasia Screening Test to evaluate aphasic symptoms.

When asked to name the SQUARE, the patient responded "rectangular." This type of response is not characteristic of persons with limited educational backgrounds; it occurs much more frequently in patients with left cerebral damage. It was necessary for the examiner to tell L.H. the name of the figure before asking him to spell the name. L.H. spelled SQUARE incorrectly twice but made different errors each time. This type of inconsistency in spelling is also seen in persons with left cerebral damage.

When he was asked to name the CROSS this man demonstrated both dysnomia and verbal perseveration by calling the figure a "square." Perseveration from the figure previously presented, even though attempts to copy the cross had intervened, are not uncommonly seen in persons with left cerebral damage.

The patient also demonstrated his limited ability to deal with simple verbal material when asked to read SEE THE BLACK DOG. Even though he had the ability to read the words, he began by reading the individual letters. He did not read the words until the examiner explicitly asked him to do so.

The errors made in enunciating MASSACHUSETTS and METHODIST EPISCOPAL are probably not indicative of left cerebral damage. It is possible that addition of the "D" sound before the beginning of EPISCOPAL is related to brain damage, but this is a very rare response and has uncertain significance concerning neuropsychological functions.

Finally, the patient became confused when asked to place his left hand to his left elbow. Initially he put his right hand to his right ear. This response probably indicates some degree of right-left confusion and also raises a question of body dysgnosia. However, except in patients with severe and pervasive dysphasia (manifested by difficulty on many items in the test), body dysgnosia is rarely observed. The examiner gave the instructions again and L.H. responded by attempting to put his right hand to his right elbow. Thus, the patient's initial mistake may have been attributable to general confusion. It is likely, however, that the responses indicated specific right-left confusion, another sign of left cerebral damage.

L.H.'s examples of writing give clear indications of dysgraphia. Initially he printed the word "clock" and the examiner asked him to write the word. His confusion in writing is apparent in both the initial "C" and the confusion in forming the "K." When he was shown the printed letters SQUARE and asked to write the word, L.H. did not get started correctly and wrote a "C" instead of an "S." When asked to write HE SHOUTED THE WARNING the patient also demonstrated confusion in forming the letters appropriately. Although his script suggests that he had had adequate background and experience in learning to write letters, he had obvious difficulty with the words HE, SHOUTED, and WARNING. These problems do not appear to be limited to spelling but represent deficits in the formation of the appropriate letters (dysgraphia).

The patient was also quite confused when attempting to solve simple arithmetic problems. He was not able to figure out how to proceed with $85 - 27 =$. He wrote the answer to the side because he was trying to get some idea of how to continue before entering the answer in the appropriate place; finally he had to discontinue his effort. The examiner then wrote an easier problem ($22 - 11 =$) for the patient to solve. Although L.H. identified this problem as involving division he proceeded to subtract correctly. L.H. insisted on writing "17 × 3" on the paper instead of trying to do the problem mentally, but even then he was not able to solve it correctly. He did answer "3 × 2" correctly except that he entered a decimal point before the "6." These results make it quite clear that the patient was distinctly and definitely confused in dealing with simple arithmetical processes (dyscalculia). All of these deficits (dysnomia, spelling dyspraxia, dysgraphia, and dyscalculia) occur much more commonly in patients with left rather than right cerebral lesions (Wheeler & Reitan, 1962).

Finally, L.H. showed definite signs of constructional dyspraxia. In his first attempt to copy the cross he omitted the right lateral extremity entirely. In his second attempt he failed to achieve symmetry, particularly of the lateral extremities. He also had great difficulty copying the key, distorting the spatial relationships of parts of the figure and totally omitting the handle. These indications of constructional dyspraxia are quite typical of right cerebral damage.

L.H. also showed further evidence of involvement of the right cerebral hemisphere. Finger tapping speed was significantly slow with the left hand (41) compared with the right (56). It is somewhat unusual for grip strength and finger tapping to dissociate in their lateralizing significance, but this does occur sometimes and appears to be a valid indication of lateralized involvement (left or right) for each hemisphere. It is entirely possible that impaired motor strength and motor speed have somewhat different pathological bases, but the etiology is unknown and in most cases the brain affects both strength and speed in a similar manner. L.H. also failed to show any improvement with his left hand (second trial) on the Tactual Performance Test, although he was capable of improving his performance when using both hands (third trial). Thus, several findings implicated the right cerebral hemisphere, including (1) primary motor speed; (2) complex manipulatory skill with the left upper extremity; and (3) constructional dyspraxia.

The overall results were consistent in suggesting cerebral damage that involved the brain generally. Typical of significant cerebral trauma, the neuropsychological test results implicated each cerebral hemisphere in a context indicating generalized brain dysfunction. Although we did not have the opportunity to follow this patient, research studies have demonstrated that improvement is likely to occur in time, especially considering the fact that L.H.'s cerebral injury had been sustained less than three weeks before the examination.

CASE #20

Name: R.C.

Age: 33

Education: 10

Sex: Male

Handedness: Right

Occupation: Auto mechanic

Background Information

Approximately nine years before this neuropsychological evaluation R.C. was involved in an accident in which he was thrown from a moving car and struck his head on the pavement. A bilateral craniotomy had to be performed to remove an epidural hematoma. It was clear that the patient had significant generalized impairment of brain functions besides the localized damage; in fact, the patient says that he "lost eight months of life" because he could not remember anything that happened for that period of time following the injury.

Within a few months after the injury R.C. began to have seizures which were frequently preceded by an onset of feeling generally ill and followed by a loss of consciousness lasting up to one hour. About three years after the head injury the aura preceding the convulsions and loss of consciousness changed to what the patient described as a "drunk" feeling, with objects spinning around him. About six months before the present examination the patient found more competent neurological treatment of his seizures and after careful adjustments of the amount and type of antiepileptic medications he had experienced no additional seizures for four months. Prior to his head injury the patient had been an automobile mechanic but because of his cognitive deficits and his frequent epileptic attacks he had not been able to work regularly since sustaining the injury.

Neurological Examination

At present the neurological examination was essentially negative. Plain x-rays of the skull showed evidence of the craniotomy done shortly after the injury. Bilateral cerebral angiograms were within normal limits. Electroencephalographic tracings showed slow wave activity in the right Sylvian area and was thought to be a result of the earlier head trauma.

The patient's neurosurgeon felt that R.C.'s cognitive abilities were deteriorating and decided to perform additional diagnostic procedures. A pneumoencephalogram showed a mild dilatation of the ventricular cavities but the ventricles were symmetrical and showed no displacement. A ventriculogram using positive contrast material demonstrated the ventricular system quite clearly and it was apparent that the anterior horns of the lateral ventricles were more dilated than other ventricular areas. On the basis of this finding it was concluded that the patient had cerebral atrophy, particularly involving the frontal lobes and probably resulting from traumatic injury that occurred more than nine years previously. Thus, the neurological evaluation described a person who had sustained a very severe head injury more than nine years earlier, experienced many severe epileptic attacks in the interim and presently showed evidence of mild generalized cerebral atrophy particularly demonstrating degeneration of the frontal lobes.

In this kind of case one would expect that any strong lateralizing findings would have resolved, at least to some extent, and the test results would demonstrate generalized impairment involving the more complex tests of higher-level brain functions rather than pronounced sensory-perceptual and motor losses and deficits on highly specific types of tasks. Of course, a generalization of this type depends upon the severity of the initial losses and in this case there were no baseline findings to use for predictions.

Neuropsychological Evaluation

This man earned Verbal (102), Performance (101), and Full Scale (102) IQ values almost exactly at the Average level, exceeding 50%–55% of his age peers. Therefore, it appears that R.C.'s general intelligence is adequate. However, on the Verbal subtests, the patient earned his lowest scores on Information (6), Arithmetic (7), and Vocabulary (8). This particular pattern suggests that R.C. probably did not get as much from his formal education as the average person with these general ability levels. In other words, his Verbal IQ might have been higher if he had profited more from his educational experiences.

Results on the Performance subtests also showed a considerable degree of variability. It is probably not surprising that the patient performed somewhat poorly on Digit Symbol (8), the Wechsler subtest generally most sensitive to brain damage. It is possible that the poor score on Block Design (6) reflects right posterior cerebral dysfunction, but it would be difficult to draw such a conclusion on the basis of the Wechsler scores alone.

The four most sensitive indicators in the HRNTB yielded clear evidence of cerebral dysfunction. The Impairment Index of 0.7 showed that approximately 70% of Halstead's tests had scores in the brain-damaged range; only the Memory component (8) of the Tactual Performance Test and the Speech-sounds Perception Test (5) were done well. The patient performed considerably worse than the average brain-damaged subject on the Category Test (79), had probably an even poorer performance on Part B of the Trail Making Test (178 sec), and was significantly into the impaired range on the Localization component (2) of the Tactual Performance Test. By comparing these scores to the adequate IQ values we have a secure basis for concluding that R.C. had experienced impairment of adaptive abilities dependent upon brain functions (Reitan, 1985).

Findings indicating lateralization of deficits were not pronounced. The patient was somewhat slow on both the Tactual Performance Test Total Time (16.8 min) and the Finger Oscillation Test (RH-42; LH-37) but the relative performances of the two hands were approximately in the normal range. R.C. also showed this relationship on measurement of grip strength with the upper extremities (RH-44.5 kg; LH-40.5 kg). He had no difficulty whatsoever with tactile finger recognition (0 errors) and performed within the normal range on the Tactile Form Recognition Test.

Note, however, that there were some findings suggesting left cerebral dysfunction and others indicating involvement of the right cerebral hemisphere. The most pronounced sign of left cerebral dysfunction probably was shown on tests of bilateral simultaneous tactile stimulation. The patient had a definite tendency to fail to perceive the stimulus to his right hand when a competing stimulus was given to the left face.

In his repetition of MASSACHUSETTS this man demonstrated an enunciatory error. The repetition of sounds at the end of the word is not a matter of slurring (as seen in many persons without left cerebral damage) but instead is rather characteristic of the type of enunciatory difficulty seen in persons with damage of the left cerebral hemisphere. The patient had a tendency to substitute an "A" for an "E" sound in repeating METHODIST EPISCOPAL, but this is a fairly common occurrence among control subjects. (The reader should note that R.C.'s ability to respond within

THE HALSTEAD-REITAN
NEUROPSYCHOLOGICAL TEST BATTERY

Patient **R.C.** Age **33** Sex **M** Education **10** Handedness **R**

WECHSLER-BELLEVUE SCALE

VIQ	102
PIQ	101
FS IQ	102

Information	6
Comprehension	14
Digit Span	9
Arithmetic	7
Similarities	12
Vocabulary	8

Picture Arrangement	11
Picture Completion	12
Block Design	6
Object Assembly	9
Digit Symbol	8

TRAIL MAKING TEST

Part A: **45** seconds
Part B: **178** seconds

STRENGTH OF GRIP

Dominant hand: **44.5** kilograms

Non-dominant hand: **40.5** kilograms

REITAN-KLØVE TACTILE FORM RECOGNITION TEST

Dominant hand: **11** seconds; **0** errors

Non-dominant hand: **9** seconds; **0** errors

REITAN-KLØVE SENSORY-PERCEPTUAL EXAM

			Error Totals
RH___LH___	Both H: RH___LH___	RH___LH___	
RH___LF___	Both H/F: RH _2_ LF___	RH _2_ LF___	
LH___RF___	Both H/F: LH___RF___	RF___LH___	
RE___LE___	Both E: RE___LE___	RE___LE___	
RV___LV___	Both V: RV___LV___	RV___LV___	

TACTILE FINGER RECOGNITION

R 1___2___3___4___5___ R **0** / **20**

L 1___2___3___4___5___ L **0** / **20**

FINGER-TIP NUMBER WRITING

R 1 **1** 2___3___4 **1** 5___ R **2** / **20**

L 1___2___3___4___5___ L **0** / **20**

HALSTEAD'S NEUROPSYCHOLOGICAL TEST BATTERY

Category Test 79

Tactual Performance Test

Dominant hand:	**7.3**
Non-dominant hand:	**5.2**
Both hands:	**4.3**

Total Time	16.8
Memory	8
Localization	2

Seashore Rhythm Test

Number Correct **21** 10

Speech-sounds Perception Test

Number of Errors 5

Finger Oscillation Test

Dominant hand:	42	42
Non-dominant hand:	37	

Impairment Index **0.7**

MINNESOTA MULTIPHASIC PERSONALITY INVENTORY

		Hs	72
		D	75
?	50	Hy	76
L	66	Pd	69
F	60	Mf	67
K	64	Pa	50
		Pt	54
		Sc	63
		Ma	50

REITAN-KLØVE LATERAL-DOMINANCE EXAM

Show me how you:	
throw a ball	R
hammer a nail	R
cut with a knife	R
turn a door knob	R
use scissors	R
use an eraser	R
write your name	R

Record time used for spontaneous name-writing:	
Preferred hand	**9** seconds
Non-preferred hand	**32** seconds

Show me how you:	
kick a football	R
step on a bug	R

REITAN-INDIANA APHASIA SCREENING TEST

Form for Adults and Older Children

Name: _____R. C._____ Age: ___33___

Copy SQUARE	Repeat TRIANGLE "Triango"
Name SQUARE	Repeat MASSACHUSETTS "Massachusesses"
Spell SQUARE	Repeat METHODIST EPISCOPAL "Mathodist Episcapal"
Copy CROSS	Write SQUARE
Name CROSS "An X;" Examiner questioned. "What the Red Cross wears." Examiner questioned again. Could not improve response.	Read SEVEN
Spell CROSS	Repeat SEVEN
Copy TRIANGLE	Repeat/Explain HE SHOUTED THE WARNING.

Name TRIANGLE
      "Diamond." Examiner questioned.
      "Triangle."
	Write HE SHOUTED THE WARNING.

Spell TRIANGLE	Compute 85 − 27 =
Name BABY	Compute 17 X 3 = "48." Additional problems used. 7 x 9 = "56"; 8 x 4 = "32"; 8 x 2 = "16."
Write CLOCK	Name KEY
Name FORK	Demonstrate use of KEY
Read 7 SIX 2	Draw KEY
Read MGW	Read PLACE LEFT HAND TO RIGHT EAR.
Reading I	Place LEFT HAND TO RIGHT EAR
Reading II	Place LEFT HAND TO LEFT ELBOW

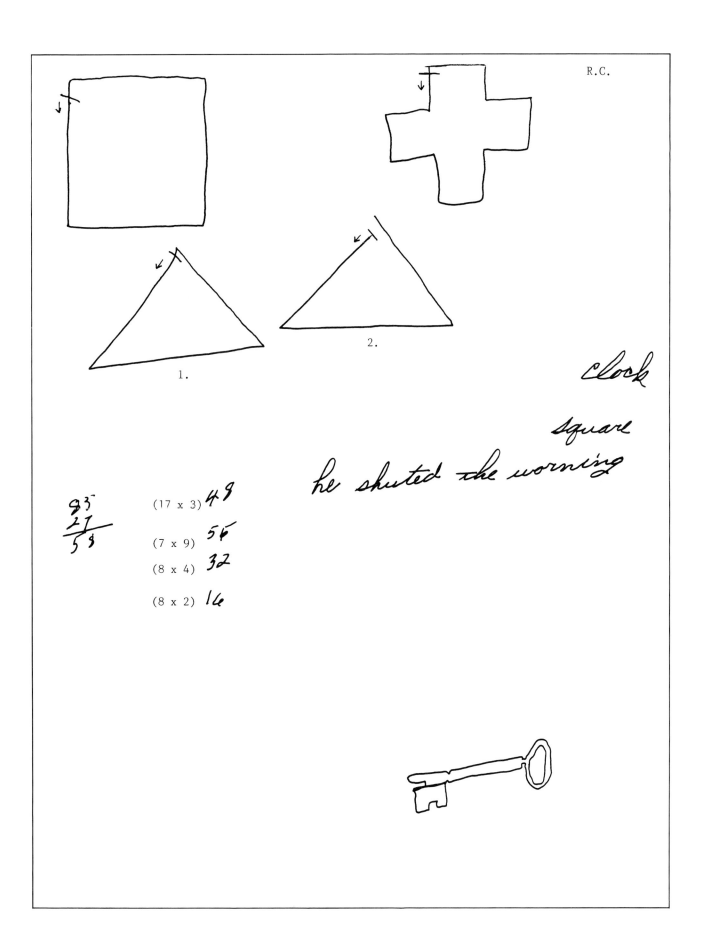

R.C.

1.

2.

clock

square

he shuted the worning

93
27
5 3

(17 x 3) 4 9

(7 x 9) 5 6

(8 x 4) 32

(8 x 2) 16

normal limits on METHODIST EPISCOPAL does not excuse his error made in repeating MASSACHUSETTS).

Finally, the patient had some difficulty in finger-tip number writing perception on his right hand, but it is possible that his attention lapsed twice when stimuli were being delivered to the right hand and was able to pay attention more carefully in every instance of stimulation to the left hand. Although these impaired findings provide some specific indications of left cerebral dysfunction, the excellent score (5) on the Speechsounds Perception Test — particularly for a person who may not have had very adequate educational training — strongly suggests that the left cerebral hemisphere is not acutely embarrassed in a biological sense.

The patient demonstrated mild difficulty in writing HE SHOUTED THE WARNING; SHOUTED as "shuted" is suspicious of left cerebral dysfunction. However, failure to drop the line after the "A" in WARNING occurs fairly frequently among normal subjects and has no particular neuropsychological significance.

The most pronounced indication of right cerebral damage was shown in the patient's drawing of the key. R.C. became somewhat confused with the notches on the stem near the handle but his major errors were the notches near the teeth (which are not symmetrical) and the confusion of the nose and the teeth. Difficulty of this kind indicates a problem in dealing with spatial relationships and is quite characteristic of persons with right cerebral damage.

It should also be noted that R.C. had particular difficulty with the triangle; he had a closure problem in both drawings. In the first drawing he was able to return to the starting point; in the second drawing, however, he did not close the figure, and we see this same kind of difficulty in his drawing of the square. We would judge, though, that the cross was within normal limits for a person who did not have particularly good skills in drawing.

Thus, the neuropsychological findings for this man indicated: (1) some definite signs of mild left cerebral dysfunction; (2) approximately equivalent definite indications of right cerebral dysfunction; and (3) a number of findings that were impaired with regard to level of performance. Other tests were done fairly well, particularly the Speechsounds Perception Test (5), the Memory component of the Tactual Performance Test (8), and the Tactile Finger Recognition Test (0 errors). These relatively good scores, in conjunction with evidence of generalized impairment on a number of brain-sensitive tests and mild positive indications of lateralized dysfunction, prevent us from postulating a focal lesion of either cerebral hemisphere. These findings are quite characteristic and typical of generalized cerebral dysfunction that is currently relatively chronic and static in nature. With this configuration of results we would not have predicted that the cerebral damage had occurred more than nine years before the examination, but the findings do suggest that the injury had been sustained some time ago (at least one to two years earlier).

Finally, results on the Minnesota Multiphasic Personality Inventory indicate that this man had some problems with the emotional aspects of adjustment. In evaluating patients who have sustained physical trauma it is necessary to consider the possibility that the responses to the MMPI cannot be interpreted in the same manner as identical responses given by patients with only psychiatric difficulties. In other words, it is entirely possible that some of the responses that contributed to R.C.'s elevated MMPI scores reflect valid symptoms of his neurological condition. It is equally possible, of course, that R.C. does have significant emotional problems of adjustment; in fact, it would be surprising if he did not have such difficulties considering the fact that his brain damage and epilepsy had disrupted his life to such an extent that he was not even able to work regularly for more than nine years.

HEAD INJURY CASE #21

Name: O.F.

Age: 35

Education: 8

Sex: Female

Handedness: Right

Occupation: None

Background Information

This 35-year-old woman was married, had one child and was apparently leading a relatively routine life until she sustained a serious head injury at the age of 27. We were not able to find out the details of the accident or the patient's immediate post-injury condition.

Since the injury O.F. had experienced two to three monthly episodes during which she developed a light-headed feeling, got dizzy, and had a major motor epileptic seizure. Following the seizure she was somewhat confused and sleepy and usually had severe generalized headaches. There was no history of other injury to the head or significant neurological illnesses. During her epileptic attacks O.F. had fallen and had scars from injuries and burns that she had sustained. She was treated with antiepileptic medication by her physician but only partial seizure control was achieved.

O.F. was divorced about six months prior to this examination and had moved in with her parents. During one seizure episode she reportedly attempted to take off her clothes in public and this precipitated her admission to a state mental institution for observation and evaluation. She was later transferred to a major medical center for a more complete evaluation. During the last year the patient had apparently had severe emotional problems, cried easily, and became increasingly frightened and insecure.

Neurological Examination

The general physical examination indicated that O.F. was definitely overweight and emotionally labile; she cried even when asked simple questions. Except for walking hesitatingly with a wide-based gait, the medical and neurological examinations were within normal limits. A definitely abnormal electroencephalogram with bilateral dysrhythmia of the posterior areas prompted O.F.'s physician to make adjustments in her antiepileptic medication. She was followed by the Epilepsy Clinic for approximately the next 15 months during which she had only one convulsive episode.

The neurological evaluation showed no evidence of a focal lesion of either cerebral hemisphere. The overall findings indicated a post-traumatic epilepsy secondary to craniocerebral trauma sustained eight years before this examination.

Neuropsychological Examination

Neuropsychological test results in a case of long-standing traumatic brain injury would be expected to principally show generalized indications of cerebral deficit. However, it is not unusual in such cases to find lateralizing indications involving both cerebral hemispheres in the context of generalized deficit. In this case we would expect the test results to be indicative of a chronic-static condition of brain dysfunction rather than show progressive pathological involvement.

This patient performed very poorly on the Wechsler Scale, earning both Verbal (63) and Performance (66) IQ values in the range of Mild Mental Retardation (exceeding less than 2% of her age peers). The scaled scores ranged from 0 (Arithmetic) to 6 (Similarities). Most of the subtest scores were 3, 4 ,or 5, indicating that the patient's intellectual functions were generally limited. There was no evidence to suggest specific impairment of any particular aspect of general intelligence or any indications that the patient had ever had normal intellectual functions.

In such an instance the reader may wonder whether further neuropsychological testing is indicated, since it is likely that the patient would perform poorly on nearly any test administered. In other words, Would it be possible to identify impaired brain functions in a person who had such limited general ability? A related question that is often asked concerns the IQ level at which it is possible to administer the Halstead-Reitan Neuropsychological Tests Battery.

There is a general correlation between IQ values and results obtained on other neuropsychological tests. Reitan (1956a) reported significant correlations in normal control groups as well as brain-damaged groups, with the pattern and configuration of correlation coefficients being essentially the same (in an overall sense) in both groups. The reliability of scores on both the Wechsler Scale and the Halstead-Reitan Battery probably decreases in patients who are not able to make much progress with the tasks. This is true because limited progress provides a limited base on which to generate a score. However, as a general guideline, one can say that if it is possible to give the Wechsler Scale to the patient it is also usually possible to administer the Halstead-Reitan Battery. In addition, the results obtained on the Halstead-Reitan Battery will generally allow the neuropsychologist to determine whether or not cerebral damage is a factor contributing to low ability levels.

Note, however, that such inferences are not supported by the adequacy of the patient's performances (i.e., a level-of-performance approach) because poor performances would usually be expected in patients with low IQ values. Instead, the determination of whether or not brain damage exists would be derived from other methods of inference, including the occurrence of specific pathognomonic performances, deviant patterns and relationships among the test results, and, especially, comparison of performances on the two sides of the body.

In O.F.'s case the four most sensitive general indicators in the Halstead-Reitan Battery were all performed quite poorly, as we would expect. Her Impairment Index was 1.0. In many patients with low IQ values a much better performance on the Tactual Performance Test would be seen. This patient's performance — a total of only 10 blocks placed in 45 minutes — is more characteristic of persons with low IQ values who have been impaired as a result of cerebral damage. On her drawing of the TPT board she was able to correctly localize only one of the shapes.

O.F. also performed much worse on the Category Test (139) than would be predicted solely on the basis of her IQ levels. She did very poorly on Part B of the Trail Making Test, requiring 300 seconds to progress up to the letter "D" and making six errors. Thus, the particularly deficient performances on these indicators of cerebral status suggest that O.F. has experienced brain damage. Although there is no evidence to indicate that she had ever developed IQ values that were higher than those presently shown, comparison with these other test results suggest that her IQ values may actually have been depressed by damage to the brain.

The test findings also have definite significance concerning the patient's general adaptive ability. The poor scores on the Seashore Rhythm Test (14 correct) and the Speech-sounds Perception

THE HALSTEAD-REITAN
NEUROPSYCHOLOGICAL TEST BATTERY

Patient __O.F.__ Age __35__ Sex __F__ Education __8__ Handedness __R__

WECHSLER-BELLEVUE SCALE

VIQ	63
PIQ	66
FS IQ	62

Information	3
Comprehension	3
Digit Span	3
Arithmetic	0
Similarities	6
Vocabulary	5

Picture Arrangement	4
Picture Completion	3
Block Design	4
Object Assembly	5
Digit Symbol	3

TRAIL MAKING TEST

Part A: __150__ seconds

Part B: Discontinued at D; 300 seconds and 6 errors

STRENGTH OF GRIP

Dominant hand: __16.5__ kilograms

Non-dominant hand: __18.0__ kilograms

REITAN-KLØVE TACTILE FORM RECOGNITION TEST

Dominant hand: __18__ seconds; __0__ errors

Non-dominant hand: __24__ seconds; __0__ errors

REITAN-KLØVE SENSORY-PERCEPTUAL EXAM – No errors

			Error Totals	
RH ___ LH ___	Both H: RH ___ LH ___		RH ___ LH ___	
RH ___ LF ___	Both H/F: RH ___ LF ___		RH ___ LF ___	
LH ___ RF ___	Both H/F: LH ___ RF ___		RF ___ LH ___	
RE ___ LE ___	Both E: RE ___ LE ___		RE ___ LE ___	
RV ___ LV ___	Both: RV ___ LV ___		RV ___ LV ___	
___ ___	___ ___			

TACTILE FINGER RECOGNITION

R 1___ 2___ 3 _1_ 4 ___ 5___ R _1_ / 20

L 1___ 2___ 3 ___ 4 _2_ 5___ L _2_ / 20

FINGER-TIP NUMBER WRITING

R 1 _3_ 2 _1_ 3 ___ 4 _2_ 5 _1_ R _7_ / 20

L 1___ 2___ 3 _1_ 4 ___ 5 _1_ L _2_ / 20

HALSTEAD'S NEUROPSYCHOLOGICAL TEST BATTERY

Category Test __139__

Tactual Performance Test

Dominant hand: __15.0 (4 blocks)__

Non-dominant hand: __15.0 (2 blocks)__

Both hands: __15.0 (4 blocks)__

Total Time	45.0 (10 blocks)	
Memory	3	
Localization	1	

Seashore Rhythm Test

Number Correct __14__ __10__

Speech-sounds Perception Test

Number of Errors __30__

Finger Oscillation Test

Dominant hand: __31__ __31__

Non-dominant hand: __29__

Impairment Index __1.0__

REITAN-KLØVE
LATERAL-DOMINANCE EXAM

Show me how you:
throw a ball	R
hammer a nail	R
cut with a knife	R
turn a door knob	R
use scissors	R
use an eraser	R
write your name	R

Record time used for spontaneous name-writing:
Preferred hand	__11__ seconds
Non-preferred hand	__13__ seconds

Show me how you:
kick a football	R
step on a bug	R

REITAN-INDIANA APHASIA SCREENING TEST

Form for Adults and Older Children

Name: _____O. F._____ Age: __35__

Copy SQUARE	Repeat TRIANGLE
Name SQUARE "Box." Examiner questioned. Then answered, "Square."	Repeat MASSACHUSETTS "Massatusses"
Spell SQUARE "S-Q-U-A-R-A-E"	Repeat METHODIST EPISCOPAL "Methobal Epistabal"
Copy CROSS	Write SQUARE
Name CROSS	Read SEVEN
Spell CROSS	Repeat SEVEN
Copy TRIANGLE	Repeat/Explain HE SHOUTED THE WARNING.
Name TRIANGLE Did not know. Couldn't guess.	Write HE SHOUTED THE WARNING.
Spell TRIANGLE "T-R-E-A-N-G-E-R-L-E"	Compute 85 − 27 =
Name BABY "Little infant"	Compute 17 X 3 =
Write CLOCK	Name KEY
Name FORK	Demonstrate use of KEY
Read 7 SIX 2 "7 − S − one − X − 2"	Draw KEY
Read MGW	Read PLACE LEFT HAND TO RIGHT EAR.
Reading I	Place LEFT HAND TO RIGHT EAR
Reading II "He is a friendly animal of a famous winter dog show."	Place LEFT HAND TO LEFT ELBOW OK, but had difficulty comprehending the instructions.

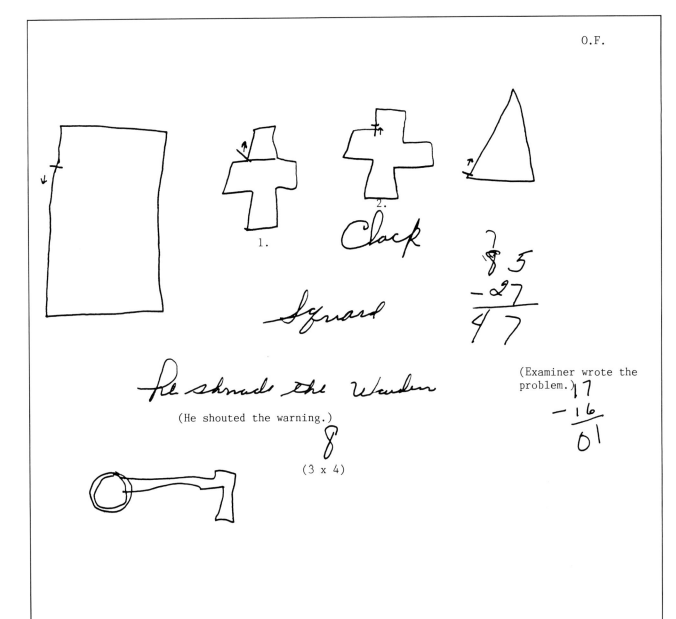

1.

Clock

2.

Square

$$
\begin{array}{r}
8\,5 \\
-27 \\
\hline
4\,7
\end{array}
$$

He shouted the Warden

(He shouted the warning.)

8

(3 x 4)

(Examiner wrote the problem.)

$$
\begin{array}{r}
17 \\
-16 \\
\hline
01
\end{array}
$$

Test (30 errors) suggest that this woman is significantly impaired in the first level of central processing (attention and concentration to specific stimulus material). Therefore, she probably cannot be expected to do even simple tasks with any degree of efficiency if they require continued attention.

In addition, the extremely poor performances on the Category Test, Part B of the Trail Making Test, and the Tactual Performance Test indicate the severity of her deficit in problem-solving situations that involve any degree of complexity. Many patients with low IQ values perform much better than O.F. on these tests, indicating some potential for efficiency in simple but useful tasks in everyday living; this woman does not have the capability to perform satisfactorily in practically any kind of situation.

Lateralizing results were present and these also indicated the likelihood of cerebral damage. Though very definitely right-handed, O.F.'s grip strength was less in the right upper extremity (16.5 kg) than the left (18.0 kg). She also was slow in finger tapping speed with both hands and particularly slow with the right hand. These signs of motor dysfunction were complemented by results on the test of finger-tip number writing perception. On this measure the patient had much more difficulty with her right hand (7 errors) than her left (2 errors).

The Aphasia Screening Test also yielded results which pointed toward damage of the left cerebral hemisphere. It is not uncommon for patients with limited educational backgrounds to name the SQUARE a box; however, when the patient is able to name the figure correctly after being questioned by the examiner, the probability that an inadequate initial response was a sign of left cerebral damage is increased.

O.F. also made errors in spelling that are more characteristic of left cerebral damage than inadequate educational background. She was able to spell the first five letters of SQUARE correctly, but then inserted an "a" before the "e." She was able to spell CROSS correctly but became confused in the proper sequence of letters when attempting to spell TRIANGLE. Spelling attempts which deviate significantly from the sounds which represent the word are characteristic of patients with left cerebral damage rather than persons with limited educational background.

The fact that O.F. was not able to give the name of the TRIANGLE cannot be counted as a specific indication of left cerebral damage; it is possible that she had never learned the name of this particular figure. When the patient gives an incorrect response to an item, as in this instance, the clinician has information he or she can use to assess whether brain functions are impaired. If the patient gives no response at all to an item the clinician has no basis for reaching a conclusion. O.F. would not even guess when asked to name the TRIANGLE; therefore, we were not able to use this item as a basis for further evaluation of dysnomia.

When asked to read 7 SIX 2 the patient obviously failed to recognize that SIX was a word representing a number. This type of mistake is often made by persons with mild dyslexia due to left cerebral damage. When persons with left cerebral damage realize that an item requires reading of words, they have an additional cue to prompt their performance. With this item, however, it is necessary to recognize that numbers are presented in the form of arabic numerals as well as letters of the alphabet.

O.F. was able to perform satisfactorily when asked to read the individual letters MGW and the first reading item, SEE THE BLACK DOG. However, when the reading became slightly more difficult she made errors, as seen in her attempt to read HE IS A FRIENDLY ANIMAL, A FAMOUS WINNER OF DOG SHOWS.

Evidence of mild central dysarthria was also manifested in the patient's attempt to enunciate METHODIST EPISCOPAL. Her difficulty (the type shown by persons with left cerebral damage) was demonstrated when she said "Methobal" instead of METHODIST, apparently confusing the sounds involved in the two words.

She did not show any signs of right-left confusion, but had difficulty understanding the instructions to place her left hand to her left elbow. However, her confusion on this item may have been related to her low general intelligence level.

Considered in total, O.F.'s responses on the Aphasia Screening Test provide definite evidence of left cerebral damage and complement the results on grip strength and finger-tip number writing perception. The patient made 30 errors on the Speech-sounds Perception Test, but we would not consider this result to be a specific indication of left cerebral damage since it very possibly may reflect her limited verbal intelligence and poor academic training.

A number of findings implicated the right cerebral hemisphere. Instead of showing improvement, the patient performed worse on the second trial of the Tactual Performance Test. Her performances on each of the three trials were distinctly defective, but she was able to show some improvement on the third trial. Therefore, the overall pattern of the three trials suggests that the left hand was significantly less efficient than the right hand, a finding that could be due to right cerebral damage. O.F. was also somewhat slower with her left hand than her right on the Tactile Form Recognition Test.

Finally, the patient's attempts to draw the square, cross, triangle, and key yield further evidence of impairment in dealing with simple spatial configurations. Her drawing of the square had the shape of a rectangle because she made her third line (the ascending line on the right side) much too long.

The drawings of the cross also reflected the type of difficulty manifested by persons with right cerebral damage. In her first attempt, O.F. did not seem to realize that she had completed the figure

and drew the final line too long. Her second drawing of the cross showed a distinct imbalance of both the lateral and vertical extremities.

The drawing of the key is difficult to evaluate because of its simplistic nature. It is possible that this woman, with her very limited abilities, has never had much skill in drawing figures and as a result was not able to do much better in this instance.

As we would expect from a person with an 8th-grade education, O.F.'s writing suggests that she has had some meaningful exposure and training in development of academic skills. Nevertheless, her inability to do arithmetic and spell correctly may reflect inadequate educational training. Therefore, it would be difficult to attribute her defective performances in writing specifically to left cerebral damage. The other findings, however, provide a convincing basis for concluding that each cerebral hemisphere has been damaged.

At this point we could question whether O.F.'s general level of intellectual and cognitive functions have been affected by her repeated epileptic seizures. Many reports in the literature contend that epileptic attacks, considered independently, do not lead to deterioration of brain functions. However, many clinicians have observed what appears to be such deterioration in patients with repeated seizures over a period of years.

Reducing the frequency of O.F.'s seizures to only one convulsive episode during the fifteen previous months could be quite advantageous in helping her retain the limited intellectual functions that she still has. Nevertheless, we can see that her present abilities are quite limited and she would be capable of performing only very simple and routine tasks in an occupational sense.

O.F.'s medical records indicated that she had not been able to work productively or care for herself and because she had no one to turn to for help, had been admitted to a state mental hospital. Despite O.F.'s minimal abilities and the fact that her cognitive functions had probably been impaired most of her life, the specific deficits she demonstrated in the neuropsychological examination, coupled with evidence of differential performances on the two sides of the body, constituted a basis for inferring the presence of brain damage, probably resulting from her serious head injury eight years ago.

CASE #22

Name: S.D.

Age: 21

Education: 6

Sex: Male

Handedness: Right

Occupation: None

Background Information

S.D.'s epilepsy began after a head injury sustained at the age of eight years. The seizures were difficult to control and the patient was admitted to the hospital at this time for neurological evaluation and adjustment of his antiepileptic medications.

When the patient was eight years old he fell about 12 feet from a building and struck the posterior part of his head on the sharp corner of a piece of wood. This injury caused a skull defect which was currently obvious as a 2 cm X 2 cm bony protuberance in the left occipital area. S.D. had an epileptic seizure shortly after this fall which was vaguely described but probably represented a major motor epileptic attack.

A post-traumatic seizure pattern developed in which the patient would be seizure-free for 30 or 40 days and then have as many as 8 to 10 episodes a day. Following these seizures he had a partial paralysis of his right arm and leg that lasted for about 30 minutes. When he was 12 years old S.D. entered a seizure-free period that lasted eight years.

At the age of 20 S.D. had another accident in which he again fell and struck the left posterior part of his head. His epileptic attacks recurred but changed in character. The seizures would now begin with a feeling of dizziness and confusion, turning of the head to the left, and tonic movements of his left arm and leg. Sometimes the attacks would progress into generalized seizures lasting

about five minutes and followed by headaches. Medication had reduced the duration of these attacks so that at the time of the present hospitalization they generally lasted a maximum of 10 to 15 seconds; however, the patient was having between 16 and 24 seizures each day.

Neurological Examination

Neurological examination was within normal limits but electroencephalograms taken over a two-month period had consistently shown a severe, generalized dysrhythmia that was maximal in the left cerebral hemisphere. A pneumoencephalogram was within normal limits. There was no evidence of progressive brain disease and the clinical problem was primarily seizure control.

Adjustment of antiepileptic medications seemed to achieve good seizure control and follow-up evaluations over a six-month period following discharge from the hospital indicated considerable improvement. The patient had only occasional episodes of "warm" feelings but no significant motor involvement or impairment of consciousness.

Neuropsychological Examination

It was apparent that this man had been significantly affected by epilepsy following the head injury at the age of eight. It had been a factor in limiting his education to the 6th grade and was the reason for his unemployed status. In his own self-evaluation (Cornell Medical Index Health

Questionnaire) the patient had a number of complaints. He said he had pains in the heart or chest area, got out of breath long before anyone else, suffered from indigestion, had pains in the back which made it difficult for him to work, was tired out completely when he attempted to work, usually got up tired and exhausted in the morning, was frequently ill, worried a great deal, and was constantly made miserable by his poor health.

S.D. also said that he got things mixed up completely when he had to do them quickly and needed to work slowly in order to avoid mistakes, was usually unhappy and depressed, was easily upset and irritated, did things on sudden impulse, found that he had to be on guard even with his friends, became angry if anyone told him what to do, and was constantly keyed-up and jittery. Results on the Minnesota Multiphasic Personality Inventory also suggested that S.D. was somewhat anxious, apprehensive, perhaps unsure of himself, and possibly depressed.

Findings of this kind are hardly surprising considering the patient's history of epilepsy and the limiting consequences with respect to his occupational status and everyday activities, such as driving a car. From a neuropsychological point of view, however, there was a question concerning the severity of deficits. Many persons who have sustained injury to the brain early in life have a limited potential for developing normal cognitive ability levels and show evidence of generalized impairment. In this case we would expect to see some effect of the limited educational background, principally affecting academic skills and certain aspects of verbal intelligence. We would not anticipate severe focal involvement of the type that frequently accompanies acutely destructive or rapidly progressive lesions; instead, the neuropsychological test results should be indicative of a chronic, static condition of biological brain disorder.

The patient earned a Verbal IQ (99) almost exactly at the Average level (exceeding about 47% of his age peers) and a Performance IQ (93) in the lower part of the Average range (exceeding about 32%). The distribution of the Verbal subtest scores suggests that S.D. does have certain deficits related to the development of verbal intelligence. His deficient scores occurred on Information (7), Arithmetic (6), Vocabulary (6) and Digit Span (7), and these results are probably associated with poor development of stored verbal information and arithmetical abilities.

The Performance subtests showed a considerable degree of variability, with the Block Design (7) and Digit Symbol (6) scores being lowest. It is not surprising to see a relatively poor score on Digit Symbol as a general indicator of brain dysfunction. The Block Design score possibly reflects specific impairment in the posterior part of the right cerebral hemisphere. The Wechsler results suggest that S.D. has experienced adverse influences of brain damage on both Verbal and Performance IQ measurements and, in fact, we suspect that he may have had considerably higher IQ values if brain damage had not interfered.

The four most sensitive indicators in the HRNTB showed evidence of mild impairment. The patient earned an Impairment Index of 0.7 (about 70% of the tests had scores in the brain-damaged range), with only the Memory component (7) of the Tactual Performance Test and the Speech-sounds Perception Test (4) having scores in the normal range. S.D. showed mild impairment on the Category Test (52) and fairly definite impairment on the Localization component (2) of the Tactual Performance Test. Although the score for Part B of the Trail Making Test did not fall beyond the cut-off point, we strongly suspect that the time required (81 seconds) reflected a mild degree of deficit. These findings suggest that S.D. had mild impairment of adaptive abilities generally considered, although he appeared to have the basic capabilities to function within normal limits.

Lateralizing findings implicated the right cerebral hemisphere to a greater extent than the left but were present for each side of the brain. On the

THE HALSTEAD-REITAN
NEUROPSYCHOLOGICAL TEST BATTERY

Patient _____ **S.D.** _____ Age __**21**__ Sex __**M**__ Education ___**6**___ Handedness ___**R**___

WECHSLER-BELLEVUE SCALE

VIQ	99
PIQ	93
FS IQ	96

Information	7
Comprehension	12
Digit Span	7
Arithmetic	6
Similarities	14
Vocabulary	6

Picture Arrangement	12
Picture Completion	9
Block Design	7
Object Assembly	12
Digit Symbol	6

TRAIL MAKING TEST

Part A: __**45**__ seconds
Part B: __**81**__ seconds

STRENGTH OF GRIP

Dominant hand: __**48.5**__ kilograms

Non-dominant hand: __**47.5**__ kilograms

REITAN-KLØVE TACTILE FORM RECOGNITION TEST

Dominant hand: __**12**__ seconds; __**0**__ errors

Non-dominant hand: __**15**__ seconds; __**0**__ errors

REITAN-KLØVE SENSORY-PERCEPTUAL EXAM — No errors

Error Totals

RH ___ LH ___	Both H:	RH ___ LH ___	RH ___ LH ___
RH ___ LF ___	Both H/F:	RH ___ LF ___	RH ___ LF ___
LH ___ RF ___	Both H/F:	LH ___ RF ___	RF ___ LH ___
RE ___ LE ___	Both E:	RE ___ LE ___	RE ___ LE ___
RV ___ LV ___	Both:	RV ___ LV ___	RV ___ LV ___

TACTILE FINGER RECOGNITION

R 1___ 2___ 3___ 4 **2** 5___   R **2** / **20**

L 1___ 2___ 3 **1** 4 **2** 5 **2**   L **5** / **20**

FINGER-TIP NUMBER WRITING

R 1___ 2___ 3___ 4___ 5___   R **0** / **20**

L 1___ 2___ 3 **1** 4___ 5___   L **1** / **20**

HALSTEAD'S NEUROPSYCHOLOGICAL TEST BATTERY

Category Test _____ **52** _____

Tactual Performance Test

Dominant hand:	**8.2**
Non-dominant hand:	**6.8**
Both hands:	**2.6**

Total Time	**17.6**
Memory	**7**
Localization	**2**

Seashore Rhythm Test

Number Correct __**18**__   **10**

Speech-sounds Perception Test

Number of Errors   **4**

Finger Oscillation Test

Dominant hand:	**35**	**35**
Non-dominant hand:	**36**	

Impairment Index   **0.7**

MINNESOTA MULTIPHASIC PERSONALITY INVENTORY

		Hs	57
		D	72
?	50	Hy	78
L	50	Pd	55
F	60	Mf	39
K	48	Pa	41
		Pt	60
		Sc	57
		Ma	58

REITAN-KLØVE LATERAL-DOMINANCE EXAM

Show me how you:

throw a ball	**R**
hammer a nail	**R**
cut with a knife	**R**
turn a door knob	**R**
use scissors	**R**
use an eraser	**R**
write your name	**R**

Record time used for spontaneous name-writing:

Preferred hand	**21** seconds
Non-preferred hand	**36** seconds

Show me how you:

kick a football	**R**
step on a bug	**R**

REITAN-INDIANA APHASIA SCREENING TEST

Form for Adults and Older Children

Name: _____S. D._____ Age: __21__

Copy SQUARE	Repeat TRIANGLE
Name SQUARE	Repeat MASSACHUSETTS
Spell SQUARE Absolutely would not attempt to spell.	Repeat METHODIST EPISCOPAL
Copy CROSS	Write SQUARE
Name CROSS	Read SEVEN
Spell CROSS Same as above.	Repeat SEVEN
Copy TRIANGLE	Repeat/Explain HE SHOUTED THE WARNING.
Name TRIANGLE	Write HE SHOUTED THE WARNING.
Spell TRIANGLE Same as above.	Compute 85 – 27 =
Name BABY	Compute 17 X 3 = Wrote "47"; given 11 x 2 and wrote "22."
Write CLOCK	Name KEY
Name FORK	Demonstrate use of KEY
Read 7 SIX 2	Draw KEY
Read MGW	Read PLACE LEFT HAND TO RIGHT EAR.
Reading I	Place LEFT HAND TO RIGHT EAR
Reading II	Place LEFT HAND TO LEFT ELBOW

85   47 22
27
58

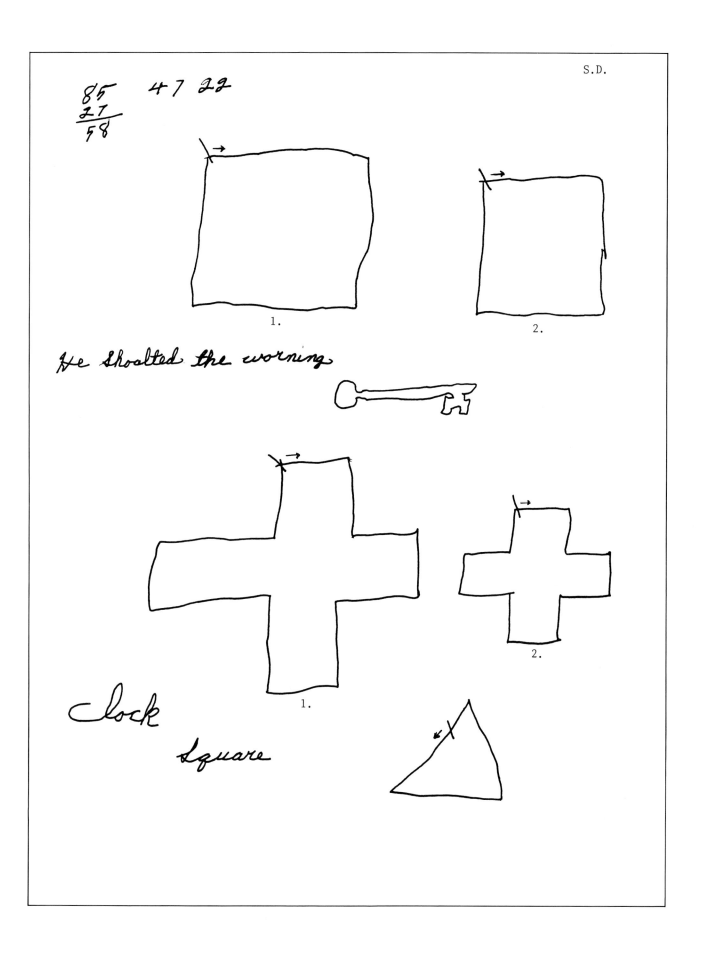

1.

2.

He shoalted the worning

clock

Square

1.

2.

Aphasia Screening Test the patient absolutely refused to try to spell simple words. He said that he was not able to spell and it appeared that he was unwilling to risk embarrassing himself. He demonstrated some spelling difficulty when asked to write the sentence HE SHOUTED THE WARNING, but neither insertion of an "L" nor substitution of a "O" for an "A" in WARNING is the usual kind of mistake made by persons with left cerebral damage. The patient's script appears to be somewhat primitive and unpracticed, in line with expectations based upon his limited educational background. S.D. showed something of the same primitive tendency in his writing of numbers.

The patient was not able to multiply 17 × 3 correctly (writing "47" as his answer) but was able to do a simpler problem. Thus, the writing, spelling and arithmetical efforts of this patient appear to correlate more closely with a limited educational background than with cerebral damage. This interpretation is probably consistent with the excellent score (4 errors) on the Speech-sounds Perception Test. Both finger tapping speed and grip strength were mildly reduced in the right as compared with the left upper extremity and, in the context of the general indicators, probably reflect some mild, chronic dysfunction of the left cerebral hemisphere.

Note that the right cerebral indicators, though not pronounced, were definite nevertheless. The patient was a little slow with his left hand (6.8 min) compared with his right (8.2 min) on the Tactual Performance Test, somewhat slow in tactile form recognition with his left hand, had definite difficulty with his left hand (5 errors) compared with his right (2 errors) in tactile finger localization, and demonstrated problems in drawing the cross and triangle that were fairly characteristic of persons with right cerebral damage. The lateral extremities of the cross were definitely deviant. The difficulty with spatial relationships was reflected not so much by the general shape of the triangle as by the starting point, comparative length of

lines, and the necessity to compensate to complete the figures.

As the reader has probably noticed, the drawing of the key was reversed in direction. We have reviewed hundreds of cases of various diagnostic categories, including persons without cerebral damage. Reversal of the direction of the key does not occur often, but it seems to occur with approximately equal frequency in all groups, including normal populations. Omission of the inside of the handle also occurs frequently and does not have pathognomonic significance for cerebral damage. Therefore, S.D.'s drawings of the cross and triangle were of considerably greater significance as indicators of cerebral dysfunction than the drawing of the key.

Finally, it should be noted that the patient made 7 mistakes in 40 trials of testing tactile finger recognition but made only 1 mistake in 40 trials of finger-tip number writing perception. The latter test is usually more difficult and a greater number of errors tends to occur on this test. We have found that normal subjects generally make no mistakes in tactile finger recognition but may make a few errors in finger-tip number writing perception. When more mistakes occur on Tactile Finger Recognition (the easier task), the results seem to have additional validity as indicators of cerebral dysfunction (as in S.D.'s case).

In summarizing this patient's neuropsychological test results we can see that the general indicators point toward mild impairment of cerebral function and the lateralizing indicators implicate each of the cerebral hemispheres (although the right hemisphere appeared to be somewhat more dysfunctional). In all probability the low score (7) on Block Design was another indicator of mild right cerebral dysfunction. These test results are completely typical of long-standing cerebral damage and not at all representative of either a recent acutely destructive insult or a rapidly progressive focal lesion.

Differentiation between chronic-static cerebral damage and recent or progressive damage depends upon the strength of the lateralized or focal indicators (that might be associated with a specific area of focal destruction) and the comparative intensity of left vs. right lateralizing signs. Evidence of specific, circumscribed deficits is much more often associated with recent, focal destruction or a progressive lesion; milder lateralizing signs — particularly when each of the hemispheres is implicated — are more typical of chronic-static involvement.

It should also be noted that persons with chronic-static cerebral damage often perform very well on some of the tests in the Battery, suggesting that the brain is not acutely embarrassed in a biological sense. In this case the most outstanding example of this type was the good score on the Speech-sounds Perception Test. Some of the subtest scores on the Wechsler Scale and the third trial of the Tactual Performance Test were other examples of good performances by this patient. The score (81 sec) on Part B of the Trail making Test would also argue against an acutely destructive or rapidly progressive focal lesion in this case.

CASE #23

Name: R.P.

Age: 29

Education: 12

Sex: Male

Handedness: Right

Occupation: Household repairman

Background Information

R.P. was a 29-year-old man who had completed high school with approximately average grades. He was working as a household utility repairman when he was involved in a moving vehicle accident and sustained a very severe head injury. R.P. apparently lost consciousness immediately after the accident, regained some degree of consciousness for a short period of time, and then lapsed into a comatose state.

Neurological Examination

When admitted to the hospital approximately six hours after the accident the patient had difficulty breathing and his respirations were irregular. His pupils were equal in size but quite constricted and reacted to light sluggishly. His eyes were slightly divergent but generally turned toward the right. Multiple scalp lacerations were evident.

A definite paresis on the left side was obvious when painful stimuli were administered. Babinski and Hoffman signs were demonstrated only on the right side and superficial abdominal reflexes were absent in all four quadrants. At times the left upper extremity assumed a position of decerebrate rigidity.

All neurological findings indicated that R.P. had experienced a very severe head injury and he was taken to surgery immediately after the initial examination in the emergency room. Bilateral burr holes revealed an acute subdural hematoma on the right side; a left parietal burr hole in the vicinity of a linear fracture showed no abnormality. The right frontal and parietal areas were irrigated and the acute subdural hematoma was evacuated.

Immediately following surgery R.P. showed a fluctuation of vital signs and later in the day bilateral angiograms were done to evaluate the condition of his brain. The results for the left cerebral hemisphere were normal but showed certain abnormalities on the right side suggesting that a very small amount of subdural hematoma might still be present. However, the amount did not seem sufficient to account for the patient's condition and the neurosurgeon thought that the abnormalities on the angiogram were probably due principally to right cerebral edema.

No further surgical intervention was recommended and R.P. slowly began to improve. However, he was frequently completely disoriented, showed signs of considerable irritability, and had episodes of loud vocalization. He gradually continued to improve and neuropsychological examination was done one and one-half months after the injury. At the time we examined him, R.P. was not able to give us any details regarding the accident. He could tell us about his prior military experience in a war zone and information regarding his family, his four children and his occupational activities, but his reports were vague and unreliable.

At the time of discharge from the hospital (two and one-half months after admission) the patient was fully oriented but showed clinical signs of intellectual deficit. He was able to be up and around but walked quite slowly and demonstrated some impairment of his right leg. He also had some motor dysfunction involving his left arm and did not appear to be able to return to gainful employment. The final diagnoses were (1) severe closed head injury with a subdural hematoma over much of the right cerebral hemisphere; (2) a linear fracture in the left parietal region; and (3) brain contusion.

Neuropsychological Evaluation

We were not able to validly administer the Minnesota Multiphasic Personality Inventory. On the first attempt R.P. was not able to coordinate the printed items with the answer sheet and had answers filled in almost randomly. We then asked him to sort the MMPI cards into groups of "true" or "false," but he distributed the cards until there was essentially no more room on the table, apparently unable to decide on any answer. Finally, he put all of the cards back in the box. We also tried reading the MMPI questions to the patient but he still had great difficulty making decisions. He did complete the Cornell Medical Index Health Questionnaire but the answers were quite inconsistent and appeared to be randomly distributed among the two alternatives. Inspection of the responses suggested that they were not valid.

As noted above, it was apparent in casual clinical observation (at this time and even one month later) that R.P. was intellectually impaired. Under these circumstances it is not surprising that the results of the neuropsychological examination revealed very profound deficits.

R.P. earned a Verbal IQ (86) in the Low Average range (exceeding about 18% of his age peers) and a Performance IQ (53) in the range of Mental Retardation (exceeding less than 1%). It is apparent from these results that the Verbal Intelligence of this man was considerably above his Performance Intelligence. He earned a Full Scale IQ (68) that was in the range of mild Mental Retardation to Borderline intelligence, but the more significant clinical conclusion would be that there was a definite difference in Verbal and Performance Intelligence levels.

Except for Object Assembly, the highest Performance subtest score was lower than the lowest Verbal subtest score. Judging from some of the better Verbal subtest scores, it would appear that at one time this man may have had general intellectual levels at least in the lower part of the normal distribution. It is difficult to make such a judgement confidently, but the scores on Information (8), Comprehension (9), and Similarities (8) would be consistent with a hypothesis suggesting that R.P. had previously had an opportunity to develop relatively normal intellectual abilities. The pronounced disparity between Verbal and Performance IQ values would certainly suggest that something adverse had occurred to impair the Performance subtest scores. In fact, in this case one might raise the possibility that right cerebral damage may have occurred.

This interpretation of the Verbal and Performance subtest disparities would be reinforced by R.P.'s performance on the Halstead-Reitan Battery. Each of the four most sensitive measures indicated the presence of significant and serious cognitive impairment. It is interesting to note that the only test not contributing to the Impairment Index of 0.9 was the Speech-sounds Perception Test (5). This good performance indicates that the patient had the basic ability to pay continuing attention to simple verbal stimulus material and make accurate discriminations. He also performed relatively well in finger tapping speed with his right hand (50).

It should be noted that R.P. showed a sharper decline in the adequacy of his performances as the tests became more complicated and required analytical or abstraction abilities. He performed extremely poorly on the Category Test (128) and Part B of the Trail Making Test (469 sec). The patient

THE HALSTEAD-REITAN
NEUROPSYCHOLOGICAL TEST BATTERY

Patient __R.P. (I)__ Age __27__ Sex __M__ Education __12__ Handedness __R__

WECHSLER-BELLEVUE SCALE
VIQ __86__
PIQ __53__
FS IQ __68__

Information __8__
Comprehension __9__
Digit Span __4__
Arithmetic __6__
Similarities __8__
Vocabulary __6__

Picture Arrangement __3__
Picture Completion __1__
Block Design __1__
Object Assembly __6__
Digit Symbol __2__

TRAIL MAKING TEST
Part A: __196__ seconds
Part B: __469__ seconds

STRENGTH OF GRIP
Dominant hand: __40.5__ kilograms
Non-dominant hand: __21.5__ kilograms

REITAN-KLØVE TACTILE FORM RECOGNITION TEST
Dominant hand: __14__ seconds; __0__ errors
Non-dominant hand: __27__ seconds; __0__ errors

REITAN-KLØVE SENSORY-PERCEPTUAL EXAM — No errors

				Error Totals		
RH___LH___	Both H:	RH___LH___	RH___LH___			
RH___LF___	Both H/F:	RH___LF___	RH___LF___			
LH___RF___	Both H/F:	LH___RF___	RF___LH___			
RE___LE___	Both E:	RE___LE___	RE___LE___			
RV___LV___	Both:	RV___LV___				

TACTILE FINGER RECOGNITION
R 1___ 2_1_ 3___ 4_1_ 5___   R _2_ / 20
L 1___ 2___ 3___ 4_1_ 5___   L _1_ / 20

FINGER-TIP NUMBER WRITING
R 1_1_ 2___ 3_1_ 4_1_ 5_1_   R _4_ / 20
L 1_1_ 2_1_ 3_1_ 4_1_ 5_1_   L _5_ / 20

HALSTEAD'S NEUROPSYCHOLOGICAL TEST BATTERY
Category Test __128__

Tactual Performance Test
Dominant hand: __15.0 (1 block)__
Non-dominant hand: __10.2 (0 blocks)__
Both hands: _____

NOT COMPLETED { Total Time _____
Memory _____
Localization _____

Seashore Rhythm Test
Number Correct __13__   __10__

Speech-sounds Perception Test
Number of Errors   __5__

Finger Oscillation Test
Dominant hand: __50__   __50__
Non-dominant hand: __23__

Impairment Index __0.9__

MINNESOTA MULTIPHASIC PERSONALITY INVENTORY

	Hs	_____	
	D	_____	
? _____	Hy	_____	
L _____	Pd	_____	PATIENT COULD
F _____	Mf	_____	NOT ADEQUATELY
K _____	Pa	_____	COMPREHEND THE QUESTIONS
	Pt	_____	
	Sc	_____	
	Ma	_____	

REITAN-KLØVE LATERAL-DOMINANCE EXAM
Show me how you:
throw a ball __R__
hammer a nail __R__
cut with a knife __R__
turn a door knob __R__
use scissors __R__
use an eraser __R__
write your name __R__

Record time used for spontaneous name-writing:
Preferred hand __10__ seconds
Non-preferred hand __162__ seconds

Show me how you:
kick a football __R__
step on a bug __R__

REITAN-INDIANA APHASIA SCREENING TEST

Form for Adults and Older Children

Name: _____R. P. (I)_____ Age: __27__

Copy SQUARE	Repeat TRIANGLE
Name SQUARE	Repeat MASSACHUSETTS
Spell SQUARE	Repeat METHODIST EPISCOPAL
Copy CROSS	Write SQUARE
Name CROSS "Square;" Examiner questioned; then OK.	Read SEVEN
Spell CROSS	Repeat SEVEN
Copy TRIANGLE	Repeat/Explain HE SHOUTED THE WARNING.
Name TRIANGLE	Write HE SHOUTED THE WARNING.
Spell TRIANGLE "T-R-I-A-G-A-L-E"	Compute 85 – 27 = (Examiner also gave additional problems.)
Name BABY	Compute 17 X 3 = (Could not do mentally. Permitted to use pencil.)
Write CLOCK	Name KEY
Name FORK	Demonstrate use of KEY
Read 7 SIX 2	Draw KEY
Read MGW	Read PLACE LEFT HAND TO RIGHT EAR.
Reading I	Place LEFT HAND TO RIGHT EAR
Reading II	Place LEFT HAND TO LEFT ELBOW

He shouted the warning

```
  98
- 53
─────
  45
```

(11 x 2)   22

```
  85
- 27
─────
  52
```

```
  17
 x 3
─────
  21
  33
─────
  54
```

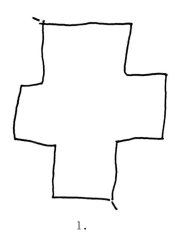

1.

clock   squre

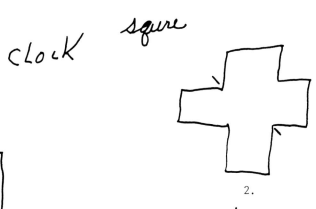

1.

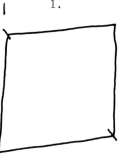

2.

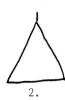

2.

1.

2.

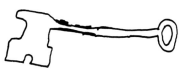

3.

was scarcely able to make any progress on the Tactual Performance Test; after working for 15 minutes with his right hand and just over two minutes with his left hand he became very discouraged and absolutely refused to continue with the task. As a result of his very minimal progress we did not ask him to draw a picture of the board. Under such circumstances we presume that both the Memory and Localization components of the Tactual Performance Test validly contribute to the Impairment Index.

Our judgment is that R.P. performed extremely poorly on the four most sensitive indicators as well as on most of the other tests in the Battery. The only tests on which he earned normal or near normal scores were those that involved verbal content. As noted previously, his abilities dropped off very sharply as the complexity of the task increased.

The lateralizing indicators showed much more significant impairment of right cerebral functions than left. His finger tapping speed was markedly reduced with the left hand compared with the right hand (23 to 50) and grip strength showed a similar relationship (21.5 kg to 40.5 kg). Note, though, that the patient's difficulty on the left side was not limited to motor functions; on the Tactile Form Recognition Test he also performed more poorly with his left hand than his right and even on measurement of speed in name writing he was extremely slow with his left hand.

Finally, even though he was able to include all four extremities, the patient had difficulty drawing the shape of a cross. His drawing of the key also deviated significantly from the correct spatial configuration, particularly concerning the size of the teeth compared with the handle.

R.P. also had some mild difficulties that may reflect left cerebral dysfunction. When he was asked to name the picture of the CROSS he perseverated by saying "square." Since this was the only instance of verbal perseveration, one might wonder whether it was a reflection of specific verbal difficulty or generalized impairment.

R.P. also demonstrated a type of confusion in spelling that is not usually a reflection of low educational level; as the reader will note, the patient omitted the "N" and added an additional "A" in TRIANGLE. He had another problem of this type when he omitted the "A" when he wrote the word SQUARE.

Finally, when asked to write HE SHOUTED THE WARNING, R.P. had difficulty in forming the "M." This latter deficit is probably more suggestive of dysgraphia than spelling dyspraxia. In any case, though, the patient showed significant problems in dealing with language symbols for communicational purposes and these findings, even though relatively mild, are quite definite in implicating the left cerebral hemisphere.

R.P. had more pronounced difficulties performing simple arithmetic problems. He made a mistake trying to compute $85 - 27 =$, possibly showing some confusion attempting to carry. The examiner gave the patient a problem in which carrying was not necessary and he was able to complete it correctly. R.P. became confused when asked to do 17×3 mentally and eventually was permitted to write the problem on the paper. He obviously did not perform this problem correctly; apparently he tried to do it in two steps but got the wrong answer. The examiner gave R.P. an easier multiplication problem (11×2) which he was able to do mentally and write the answer on the paper.

These findings suggest that R.P. was able to do very simple arithmetic correctly but when the problem became just a little more complicated he became confused and had significant difficulties. Although we would interpret these results as possible representations of dyscalculia, we would again note that they probably reflect the fact that R.P.'s performances on very simple tasks are considerably better than on tasks that are somewhat more complicated.

Despite his good performance on the Speech-sounds Perception Test, there is no doubt that R.P.

has some evidence of mild left cerebral dysfunction in addition to the right cerebral hemisphere deficits. The good score on the Speech-sounds Perception Test is significant because it strongly suggests that R.P. did not have a brain disease that would lead to progressive deterioration. In other words, this finding is a major factor in our conclusion that the test results reflect an insult to the brain from an external source rather than an internal disease process. In the face of such serious deficits on other measures, such a good score could not have been achieved unless the biological condition of the brain was relatively stable.

It is interesting to note that R.P. made no mistakes on the tests of bilateral simultaneous sensory stimulation and had very little difficulty with tests of tactile finger recognition; he obviously had the basic ability to pay attention to simple stimulus material. On the Finger-tip Number Writing Perception Test he had more difficulty, making more errors on each hand than would be expected from a person with an undamaged brain. This latter finding should be noted as a deviation from normal expectancy and suggests damage of both cerebral hemispheres. A relative absence of sensory-perceptual deficits (and even motor dysfunction) compared to a degree of impairment shown on more complex tests tends to occur more frequently in cases of head injury than intrinsic tumors and strokes (Hom & Reitan, 1982).

In summary, this man showed significant motor deficits and less pronounced tactile-perceptual losses with his left upper extremity. His Performance intelligence was strikingly reduced compared to his Verbal intelligence. He earned extremely poor scores on the Category Test, the Trail Making Test and the Tactual Performance Test, suggesting that he was particularly impaired in his ability to deal with (1) complex tasks requiring simultaneous attention to several elements of the situation; and (2) situations in which he had to define the nature of the problem as a basis for its solution.

Results of this kind are entirely consistent with findings expected in instances of severe head injury. It is not uncommon to find that one cerebral hemisphere is considerably more impaired than the other, even if the injury was not penetrating or open. In this case the surgical findings of an extensive subdural hematoma correlated significantly with the neuropsychological findings, although (as one would expect in cases of head injury) there was also some evidence of generalized impairment and even some specific signs of left cerebral damage.

This case is probably somewhat deviant from what we normally expect in cases of closed head injury because the evidence of right cerebral damage (with relation to the findings of left cerebral damage) was so pronounced. The relatively good performances on the Sensory-perceptual Examination are fairly typical of many head-injured persons and the excellent score on the Speech-sounds Perception Test strongly suggests that this patient's brain is relatively stabilized in a biological sense (even though it is definitely damaged and impaired).

The ability to draw simple spatial configurations with relation to the motor deficits on the left side and the serious impairment of higher-level abilities (i.e., relative sparing of the ability to deal with simple spatial configurations even though there was some evidence of impairment) is also fairly typical of craniocerebral trauma. However, it is also entirely possible that in this case the major structural damage was in the right frontal area and therefore spared R.P.'s figure-drawing ability as well as his sensory-perceptual skills. The neurosurgeon's observations did not suggest differential involvement of the frontal and parietal areas.

We examined this patient on two additional occasions, approximately five months and 19 months after the first testing. Because R.P. did not have any physical therapy, occupational therapy or rehabilitational program available to him, any improvement would be related to a spontaneous recovery process of the brain, facilitated only by normal and routine activities.

As noted, the second neuropsychological examination was conducted five months after the first testing (seven months post-injury). Even though the evidence of cerebral damage was severe and quite striking on the first examination, we would expect some improvement of cognitive deficits, particularly in the areas which initially showed impairment.

We will first evaluate the test results in terms of residual indications of brain impairment and then compare the results of the two examinations.

R.P. earned Verbal, Performance, and Full Scale IQ values that were all in the lower part of the Average range. Even though he was probably so impaired on the first examination that he would not be as likely to gain as much from practice effect as the normal subject, some gains due to familiarity with the tests might be expected. The Verbal subtests did not show any significant variability. Digit Span was the lowest score (6) and the other scores ranged from 8 to 11. In general, the Performance subtests were within the same range, with scores ranging from 8 to 12. There does not appear to be any basis for inferring differential performances on the Verbal and Performance subtests, and there are no indications of specific deficits that might be associated with cerebral damage.

Although the Wechsler Scale showed essentially negative findings, the four most sensitive indicators on the Halstead-Reitan Battery consistently yielded evidence of impairment (despite any practice-effect that might have occurred). The Impairment Index (0.7), the Category Test (96), Part B of the Trail Making Test (111 sec), and the Localization component of the Tactual Performance Test (2) all indicated deficient performances. Therefore, a consideration of the results on these four measures relative to the IQ values would be

a convincing basis for hypothesizing the presence of some impairment of brain function.

We will next evaluate the lateralizing indicators. There were a number of results suggesting right cerebral hemisphere damage. On the Tactual Performance Test the patient performed poorly with his left hand (11.0 min) compared with his right (12.2 min) although the results indicated a generally poor overall performance. R.P. was within the normal range on the Memory component of the TPT (6) but, as indicated previously, distinctly impaired on the Localization component (2). He also showed a mild degree of deficit in finger tapping speed with his left hand (45) compared with his right (55).

It is important to note that the left-sided deficits were not restricted to motor performances; on the Tactile Form Recognition Test R.P. had some difficulty with his left hand (16 sec) compared with his right (11 sec). He also demonstrated a very mild tendency to imperceive a visual stimulus toward his left side when it was given with a competing stimulus on the right side.

The drawing of the cross did not show any particular deficits. One could question the symmetry (particularly of the lateral extremities) but if this cross were viewed independently and without reference to other results, it would probably be considered to be within normal limits.

R.P.'s drawing of the key, however, was unequivocal in its significance and definitely suggested certain difficulties in dealing with spatial relationships. The somewhat unsteady lines are seen in many patients' drawings and are probably not a valid indication of brain dysfunction. The general configuration of the key in this drawing is not adequately representative of the stimulus figure; there are difficulties with the handle and the line representing the stem within the area of the teeth was not properly continuous. Of all the problems with the key, the most significant probably relates to the notches on the stem. R.P. showed

THE HALSTEAD-REITAN
NEUROPSYCHOLOGICAL TEST BATTERY

Patient ___R.P. (II)___ Age __27__ Sex __M__ Education __12__ Handedness __R__

WECHSLER-BELLEVUE SCALE

VIQ	94
PIQ	97
FS IQ	95

Information	8
Comprehension	8
Digit Span	6
Arithmetic	9
Similarities	11
Vocabulary	10

Picture Arrangement	8
Picture Completion	12
Block Design	10
Object Assembly	8
Digit Symbol	8

TRAIL MAKING TEST

Part A: __54__ seconds
Part B: __111__ seconds

STRENGTH OF GRIP

Dominant hand: __45.0__ kilograms
Non-dominant hand: __40.5__ kilograms

REITAN-KLØVE TACTILE FORM RECOGNITION TEST

Dominant hand: __11__ seconds; __0__ errors
Non-dominant hand: __16__ seconds; __0__ errors

REITAN-KLØVE SENSORY-PERCEPTUAL EXAM

				Error Totals	
RH___ LH___	Both H:	RH___ LH___		RH___ LH___	
RH___ LF___	Both H/F:	RH___ LF___		RH___ LF___	
LH___ RF___	Both H/F:	LH___ RF___		RF___ LH___	
RE___ LE___	Both E:	RE___ LE___		RE___ LE___	
RV___ LV___	Both:	RV___ LV___		RV___ LV __2__	
___ ___				___	
___ ___				___ __2__	

TACTILE FINGER RECOGNITION

R 1___ 2___ 3___ 4 __2__ 5___   R __2__ / __20__

L 1___ 2___ 3___ 4___ 5___   L __0__ / __20__

FINGER-TIP NUMBER WRITING

R 1 __1__ 2___ 3___ 4___ 5___   R __1__ / __20__

L 1___ 2___ 3___ 4___ 5___   L __0__ / __20__

NO APHASIC SYMPTOMS

HALSTEAD'S NEUROPSYCHOLOGICAL TEST BATTERY

Category Test		96

Tactual Performance Test

Dominant hand:	12.2	
Non-dominant hand:	11.0	
Both hands:	5.5	
	Total Time	28.7
	Memory	6
	Localization	2

Seashore Rhythm Test

Number Correct	15		10

Speech-sounds Perception Test

Number of Errors		10

Finger Oscillation Test

Dominant hand:	55	55
Non-dominant hand:	45	

Impairment Index __0.7__

REITAN-KLØVE
LATERAL-DOMINANCE EXAM

Show me how you:

throw a ball	R
hammer a nail	R
cut with a knife	R
turn a door knob	R
use scissors	R
use an eraser	R
write your name	R

Record time used for spontaneous name-writing:

Preferred hand	3	seconds
Non-preferred hand	10	seconds

Show me how you:

kick a football	R
step on a bug	R

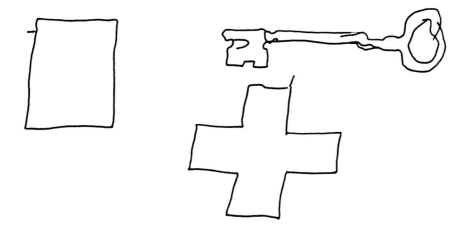

$$85 - 27 = 58$$

51   CLOCK

SQUARE   (1)

square (2)

He shouted the warning

some confusion in his attempt to achieve a mirror-image of the notches, particularly those close to the handle. With all of these aberrations, we would definitely not consider this key to be within normal limits.

The drawing of the square also raises a question about the patient's ability to deal with spatial relationships. Note that R.P. began on the left side, drawing a vertical line in downward direction. He then proceeded across with the bottom horizontal line but then made a mistake by extending the upward vertical line on the right side too far. At that point he was obliged to draw the top line in a horizontal plane and compensate for the closure by returning to the starting point. Although this kind of mistake does not greatly affect the appearance of the figure, it is frequently seen in persons with relatively mild impairment of spatial relationships. In total, then, there were several specific indicators of right cerebral dysfunction.

Conversely, there was little evidence to implicate the left cerebral hemisphere. On the Tactile Finger Recognition Test the patient made two mistakes in 20 trials on his right hand and no mistakes on his left hand. However, he had absolutely no evidence of aphasia.

In summary, R.P. showed definite impairment on measures of higher-level aspects of brain functions and relatively mild indications of right cerebral damage. This second set of test results has a pattern essentially the same as the one seen on the first examination, in which there were severe deficits involving the right cerebral hemisphere, very serious losses of higher-level functions, and mild indications of left cerebral involvement.

The results of the second examination still deviate significantly from normal and could not be interpreted as representative of a normal brain. If these results had been obtained on the first testing they would probably have been interpreted as suggesting only relatively mild cerebral damage. However, the practical implications of the findings, particularly the very poor score on the Category Test,

would be relatively serious; this man is probably restricted in his ability to deal with complex problems that require analysis, definition, and reasoning through to a solution as the problem evolves.

As we noted, we expect the greatest improvement to occur on the tests that initially showed the greatest deficit. This improvement does not occur as much on the Impairment Index (and perhaps the Category Test) as on other measures. This occurs because the Impairment Index and the Category Test are very sensitive indicators of cognitive functions and often reveal evidence of significant impairment even in cases of relatively mild cerebral damage. However, other tests that have more focal significance and are not as specifically sensitive to cerebral damage (wherever it may have occurred) often show substantial improvement when the patient is re-examined.

In this case, the Impairment Index changed from 0.9 to 0.7 and the performance on the Category Test (although not as deficient as initially) improved only from 128 errors to 96 errors. Part B of the Trail Making Test, which was performed very poorly on the initial examination (469 sec) improved to 111 seconds. On the first examination the patient was grossly impaired on the Tactual Performance Test (despite an improved performance on the third trial) and on the second testing he still performed worse than the average brain-damaged person. His Memory score (6) was within the normal range but his Localization score (2) (which is generally more sensitive to cerebral damage than the Memory score) was clearly impaired.

On the first testing R.P.'s Performance IQ of 53 had been noted to be especially deficient, particularly with relation to his Verbal IQ of 86. Therefore, we would expect a much greater increment on Performance IQ than on Verbal IQ. On the second examination R.P.'s Performance IQ was a few points higher than his Verbal IQ; it improved from a score of 53 to 97. R.P.'s Verbal IQ increased from 86 to 94. There is no doubt that the improved Performance IQ was due to spontaneous recovery and even the Verbal IQ change was probably greater than would be expected on the basis of positive practice-effect.

Because R.P. demonstrated pronounced deficits in motor function on the left side of the body at the time of the initial examination, we would now expect to see definite improvement on the left side of the body with relatively lesser changes on the right side. Finger tapping speed improved five points with the right hand and 22 points with the left hand, with the pattern approaching a relationship showing only mild deficit with the left hand compared with the right.

Grip strength in the left upper extremity had been markedly diminished at the time of the first examination, being only about half as strong as the right hand. The patient demonstrated a 4.5 kg gain in strength with his right upper extremity and 19 kg with his left.

R.P. had been extremely slow in writing his name with his left hand (162 sec). On the second examination he had reduced the writing time with his right hand from 10 seconds to 3 seconds and from 162 seconds to 10 seconds with the left hand. Although he showed some improvement in Tactile Form Recognition (especially with his left hand) he still continued to show evidence of mild right cerebral dysfunction.

On the second examination R.P. drew a considerably better cross and his key may have improved somewhat. He tried to put more detail into the key but found his effort to represent neuropsychological deficit, probably because of the complexity of this figure. Although R.P. had previously had mild difficulty dealing with language symbols for communicational purposes and definite confusion in slightly complex arithmetical processes, he had no such manifestations at the present time. Thus, it is clear that many of R.P.'s deficits — particularly those that deal with more specific and simple tasks rather than those that represent general functions or require definition of the nature

of the problem before it can be solved — were considerably improved.

As noted, the patient still showed a pattern of results that tended to implicate the right cerebral hemisphere. Compared with normal standards, he also performed poorly on complex problem-solving tasks; simple tasks were performed somewhat better. On the second examination R.P. actually performed worse on the Speech-sounds Perception Test than he did initially, but for a person with a Verbal IQ of 94 a score of 10 errors is essentially within the normal relationship.

It is worth studying the natural manifestations of spontaneous improvement following traumatic insult to the brain in order to learn how the healing process occurs in a natural manner, unaffected by the notions (or prejudices) of remediation that represent either current scientific thinking or prevailing theories. One of the problems that has impeded progress in understanding appropriate methods of approach in rehabilitation has been the dependence upon the theories and expectations of man rather than upon the wisdom of nature.

One year after the second examination R.P. was examined a third time. We would expect him to show some continued improvement although the results of the second examination were probably approaching the point at which any residual impairment would be chronic.

We will first consider the results of the third examination independently, before referring to the findings of the previous examinations.

R.P. earned both Verbal and Performance IQ values that were near the Average level, yielding a Full Scale IQ of 101. The Verbal subtests did not show any significant variability, at least when considered among the types of patients seen in a hospital setting.

The Performance subtests, however, might raise the possibility of a mild degree of impairment. The Digit Symbol subtest, which is generally the most sensitive of the Wechsler variables to brain damage, was tied with Picture Arrangement for

THE HALSTEAD-REITAN
NEUROPSYCHOLOGICAL TEST BATTERY

Patient __R.P. (III)__ Age __29__ Sex __M__ Education __12__ Handedness __R__

WECHSLER-BELLEVUE SCALE

VIQ	99
PIQ	104
FS IQ	101

Information	9
Comprehension	11
Digit Span	6
Arithmetic	9
Similarities	11
Vocabulary	11

Picture Arrangement	8
Picture Completion	12
Block Design	10
Object Assembly	12
Digit Symbol	8

TRAIL MAKING TEST

Part A: __31__ seconds
Part B: __71__ seconds

STRENGTH OF GRIP

Dominant hand: __51.0__ kilograms

Non-dominant hand: __47.5__ kilograms

REITAN-KLØVE TACTILE FORM RECOGNITION TEST

Dominant hand: __10__ seconds; __0__ errors

Non-dominant hand: __14__ seconds; __0__ errors

REITAN-KLØVE SENSORY-PERCEPTUAL EXAM — No errors

				Error Totals	
RH ___ LH ___	Both H:	RH ___ LH ___		RH ___ LH ___	
RH ___ LF ___	Both H/F:	RH ___ LF ___		RH ___ LF ___	
LH ___ RF ___	Both H/F:	LH ___ RF ___		RF ___ LH ___	
RE ___ LE ___	Both E:	RE ___ LE ___		RE ___ LE ___	
RV ___ LV ___	Both:	RV ___ LV ___		RV ___ LV ___	
___ ___		___ ___			
___ ___		___ ___			

TACTILE FINGER RECOGNITION

R 1___ 2___ 3___ 4 _3_ 5___ R __3__ / 20

L 1___ 2___ 3___ 4___ 5___ L __0__ / 20

FINGER-TIP NUMBER WRITING

R 1___ 2___ 3 _1_ 4 _1_ 5___ R __2__ / 20

L 1 _1_ 2___ 3___ 4 _1_ 5___ L __2__ / 20

HALSTEAD'S NEUROPSYCHOLOGICAL TEST BATTERY

__Category Test__ __88__

Tactual Performance Test

Dominant hand:	__11.7__	
Non-dominant hand:	__9.3__	
Both hands:	__6.4__	

Total Time	27.4
Memory	7
Localization	0

Seashore Rhythm Test

Number Correct __22__ __10__

Speech-sounds Perception Test

Number of Errors __3__

Finger Oscillation Test

Dominant hand:	__52__	__52__
Non-dominant hand:	__44__	

__Impairment Index__ __0.6__

MINNESOTA MULTIPHASIC PERSONALITY INVENTORY

		Hs	52
		D	58
?	50	Hy	62
L	70	Pd	60
F	50	Mf	53
K	70	Pa	56
		Pt	56
		Sc	53
		Ma	53

REITAN-KLØVE LATERAL-DOMINANCE EXAM

Show me how you:

throw a ball	R
hammer a nail	R
cut with a knife	R
turn a door knob	R
use scissors	R
use an eraser	R
write your name	R

Record time used for spontaneous name-writing:

Preferred hand	8	seconds
Non-preferred hand	16	seconds

Show me how you:

kick a football	R
step on a bug	R

REITAN-INDIANA APHASIA SCREENING TEST

Form for Adults and Older Children

Name: _____ R. P. (III) _____ Age: 29

Copy SQUARE	Repeat TRIANGLE
Name SQUARE	Repeat MASSACHUSETTS
Spell SQUARE	Repeat METHODIST EPISCOPAL
Copy CROSS	Write SQUARE
Name CROSS	Read SEVEN
Spell CROSS	Repeat SEVEN
Copy TRIANGLE	Repeat/Explain HE SHOUTED THE WARNING.
Name TRIANGLE	Write HE SHOUTED THE WARNING.
Spell TRIANGLE "T–R–I–A–G–L–E"	Compute 85 – 27 =
Name BABY	Compute 17 X 3 =
Write CLOCK	Name KEY
Name FORK	Demonstrate use of KEY
Read 7 SIX 2	Draw KEY
Read MGW	Read PLACE LEFT HAND TO RIGHT EAR.
Reading I	Place LEFT HAND TO RIGHT EAR
Reading II	Place LEFT HAND TO LEFT ELBOW

$$\begin{array}{r} 85 \\ -27 \\ \hline 58 \end{array}$$

51

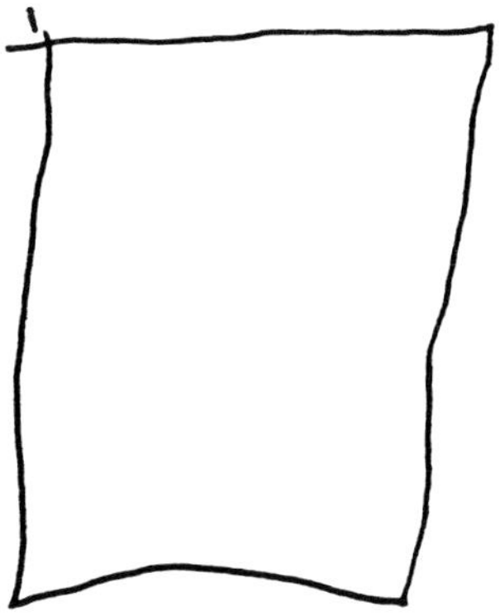

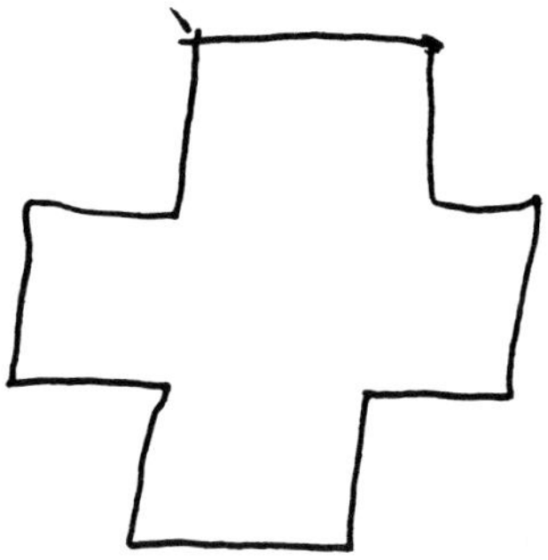

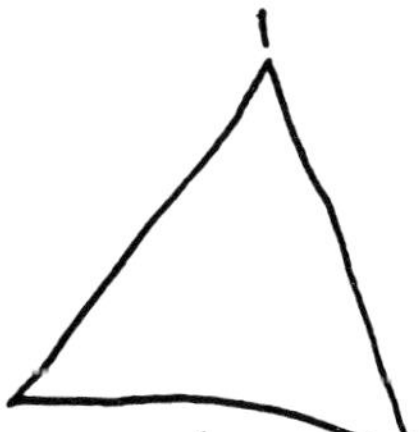

1.

clock

clock

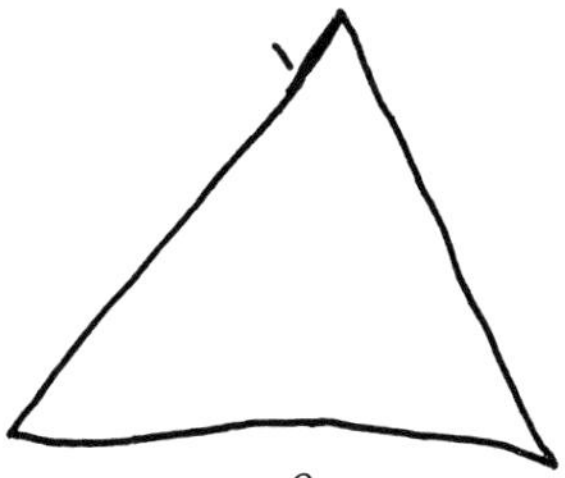

2.

square

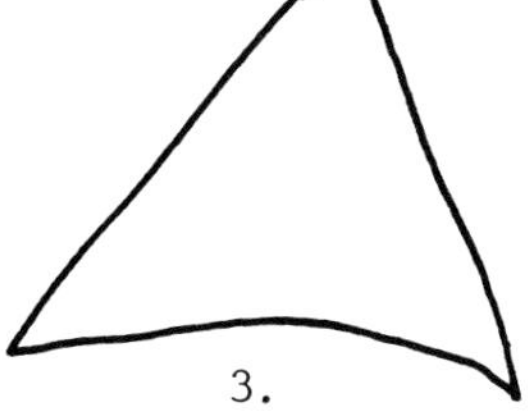

3.

he shouted the warning

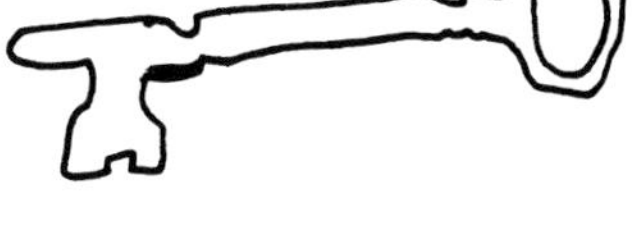

having the lowest score (8). Block Design was the next lowest score (10). Among the Performance subtests, Picture Arrangement and Block Design are the best indicators of right cerebral dysfunction; therefore, this particular pattern might suggest some impairment. However, as we have frequently found with the Wechsler subtests, it is difficult to draw definite conclusions.

The four most sensitive indicators in the HRNTB continued to show a degree of impairment. On this examination the patient performed better on the Trail Making Test (71 sec), suggesting that his quickness and alertness in dealing with fairly well-defined stimulus material has continued to improve. However, on a more complicated task, the Category Test, he showed only slight improvement. On his drawing of the Tactual Performance Test board he was not able to correctly localize any of the shapes, actually performing somewhat worse than he did on the second examination. The Total Time required to complete the Tactual Performance Test was only slightly better this time than on the second examination and all of the improvement is attributable to a better performance with the left upper extremity.

Also note that R.P. did better on the Seashore Rhythm Test (22 correct) and significantly improved his performance on the Speech-sounds Perception Test (3 errors). It would appear that the subject currently has good ability to pay close and continuing attention to specific stimulus material and almost certainly has reached the point where he should be able to work effectively at a job that does not require analysis, reasoning, and definition of problems.

In summary, the test results indicate that some general deficits remain, particularly in the areas of abstraction and reasoning, incidental memory, and the ability to solve complex psychomotor tasks.

Only very mild lateralizing findings were present on the third examination. The drawing of the cross deviated slightly from normal expectancy, particularly in the appositional symmetry of the

extremities. In addition, the patient had to effect compensation in his drawings of the second and third triangles in order to improve their representation of the model. He continued to have some difficulty drawing the key but we could not be confident that this drawing of the key, considered by itself, was definitely pathognomonic.

The patient was not quite as efficient with his left hand on the Tactual Performance Test as would be expected, but the more important finding probably related to the slowness in both performances. Finger tapping speed with the left hand was perhaps very mildly reduced when compared with the right hand and the patient continued to show some impairment with the left hand in Tactile Form Recognition. He also made a mistake in spelling TRIANGLE and continued to have some problems with Tactile Finger Recognition with his right hand.

In summary, the results of the third examination show mild deviation from normal expectancy but have almost reached the point where one would be reluctant to implicate the right cerebral hemisphere to a greater extent than the left. The remaining deficits continue to represent the pattern of particular difficulty with complex tasks that require definition of the nature of the problem before any progress toward its solution can be made.

Both the Cornell Medical Index Health Questionnaire and the Minnesota Multiphasic Personality Inventory were also administered. On the Cornell Medical Index the patient denied any difficulties, indicating only that he had suffered a prior head injury, had been unconscious and had undergone a serious operation. All other possible problems were denied. Results on the MMPI might suggest that the patient was a little defensive and interested in presenting a good image, but the profile was essentially within the normal range.

The three examinations on this man illustrate fairly characteristically the deficits that may be experienced following craniocerebral trauma as well as the process of spontaneous recovery. A great deal of improvement had occurred between the first and the second testings, but much less spontaneous improvement occurred between the second and the third testings. This confirmed our impression that the recovery process was almost complete by the time of the second testing. Although we do not have additional examinations of this patient, we would estimate that the results of the third examination would reflect his permanent cognitive status.

CASE #24

Name: G.C.

Age: 19

Education: 12

Sex: Male

Handedness: Right

Occupation: Student

Background Information and Neurological Examination

G.C. was a freshman in college when he sustained a head injury in an automobile accident. He had recovered uneventfully from the usual childhood illnesses and had always been in good health.

Upon admission to the hospital after the auto accident G.C.'s vital signs were within normal limits but he was deeply obtunded and could be roused only by painful stimuli. It was apparent that he had a right hemiparesis with right facial involvement. Extraocular movements were full, pupils were equal and normally reactive, and there was no evidence of papilledema. Deep tendon reflexes were slightly hyperactive on the right and Babinski signs were present bilaterally. Cerebral angiography was within normal limits and showed no evidence of intracranial mass. However, a lumbar puncture revealed moderately bloody spinal fluid, indicating the probability of cerebral contusion and traumatic subarachnoid hemorrhage.

The patient was placed in the Intensive Care Unit to monitor his condition constantly. He was unconscious for about five days and in a state of impaired consciousness for an additional two weeks. An electroencephalogram done three days after the injury was only minimally abnormal, but another EEG done 12 days later showed diffuse abnormality with maximal involvement in the posterior part of the left cerebral hemisphere. The tracings were interpreted as compatible with contusion of the middle and posterior part of the left cerebral hemisphere. Serial echoencephalograms were all within normal limits.

Within two weeks following the injury the patient was conversant though mildly impaired in spatial and temporal orientation. The neurosurgeon felt that G.C.'s speech was fairly intact although there might be a mild dysphasia. The patient received physical therapy for the paresis of his right arm and leg. The right facial weakness persisted.

Eighteen days following the injury G.C. was discharged to the care of his parents. It was clear from his history information that the patient had sustained a significant closed head injury with probable contusion of the left cerebral hemisphere.

Neuropsychological Examination

Neuropsychological examination was done 51 days post-injury. On the Cornell Medical Index Health Questionnaire G.C. denied any symptoms except that he had been knocked unconscious, part of his body was paralyzed, and there was a constant numbness or tingling in parts of his body. When questioned directly about the nature of his problem, though, he described his head injury, said that his entire right side had been partially paralyzed, his ability to talk had been impaired and his memory was "not so good," but that he was improving. The patient felt that he had essentially regained his pre-injury status.

G.C. earned a Verbal IQ (107) that exceeded 68% of his age peers and a Performance IQ (96)

11 points lower, exceeding 39%. The results indicate that the patient had the advantage of an essentially normal development of intelligence, a conclusion supported by the fact that he was a college student. However, the low score on Digit Span (4) was quite inconsistent with the other Verbal subtest scores and suggests a problem of some kind, even though it may not be due to brain damage.

The distribution of Performance subtest scores might raise a question of cerebral impairment, considering the fact that Digit Symbol (the most sensitive of all the Wechsler subtests to brain damage) was low, earning a score of 7. In addition, it is not uncommon to observe a low Picture Arrangement score in cases of head injury, possibly due to compression and damage of the right anterior temporal pole, a finding observed in many studies. From the results on the Wechsler Scale we see that this young man may have had difficulties and problems, although the findings are not unequivocal in implicating brain damage.

Results on the four most sensitive measures in the HRNTB yielded a mixed picture. The Impairment Index (0.3) was within normal limits and the Category Test (20) was done extremely well. However, the Localization component (4) of the Tactual Performance Test was in the mildly impaired range and the score on Part B of the Trail Making Test (146 sec) was strikingly deviant and appears to require an explanation besides chance variation. At this point, however, one could not definitely conclude that the patient had sustained any cerebral damage.

We can see that C.G. was able to do quite well on a number of tests. It is apparent from the adequate scores on the Seashore Rhythm (26 correct) and Speech-sounds Perception Tests (5 errors) that the first level of central processing (alertness and attention) were intact. The patient also performed well on tests of tactile finger localization and finger-tip number writing perception. He adapted

well to the requirements of the Tactual Performance Test and completed the task with normal improvement on successive trials and an adequate overall time (12.1 min). His Memory score (9) was excellent even though, as noted above, he performed somewhat worse on the Localization score. Many of the results for this man were within normal limits, but there were unexpectedly poor performances as well.

Up to this point in the evaluation of the test results we have depended upon inferences derived from level of performance and variation in adequacy of performances (patterns and relationships among ability levels). We will now evaluate specific deficits and comparisons of performances on the two sides of the body in order to gain additional information.

The Aphasia Screening Test provides the principal information concerning specific deficits. G.C. had certain difficulties dealing with simple language material for communicational purposes that are quite characteristic of persons with left cerebral damage. For example, he initially omitted the "E" when spelling SQUARE, a mistake not uncommon in persons with limited educational backgrounds. It is conceivably possible that G.C. had never learned to spell very well (despite being in college) but after he thought very carefully he was able to correct his error. This kind of response implies that the patient had sustained some kind of spelling deficit rather than never learning to spell.

G.C. demonstrated a similar problem when asked to read 7 SIX 2. Instead of responding quickly (as most normal subjects do), he considered the task very deliberately to determine that he was interpreting the symbols correctly. He did not make an actual error, but it was apparent that he needed to study the stimulus material carefully. On the second reading item he read FRIENDLY as "friend," acted somewhat confused and hesitated for a moment, then corrected himself and was able to read the rest of the sentence correctly. Although this is not a very serious error, it is exactly the way

THE HALSTEAD-REITAN
NEUROPSYCHOLOGICAL TEST BATTERY

Patient ___G.C.___ Age __19__ Sex __M__ Education __12__ Handedness __R__

WECHSLER-BELLEVUE SCALE

VIQ	107
PIQ	96
FS IQ	102

Information	12
Comprehension	12
Digit Span	4
Arithmetic	10
Similarities	14
Vocabulary	10

Picture Arrangement	8
Picture Completion	12
Block Design	12
Object Assembly	10
Digit Symbol	7

TRAIL MAKING TEST

Part A: __56__ seconds
Part B: __146__ seconds

STRENGTH OF GRIP

Dominant hand: __37.5__ kilograms

Non-dominant hand: __42.5__ kilograms

REITAN-KLØVE TACTILE FORM RECOGNITION TEST

Dominant hand: __0__ errors

Non-dominant hand: __0__ errors

REITAN-KLØVE SENSORY-PERCEPTUAL EXAM — No errors

			Error Totals	
RH___ LH___	Both H: RH___ LH___	RH___ LH___		
RH___ LF___	Both H/F: RH___ LF___	RH___ LF___		
LH___ RF___	Both H/F: LH___ RF___	RF___ LH___		
RE___ LE___	Both E: RE___ LE___	RE___ LE___		
RV___ LV___	Both: RV___ LV___	RV___ LV___		

TACTILE FINGER RECOGNITION

R 1___ 2___ 3___ 4___ 5___ R __0__ / 20

L 1___ 2___ 3___ 4___ 5___ L __0__ / 20

FINGER-TIP NUMBER WRITING

R 1___ 2___ 3___ 4 __1__ 5___ R __1__ / 20

L 1___ 2___ 3___ 4___ 5___ L __0__ / 20

HALSTEAD'S NEUROPSYCHOLOGICAL TEST BATTERY

Category Test	20

Tactual Performance Test

Dominant hand:	5.9
Non-dominant hand:	4.2
Both hands:	2.0

Total Time	12.1
Memory	9
Localization	4

Seashore Rhythm Test

Number Correct __26__   5

Speech-sounds Perception Test

Number of Errors   5

Finger Oscillation Test

Dominant hand:	48	48
Non-dominant hand:	45	

Impairment Index   0.3

MINNESOTA MULTIPHASIC PERSONALITY INVENTORY

		Hs	44
		D	39
?	50	Hy	56
L	40	Pd	46
F	48	Mf	53
K	46	Pa	56
		Pt	52
		Sc	48
		Ma	63

REITAN-KLØVE LATERAL-DOMINANCE EXAM

Show me how you:

throw a ball	R
hammer a nail	R
cut with a knife	R
turn a door knob	R
use scissors	R
use an eraser	R
write your name	R

Record time used for spontaneous name-writing:

Preferred hand	7 seconds
Non-preferred hand	25 seconds

Show me how you:

kick a football	R
step on a bug	R

REITAN-INDIANA APHASIA SCREENING TEST

Form for Adults and Older Children

Name: _____ G. C. _____ Age: __19__ Date: _____

Copy SQUARE	Repeat TRIANGLE
Name SQUARE	Repeat MASSACHUSETTS "Massachusess"
Spell SQUARE "S-Q-U-A-R," thought carefully, then corrected the spelling.	Repeat METHODIST EPISCOPAL "Methodist Episcobal"
Copy CROSS	Write SQUARE
Name CROSS	Read SEVEN
Spell CROSS	Repeat SEVEN
Copy TRIANGLE	Repeat/Explain HE SHOUTED THE WARNING.
Name TRIANGLE	Write HE SHOUTED THE WARNING.
Spell TRIANGLE	Compute 85 – 27 =
Name BABY	Compute 17 X 3 = "41" 12 x 5 = "60"
Write CLOCK	Name KEY
Name FORK	Demonstrate use of KEY
Read 7 SIX 2 "Seven, then the word six, then the numeral two."	Draw KEY
Read MGW	Read PLACE LEFT HAND TO RIGHT EAR. "Place left hand to the right ear." corrected spontaneously.
Reading I	Place LEFT HAND TO RIGHT EAR
Reading II "He is a friend" (hesitated), corrected himself, and read the rest correctly.	Place LEFT HAND TO LEFT ELBOW

G.C.

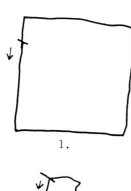

1.

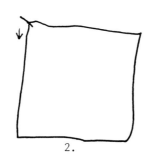

2.

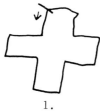

1.

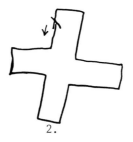

2.

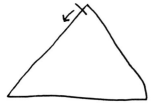

clock

square

he shouted the warning

85
27
5 8

41
60

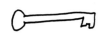

many persons with limited ability proceed. In fact, these types of mistakes on the Aphasia Screening Test would be sufficient to implicate a mild degree of impairment in dealing with verbal symbols. G.C. also had some difficulty reading PLACE LEFT HAND TO RIGHT EAR, gratuitously inserting "the". Again, his spontaneous correction documented the fact that he had made an error. His enunciation of MASSACHUSETTS and METHODIST EPISCOPAL were within normal limits and his computational error was the type that frequently occurs among normal subjects.

Careful evaluation of the patient's drawings yields further evidence of mild cerebral damage. In the first drawing of the square the subject drew the second line too long and had to compensate to complete the figure properly. He had the same kind of problem in his second attempt to draw the cross and, in addition, did not manage to balance the extremities quite as well as he should have. The drawing of the key is difficult to interpret because the patient did not include any details.

Measures of lateral dominance indicated that the patient was strongly right-handed. His grip strength, however, was distinctly less for his right upper extremity (37.5 kg) than his left (42.5 kg). Also note that the patient was a little slow in finger tapping speed with his right hand (48) compared with his left (45), although this score was almost within normal limits. Slight impairment of the right upper extremity on both of these measures has a complementary effect and, in the context of mild difficulty dealing with language symbols for communicational purposes, suggests mild left cerebral impairment.

If one were dependent exclusively on a level-of-performance approach it is likely that a conclusion of normal brain functions would be reached despite the poor score on Part B of the Trail Making Test. Many clinicians, observing the good scores on several tests, would reason that some variability in results was expected and the Trail Making Test was merely reflecting the extreme end of this range. However, when we evaluate the specific difficulties on simple spelling and reading tasks on the Aphasia Screening Test and note the mild impairment of motor functions of the right upper extremity, we can see that the overall picture strongly points to mild but nonetheless definite brain damage. Even the poor score on the Picture Arrangement subtest (8) and the mild problem drawing the figures in the Aphasia Screening Test are significant, indicating mild right cerebral hemisphere dysfunction.

It is unusual to find dysphasia and lateralized motor dysfunction in a persons with a normal Impairment Index and such a good score on the Category Test, but be aware that the good scores do not limit the conclusion of mild brain damage based upon right-left differences, specific deficits, poor performances on certain sensitive tests, and the overall configuration of the test results.

Originally this case was evaluated "blindly," before referring to the history information, and it was noted that although the pattern of results was unusual it was nevertheless unequivocal in its implication of brain damage. A considerable degree of experience is necessary to be able to recognize such a configuration of mild impairment and know that it definitely and unequivocally indicates residual cerebral damage, but for the alert and astute clinician the information is available in the test results.

Considering his history information, this man showed a remarkable recovery following his injury. His right hemiparesis was obvious approximately five weeks earlier when he was discharged from the hospital but at the present time he performed very well with his right upper extremity on the complex manipulatory tasks required by the Tactual Performance Test and had only a mild degree of impairment in finger tapping speed and grip strength. Although the neurosurgeon had felt that the patient had fairly intact speech and no evidence of gross aphasia, it is likely that G.C. had much more difficulty using language symbols for communicational purposes several weeks ago than he did on this neuropsychological examination. The patient's own observation that his skill in verbal communication was impaired is such an indication.

Although we did not have the opportunity to follow this man and chart his progress in college, it appeared likely that he would have considerably more difficulty dealing with the verbal and language requirements of his schoolwork than he did previously. A considerable clinical service could have been provided by closely coordinating the patient's remaining deficits with his academic requirements, so that he would not be taking classes too difficult for him and causing him to fail. He should also receive counseling from a therapist who understands the neuropsychological basis of his deficits and could help G.C. gain better insight into the difficulties that he will encounter. In addition, his impaired abilities in concentrating when confronted with tasks that involve several elements (Part B of the Trail Making Test) constituted another problem that would probably be inhibiting when G.C. attempted to do college work. Even though G.C. appeared to have made remarkable and rapid improvement, his residual deficits could be significant in limiting his academic progress and be very emotionally upsetting in the future unless the patient gains some understanding of the nature of his problems through counseling.

CASE #25

Name: C.S.

Age: 32

Education: 9

Sex: Male

Handedness: Right

Occupation: Railroad conductor

Background Information

C.S., a chronic alcoholic for several years, was involved in an automobile accident when he was 30 years old. He sustained a depressed skull fracture in the left parietal area (which had to be elevated surgically) and was unconscious for approximately six weeks following the accident.

Twenty-one months after the accident C.S. was admitted to a major medical center because he had recently experienced a major motor seizure. His physician attributed the seizure to the prior brain injury. In addition to controlling the seizures it was hoped that C.S. could also receive rehabilitation therapy for his residual speech and language deficits, a right hemiparesis, and a "memory loss" that had lead to impaired efficiency in occupational and everyday activities.

It is not uncommon for patients with significant neuropsychological impairment (especially when the deficits include the areas of abstraction, reasoning, and logical analysis) to identify their problem as "memory loss." This same characterization of neuropsychological dysfunction is frequently given by neuropsychologists who fail to do a complete neuropsychological examination and, as a result, do not learn about the patient's specific deficits.

Neurological Examination

At the time of admission C.S. was oriented to time, person, and place but had some difficulty with memory of past events. He could not recall the accident or any activities that occurred two days preceding it. The neurologist noted that C.S. demonstrated some stuttering and an element of dysarthria. The patient's muscle stretch reflexes were hyperactive on the right side of the body; there was no extensor toe sign (Babinski reflex). The patient also demonstrated some evidence of dystereognosis. The neurologist also noted C.S.'s apparent lack of concern about his disabilities.

Skull x-rays indicated a defect in the left parietal region associated with the depressed skull fracture and surgical treatment. The electroencephalogram revealed a significant asymmetry of the Alpha rhythm showing a suppression of activity on the left side compared to the right. The EEG abnormality principally involved the left parietal area but also extended into the temporal region. A pneumoencephalogram demonstrated moderate dilatation of all the ventricles, essentially equivalent and comparable on both sides.

C.S. was hospitalized for approximately five months for intensive rehabilitation and no seizures were observed during that time. The neuropsychological evaluation was done during the third month of hospitalization (two years post-injury). The patient had been actively involved in speech therapy and physical therapy, felt that he was profiting from these activities, and had no particular complaints.

Neuropsychological Examination

C.S. earned relatively low IQ values. His Verbal IQ (88) exceeded only about 21% of his age peers and his Performance IQ (60) exceeded less than 1%. Although his Verbal subtest scores were consistently below the average level, a number of the scores suggested that at one time C.S. may possibly have done somewhat better. Scores on Information, Comprehension and Vocabulary were slightly higher than scores on the other Verbal subtests.

Scores on the Performance subtests were consistently far below average (two standard deviations or more) and the resulting Performance IQ was strikingly deficient. Since none of his Verbal subtest scores were nearly as low as his highest Performance subtest score, it appears that the patient's verbal intelligence was better than his performance intelligence. Note, though, that the pattern of scores did not simulate results that would be expected from a person with a lateralized cerebral lesion; instead, C.S.'s individual subtest scores showed no particularly striking pattern and his results were similar to those seen in persons with generalized, chronic cerebral damage.

The patient performed poorly on all four of the most sensitive indicators in the Halstead-Reitan Battery. He earned an Impairment Index of 1.0, did quite poorly on Part B of the Trail Making Test (153 sec), made 76 errors on the Category Test and was able to localize only two figures in his drawing of the Tactual Performance Test. These scores strongly suggest that C.S. has significant generalized impairment of abilities dependent upon brain functions.

We should note, however, that C.S.'s score on the Seashore Rhythm Test (25 correct) was definitely better than his scores on the four most sensitive indicators. Despite his relatively low IQ, he

performed at the average level for brain-damaged subjects on the Speech-sounds Perception Test (14 errors).

The reader should keep in mind that the correlation between Verbal IQ and the Speech-sounds Perception Test score is generally high (Reitan, 1956a) and C.S.'s score on the latter test was particularly good in consideration of his Verbal IQ. Therefore, his scores on the Speech-sounds Perception and Rhythm Tests, which reflect ability to pay attention to specific and well-defined stimulus material, were considerably better than many of his other performances. Such results would suggest that C.S.'s brain impairment is relatively chronic and stabilized in a biological sense.

Lateralizing indicators consistently implicated the left cerebral hemisphere to a much greater extent than the right. C.S.'s difficulties principally involved the right side of his body. Although he was strongly right-handed (and had been before his injury) his finger tapping speed and grip strength were both strikingly reduced with the right upper extremity compared with the left. Thus, right-sided motor impairment was definitely established.

C.S. also had distinct sensory-perceptual losses on the right side. On the Tactile Form Recognition Test he was much slower and made more mistakes on his right hand (42 sec, 3 errors) than his left (12 sec, 0 errors). In addition, he had difficulty perceiving tactile and auditory stimuli on the right side when a competing stimulus was administered simultaneously on the left side. The consistency of the latter results was perfect except when the left hand and right face were in competition; in that instance the patient had some difficulty on each side, reflecting the fact that the face is more sensitive than the hand and, even with left hemisphere damage, the face competed equally with the hand in terms of tactile perception.

On the Tactile Finger Recognition Test C.S. also had much more difficulty with his right hand

THE HALSTEAD-REITAN
NEUROPSYCHOLOGICAL TEST BATTERY

Patient _____ **C.S.** _____ Age __**32**__ Sex __**M**__ Education __**9**__ Handedness __**R**__

WECHSLER-BELLEVUE SCALE

VIQ	88
PIQ	60
FS IQ	73

Information	8
Comprehension	9
Digit Span	6
Arithmetic	7
Similarities	6
Vocabulary	8

Picture Arrangement	4
Picture Completion	3
Block Design	3
Object Assembly	0
Digit Symbol	4

TRAIL MAKING TEST

Part A: __**116**__ seconds
Part B: __**153**__ seconds

STRENGTH OF GRIP

Dominant hand: __**14.5**__ kilograms
Non-dominant hand: __**35.0**__ kilograms

REITAN-KLØVE TACTILE FORM RECOGNITION TEST

Dominant hand: __**42**__ seconds; __**3**__ errors
Non-dominant hand: __**12**__ seconds; __**0**__ errors

REITAN-KLØVE SENSORY-PERCEPTUAL EXAM

			Error Totals
RH___ LH___	Both H:	RH **2** LH___	RH **2** LH___
RH___ LF___	Both H/F:	RH **3** LF___	RH **3** LF___
LH___ RF___	Both H/F:	LH **1** RF **1**	RF **1** LH **1**
RE___ LE___	Both E:	RE **2** LE___	RE **2** LE___
RV___ LV___	Both:	RV___ LV___	RV___ LV___

TACTILE FINGER RECOGNITION

R 1 **1** 2 **2** 3 **2** 4 **4** 5 **2**   R **11** / **20**

L 1___ 2 **1** 3 **2** 4 **1** 5___   L **4** / **20**

FINGER-TIP NUMBER WRITING

R 1 **3** 2 **2** 3 **4** 4 **2** 5 **3**   R **14** / **20**

L 1 **3** 2 **2** 3 **2** 4 **3** 5 **2**   L **12** / **20**

HALSTEAD'S NEUROPSYCHOLOGICAL TEST BATTERY

Category Test		76

Tactual Performance Test

Dominant hand:	**15.0 (2 blocks)**
Non-dominant hand:	**7.9**
Both hands:	**7.2**

Total Time	**30.1 (22 blocks)**
Memory	**4**
Localization	**2**

Seashore Rhythm Test

Number Correct __**25**__   **6**

Speech-sounds Perception Test

Number of Errors   **14**

Finger Oscillation Test

Dominant hand:	**28** **28**
Non-dominant hand:	**43**

Impairment Index   **1.0**

MINNESOTA MULTIPHASIC PERSONALITY INVENTORY

			Hs	67
			D	68
?	50		Hy	67
L	53		Pd	66
F	53		Mf	65
K	42		Pa	67
			Pt	52
			Sc	63
			Ma	60

REITAN-KLØVE LATERAL-DOMINANCE EXAM

Show me how you:

throw a ball	R
hammer a nail	R
cut with a knife	R
turn a door knob	R
use scissors	R
use an eraser	R
write your name	R

Record time used for spontaneous name-writing:

Preferred hand	**18** seconds
Non-preferred hand	**16** seconds

Show me how you:

kick a football	R
step on a bug	R

REITAN-INDIANA APHASIA SCREENING TEST

Form for Adults and Older Children

Name: _____C. S._____ Age: __32___

Copy SQUARE	Repeat TRIANGLE
Name SQUARE "Block"	Repeat MASSACHUSETTS "Masschusetts"
Spell SQUARE	Repeat METHODIST EPISCOPAL
Copy CROSS	Write SQUARE
Name CROSS "Red Cross button"	Read SEVEN
Spell CROSS	Repeat SEVEN
Copy TRIANGLE	Repeat/Explain HE SHOUTED THE WARNING.
Name TRIANGLE	Write HE SHOUTED THE WARNING.
Spell TRIANGLE	Compute 85 – 27 = See attempts. Finally correct on third trial.
Name BABY	Compute 17 X 3 = Could not do.
Write CLOCK	Name KEY
Name FORK	Demonstrate use of KEY
Read 7 SIX 2	Draw KEY
Read MGW	Read PLACE LEFT HAND TO RIGHT EAR.
Reading I	Place LEFT HAND TO RIGHT EAR
Reading II	Place LEFT HAND TO LEFT ELBOW Initially placed left hand to right elbow. Corrected after questioned by examiner.

1.

2.

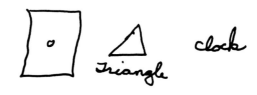

Triangle   clock

Square   cross

seven

1. $\begin{array}{r} 85 \\ 27 \\ \hline 18 \\ 63 \\ \hline 48 \end{array}$

2. $27\overline{)85}$

3. $\begin{array}{r} 85 \\ 27 \\ \hline 58 \end{array}$

he shouted a warning

(11 errors) than his left (4 errors). The more complex task of finger-tip writing perception did not show such strikingly lateralized findings, probably because of the patient's generalized impairment (Fitzhugh, Fitzhugh, & Reitan, 1961). C.S. also had a considerable amount of trouble on the Tactual Performance Test when using his right upper extremity; in 15 minutes he was able to place only two blocks. We see, then, that the results of tests that provide a direct comparison of performances on the two sides of the individual's body strongly indicated that C.S. had more significant impairment of the left cerebral hemisphere than the right.

Note, though, that C.S. did not show any evidence of specific and severe language deficits on the Aphasia Screening Test. From his efforts to name the SQUARE and the CROSS we would judge that he had some mild difficulty using language for communicational purposes. He did not enunciate MASSACHUSETTS perfectly, but it would be difficult to attribute his error to left cerebral damage.

C.S. did show definite evidence of dyscalculia; he was quite confused in his various attempts to subtract 27 from 85 (see the recorded results). He finally was able to solve the problem but only after more confusion that included an attempt to divide 85 by 27. As the reader will recall, dyscalculia occurs about four times more frequently in persons with left cerebral damage than right cerebral damage (Wheeler & Reitan, 1962).

The patient also had mild difficulty responding to the examiner's request to place his left hand to his left elbow. Initially he placed his left hand to his right elbow; after the examiner asked him to consider the request more carefully C.S. was able to perform the task correctly.

Although these indications of left cerebral damage are unequivocal in their significance they are not nearly as strong as the evidence of motor and sensory-perceptual deficits on the right side.

Results of this kind suggest that the patient probably has shown a degree of recovery of dysphasia, even though lateralized deficits of lower-level functions are still present.

We also see that C.S. had a few difficulties that implicated the right cerebral hemisphere. Although his drawings of the cross and key were much smaller than the stimulus figures, they strongly suggested that he had some problems dealing with spatial configurations. In addition, recall that his Performance IQ was much lower than his Verbal IQ.

Results on the Minnesota Multiphasic Personality Inventory suggested that C.S. also had concerns of an emotional and affective nature. This is hardly surprising considering the fact that the neuropsychological testing was done two years after the injury was sustained and during that time the patient had been faced with significant neuropsychological deficits that impeded his prospect of effecting an adequate adjustment.

We previously mentioned that this man had a history of alcoholism for several years in addition to a serious closed head injury that rendered him unconscious for about six weeks. In such cases it is often difficult to differentiate between the neuropsychological impairment caused by chronic alcoholism and the deficits due to traumatic brain injury. Although such a differentiation can sometimes be made, it is not possible in the majority of cases.

Sometimes the patient demonstrates very mild, though definite, lateralizing signs (resulting from a head injury) as well as severe losses on the general indicators of cognitive functioning. In such cases the mild lateralizing deficits are not sufficiently strong to account for the serious generalized impairment and the interpreter can deduce that the head injury was probably not severe enough to account for the serious generalized dysfunction. One can then postulate that the serious general losses resulted from a long-term, continuing, deteriorative influence (such as chronic alcoholism).

Most patients in whom such a judgment can be drawn, however, are older than C.S. and have a history of alcoholism that extends over decades. Even in such cases, though, the patient may have sustained a very severe head injury which compromised the general indicators of brain functions in addition to demonstrating specific signs of focal or lateralized deficit.

In general, it is likely that the effects of craniocerebral trauma will be more severe and pronounced in persons who are chronic alcoholics because they will show the additive effect of multiple sources of brain insult. However, in individual instances, as in this man's case, it is often difficult to differentiate between the adverse effects of alcoholism and head injury, even though both conditions may have contributed to the neuropsychological dysfunction.

CASE #26

Name: M.V.

Age: 55

Education: 14

Sex: Female

Handedness: Right

Occupation: Housewife

Background Information

Other than a long history of chronic alcoholism M.V.'s health had always been good. One day she was alone in her house and apparently fell and struck her head on a heavy piece of furniture. She believes that she was unconscious only briefly but several hours following the injury she became confused and developed a left hemiparesis.

Her husband, a physician, came home about four hours after the accident occurred and noted that M.V.'s right pupil was larger than her left pupil and that she had a marked hemiparesis, hyperactive reflexes and a Babinski sign on the left side. These symptoms, as well as the confusion, persisted four hours later (eight hours after the injury) and she was seen by a neurosurgeon who admitted her to the hospital.

Neurological Examination

At the time of admission M.V. was quite confused and very lethargic. Although examination of the fundi did not show any evidence of papilledema or hemorrhage, her right pupil was still dilated and did not react to light. She showed a complete loss of third cranial nerve function on the right side. There was a slight left facial paresis, a 3 cm–4 cm area of swelling over the right occipital region, and a large area of ecchymosis over the right mastoid area and extending down into the neck (Battle's sign). M.V. was able to move both left upper and lower extremities although they were

definitely paretic. Hyperactive reflexes and a Babinski sign were still present on the left side.

Bilateral cerebral angiograms done shortly after admission to the hospital showed a large mass in the right temporal area. A right subtemporal craniectomy revealed a subdural hematoma which was evacuated. However, because the neurosurgeon felt that the brain was still under considerable tension following this procedure, a small cortical incision was made and a huge intracerebral hematoma in the right inferior temporal area was found and evacuated. Tissue of the area taken for biopsy was compatible with acute hematoma and showed no evidence of pre-existing disease.

The patient tolerated surgery well and 24 hours after the injury had occurred she was awake and talking, although she had a mild dysarthria and a slight deviation of her tongue to the left. The third cranial nerve paresis had almost completely resolved and the left hemiparesis had definitely improved. There was no appreciable weakness of her left upper or lower extremity. M.V.'s pupils were equal and responded to light and there was no imbalance of the extraocular muscles.

On the second post-operative day the patient started becoming confused and had visual hallucinations. Her wound was healing satisfactorily and her neurological examination was within normal limits, but she continued to have marked confabulation and periods of confusion and disorientation. The neurological and psychiatric opinion was that M.V. showed evidence of Korsakoff's syndrome. Although liver function tests were within normal limits, her physicians believed that the combination of chronic alcoholism and the brain injury was responsible for her continuing disorientation and confabulation (even though she had recovered from deficits initially shown on the neurological examination).

Electroencephalography done nine days and fifteen days following the injury showed generalized slow wave activity maximal in the right Sylvian area and a generalized dysrhythmia maximal in the left Sylvian area. Although she occasionally had brief lucid intervals, M.V.'s confabulation was present for most of the 26 days she was hospitalized.

Neuropsychological Examination

The first neuropsychological examination was done 10 days after the injury. As might be expected, this woman was somewhat difficult to test; we had to discontinue testing when she was in a period of extreme confusion and the Battery was administered over a period of several days. Nevertheless, it was possible to obtain enough valid data to draw meaningful clinical conclusions about the patient's neuropsychological status. She was not able to make any reliable progress on tests such as the Minnesota Multiphasic Personality Inventory because she had no efficiency or organization of her activities when left alone.

It is not unusual for brain-damaged persons to be unable to maintain organized and efficient behavior on their own initiative. This is the reason that many of the psychological tests that have been developed for normal persons cannot be administered appropriately to brain-damaged persons. The examiner frequently must maintain close contact with the subject, item by item, in order to elicit valid performances.

Even following standard procedure was difficult in this case. For example, M.V. was completely confused by the Seashore Rhythm Test and was able to make no progress, although when she took the Speech-sounds Perception Test she was able to pay close attention and follow instructions throughout the entire test. The Tactual Performance Test was extremely difficult and frustrating for M.V.; after working for 5.2 minutes with her right hand and placing two blocks, she suddenly tore off the blindfold and refused to continue taking the test. When she removed the blindfold she saw the board and blocks so we did not try to complete the test or have the patient do the drawing of the board.

The patient earned Verbal (106), Performance (104), and Full Scale (104) IQ values in the upper part of the Average range, exceeding 61% to 66% of her age peers. The subtest distribution definitely suggests that M.V. has experienced some degree of impairment of certain aspects of both Verbal and Performance intelligence. Among the Verbal subtests that appear to be particularly resistive to impairment (Information, Comprehension, Similarities, and Vocabulary), all except Comprehension had scores a standard deviation or more above the mean. As we have noted previously, the Digit Span score is usually low in a hospitalized population regardless of the presence or absence of brain damage.

It is possible that this woman had not had much need to perform arithmetical problems and the low score on Arithmetic (7) was a reflection of such circumstances, but we should also note that the Arithmetic subtest is probably the most sensitive of the Verbal subtests to brain damage. Therefore, it is possible that the patient is demonstrating some degree of impairment on the Arithmetic (and possibly Comprehension) subtest.

The results on the Performance subtests are much more definitive. The lowest scores are on Picture Arrangement (4), Block Design (6), and Digit Symbol (6). While the latter of these tests is often impaired in persons with generalized cerebral damage, Picture Arrangement and Block Design most reliably reflect right hemisphere involvement. The pattern of results shown by this woman

THE HALSTEAD-REITAN
NEUROPSYCHOLOGICAL TEST BATTERY

Patient ___M.V. (I)___ Age __55__ Sex __F__ Education __14__ Handedness __R__

WECHSLER-BELLEVUE SCALE

VIQ	106
PIQ	104
FS IQ	104
Information	13
Comprehension	8
Digit Span	6
Arithmetic	7
Similarities	13
Vocabulary	14
Picture Arrangement	4
Picture Completion	8
Block Design	6
Object Assembly	10
Digit Symbol	6

TRAIL MAKING TEST

Part A: __50__ seconds
Part B: __257__ seconds

STRENGTH OF GRIP

Dominant hand: __19.0__ kilograms
Non-dominant hand: __16.5__ kilograms

REITAN-KLØVE TACTILE FORM RECOGNITION TEST

Dominant hand: __14__ seconds; __0__ errors
Non-dominant hand: __23__ seconds; __0__ errors

REITAN-KLØVE SENSORY-PERCEPTUAL EXAM

				Error Totals	
RH___ LH___	Both H:	RH___ LH___		RH___ LH___	
RH___ LF___	Both H/F:	RH___ LF___		RH___ LF___	
LH___ RF___	Both H/F:	LH___ RF___		RF___ LH___	
RE _3_ LE___	Both E:	RE _4_ LE _0_		RE _4_ LE___	
RV___ LV___	Both:	RV___ LV___		RIGHT EAR DEAFNESS	
___ ___		___ ___			
___ ___		___ ___			

TACTILE FINGER RECOGNITION

R 1___ 2___ 3___ 4___ 5___   R __0__ / __20__

L 1___ 2___ 3___ 4___ 5 _1_   L __1__ / __20__

FINGER-TIP NUMBER WRITING

R 1 _2_ 2___ 3___ 4___ 5___   R __2__ / __20__

L 1 _2_ 2___ 3___ 4___ 5___   L __2__ / __20__

NO EVIDENCE OF APHASIA (SEE DRAWINGS)

HALSTEAD'S NEUROPSYCHOLOGICAL TEST BATTERY

Category Test   127

Tactual Performance Test

Dominant hand:	**5.2 (2 blocks)**
Non-dominant hand:	Not Done
Both hands:	Not Done

Total Time	—
Memory	Not Done
Localization	Not Done

Seashore Rhythm Test

Number Correct   Could Not Do   —

Speech-sounds Perception Test

Number of Errors   8

Finger Oscillation Test

Dominant hand:	40	40
Non-dominant hand:	14	

Impairment Index   1.0 (Est.)

REITAN-KLØVE
LATERAL-DOMINANCE EXAM

Show me how you:

throw a ball	**R**
hammer a nail	**R**
cut with a knife	**R**
turn a door knob	**R**
use scissors	**R**
use an eraser	**R**
write your name	**R**

Record time used for spontaneous name-writing:

Preferred hand	__8__ seconds
Non-preferred hand	__33__ seconds

Show me how you:

kick a football	**R**
step on a bug	**R**

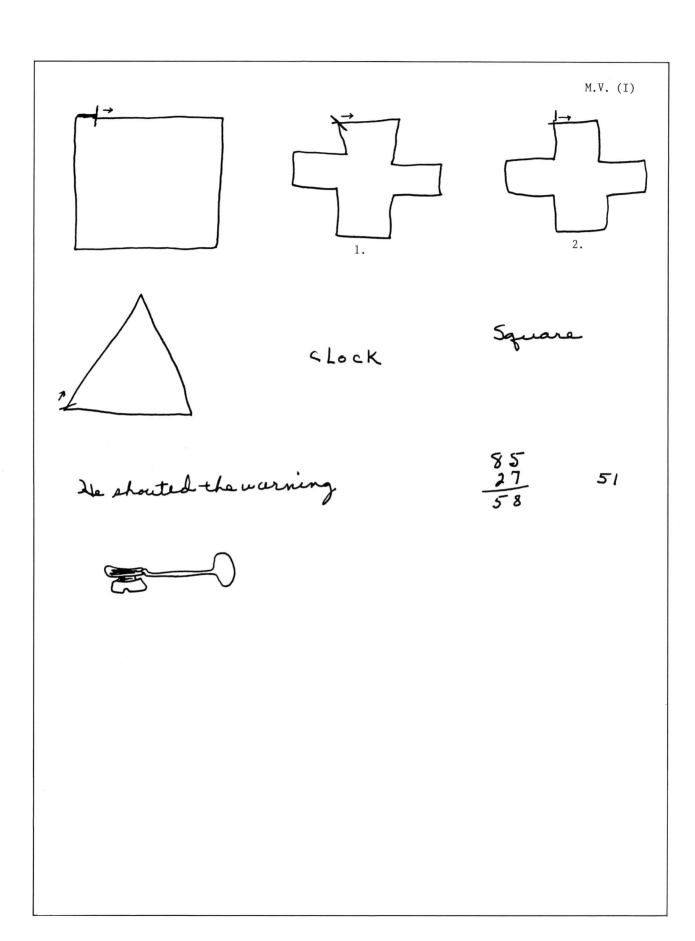

1.

2.

cLock

Square

He shouted the warning

$$\begin{array}{r} 85 \\ 27 \\ \hline 58 \end{array}$$

51

are not only suggestive of brain damage in general but would definitely raise a question about more significant involvement of the right cerebral hemisphere. (The reader should be aware that the relatively high Performance IQ compared to the Verbal IQ is a function of the age adjustment used with the Wechsler-Bellevue Scale).

Compared to the IQ values, there was much more significant evidence of neuropsychological deficit on the four most sensitive measures in the HRNTB. Because the patient did not complete the Tactual Performance Test and was not able to do the Seashore Rhythm Test it was necessary to estimate the Impairment Index. Since it seemed likely that her performances on the tests she did not do would have been impaired, we estimated the Impairment Index to be 1.0.

M.V. had great difficulty with the Category Test (127) and performed very poorly on Part B of the Trail Making Test (257 sec). In fact, among Halstead's tests and the Trail Making Test, M.V.'s only satisfactory score was on the Speech-sounds Perception Test (8). This score indicates that at certain times (or perhaps with certain test content) she was able to maintain concentrated attention over a period of time.

It is difficult to postulate why the patient was not able to do the Seashore Rhythm Test. It would be tempting to conclude that the non-verbal content was the critical factor, but such a conclusion is not borne out as showing a significant differential result in comparison of groups of subjects with lateralized lesions.

In summary, the test findings are quite clear in indicating that this woman has significant and serious impairment of higher-level neuropsychological functions.

The lateralizing indicators included (1) the Picture Arrangement score; (2) the Block Design score; (3) impairment of finger tapping speed with the left hand; (4) some degree of deficit in Tactile Form Recognition with the left hand; and (5) very mild difficulties in copying the cross and key. The

strongest and most definite of these indicators involved finger tapping speed, although the slowness of response with the left hand in tactile form discrimination was definite and provided evidence of both a tactile-perceptual as well as motor deficit on the left side.

Each of the patient's drawings of the cross demonstrates a similar deviation from a perfectly normal performance. The first attempt, with the plane of the lateral extremities being different, is probably more blatantly deviant. Obviously, these are not grossly defective drawings, but they are quite characteristic of the type of difficulty shown by persons with right cerebral damage. Although the key was not drawn in much detail, it also suggests right cerebral dysfunction. Note that the critical error in the drawing of the key relates to the notches in the stem near the teeth. Therefore, we see that the positive findings relating to right cerebral damage are consistent and definite.

The patient showed no evidence of difficulty on the Aphasia Test, although she was quite detailed and even loquacious in her verbal explanations.

It is interesting to find that M.V. had relatively little difficulty on the Sensory-perceptual Examination. She did not respond readily to auditory stimuli delivered to the right ear regardless of whether the stimulus was given unilaterally or bilaterally and this was probably due to a peripheral hearing loss. However, most of her responses were accurate in Tactile Finger Recognition and Fingertip Number Writing Perception.

In comparing groups of subjects with lateralized cerebral lesions (cerebral vascular lesions, intrinsic tumors, and head injuries), Hom and Reitan (1982) found that the subjects with head injuries had less difficulties on the sensory-perceptual tasks than the other two groups. We must also note that this group also demonstrated less evidence of impairment in finger tapping speed.

Although M.V. was impaired in finger tapping speed with her left hand, the fact that she was able to perform relatively well on the sensory-perceptual tests would lean the interpretation in the direction of head trauma rather than certain other types of lateralized lesions.

Some of the test findings in this case were somewhat surprising: (1) the generalized brain functions were significantly impaired; (2) the indications of right cerebral hemisphere dysfunction were definite (though not pervasive); and (3) there were no specific indications of left cerebral damage. When lateralizing indications principally implicate one cerebral hemisphere and general indicators show evidence of severe impairment, there are usually at least some isolated results which implicate the other cerebral hemisphere.

In this case we followed our usual procedure of testing the patient without referring to the history or neurological findings beforehand. However, after the neuropsychological testing had been completed we learned that M.V.'s neurological and psychiatric evaluations had indicated that her clinical condition represented an interaction of chronic alcoholism and the head injury and a diagnosis of Korsakoff's syndrome had been made. We were interested in obtaining a follow-up examination because it seemed likely that the patient would show a substantial degree of improvement.

The main basis for the diagnosis of Korsakoff's syndrome was the patient's episodes of confusion, disorientation and confabulation. These symptoms might be related to the indications of general neuropsychological deficit, but the rest of the neuropsychological picture did not suggest gross or severe brain damage. In fact, in time M.V. may show improvement in some of her areas of deficit (e.g., finger tapping speed).

Six weeks after the initial examination (approximately eight weeks after the injury) we had the opportunity to re-examine this woman.

On the second neuropsychological examination M.V. showed substantial improvement, although some deficits were still present and the general pattern of test results was the same. Both

Verbal (114) and Performance (113) IQ values were now in the High Average range, exceeding just over 80% of her age peers. Although there may have been some degree of positive practice-effect, it is important to note that practically no changes occurred on any subtests except those that had initially been identified as impaired. The same pattern of results was present, with Digit Span (7) and Arithmetic (9) being the lowest of the Verbal subtests and Picture Arrangement (7), Block Design (6), and Digit Symbol (7) having the lowest scores of the Performance subtests.

The patient continued to show evidence of significant impairment on the four most sensitive indicators. The Impairment Index (.9), which represents *consistency* of deficit rather than *severity* of deficit, indicated that approximately 90% of the tests had scores in the brain-damaged range; only the Speech-sounds Perception Test score (5) was in the normal range. Thus, it is clear that M.V. was generally impaired in her basic adaptive abilities despite her relatively adequate IQ values.

M.V. showed a great deal of improvement on the Category Test (74) and Part B of the Trail Making Test (112 sec), suggesting that she is considerably more alert, can deal with complex situations more effectively, and has improved abstraction and reasoning abilities. Nevertheless, the performances on the Category Test and the Tactual Performance Test (including the Memory [3] and Localization [0] components) were impaired. M.V. did well on the Speech-sounds Perception Test (5) but, as she did on the initial examination, performed very poorly on the Seashore Rhythm Test (26 errors). The reason for this deficient performance, in terms of a neuropsychological explanation, is not apparent.

Results from the Minnesota Multiphasic Personality Inventory were essentially within the normal range, although this woman might be viewed as somewhat rigid and concerned about the image that she projects to others. Even though the MMPI did not suggest significant emotional problems, it

THE HALSTEAD-REITAN
NEUROPSYCHOLOGICAL TEST BATTERY

Patient ___M.V. (II)___ Age __55__ Sex __F__ Education __14__ Handedness __R__

WECHSLER-BELLEVUE SCALE
VIQ	114
PIQ	113
FS IQ	114
Information	13
Comprehension	12
Digit Span	7
Arithmetic	9
Similarities	14
Vocabulary	14
Picture Arrangement	7
Picture Completion	13
Block Design	6
Object Assembly	10
Digit Symbol	7

TRAIL MAKING TEST
Part A: __47__ seconds
Part B: __112__ seconds

STRENGTH OF GRIP
Dominant hand: __23.0__ kilograms
Non-dominant hand: __21.5__ kilograms

REITAN-KLØVE TACTILE FORM RECOGNITION TEST
Dominant hand: __11__ seconds; __0__ errors
Non-dominant hand: __16__ seconds; __0__ errors

REITAN-KLØVE SENSORY-PERCEPTUAL EXAM — No errors

			Error Totals	
RH___LH___	Both H: RH___LH___	RH___LH___		
RH___LF___	Both H/F: RH___LF___	RH___LF___		
LH___RF___	Both H/F: LH___RF___	RF___LH___		
RE___LE___	Both E: RE___LE___	RE___LE___		
RV___LV___	Both: RV___LV___	RV___LV___		

TACTILE FINGER RECOGNITION
R 1__2__3__4__5__ R __0__ / __20__
L 1__2__3__4__5__ L __0__ / __20__

FINGER-TIP NUMBER WRITING
R 1__2__3__4__5__ R __0__ / __20__
L 1__2__3__4__5__ L __0__ / __20__

NO APHASIC SYMPTOMS

HALSTEAD'S NEUROPSYCHOLOGICAL TEST BATTERY

Category Test __74__

Tactual Performance Test
Dominant hand:	13.6
Non-dominant hand:	13.6
Both hands:	10.0

Total Time	37.2
Memory	3
Localization	0

Seashore Rhythm Test
Number Correct __4__ __10__

Speech-sounds Perception Test
Number of Errors __5__

Finger Oscillation Test
Dominant hand: __41__ __41__
Non-dominant hand: __34__

Impairment Index __0.9__

MINNESOTA MULTIPHASIC PERSONALITY INVENTORY

		Hs	48
		D	49
?	50	Hy	52
L	70	Pd	57
F	46	Mf	49
K	70	Pa	53
		Pt	48
		Sc	51
		Ma	38

REITAN-KLØVE LATERAL-DOMINANCE EXAM

Show me how you:
throw a ball	R
hammer a nail	R
cut with a knife	R
turn a door knob	R
use scissors	R
use an eraser	R
write your name	R

Record time used for spontaneous name-writing:
Preferred hand	__7__ seconds
Non-preferred hand	__18__ seconds

Show me how you:
kick a football	R
step on a bug	R

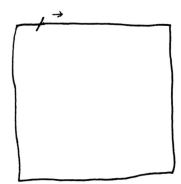

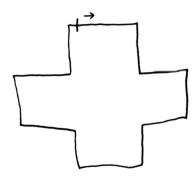

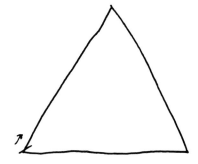

clock

square

He shouted the warning

$$\begin{array}{r} 8\,5 \\ 2\,7 \\ \hline 5\,8 \end{array}$$

51

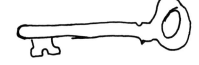

is clear that the generalized impairment of higher-level neuropsychological functions is very pronounced and will undoubtedly be reflected by impaired performances in everyday life.

Lateralizing signs were not as evident as they were on the first examination, primarily because of substantial improvement in finger tapping speed with the left hand. On the Tactual Performance Test the patient had identical scores with each hand (13.6 min), demonstrating that she was unable to make any improvement on the second trial. Therefore, the comparison of performances on the two sides of the body on these measures, together with the results on the Tactile Form Recognition Test, suggest involvement of the middle part of the right cerebral hemisphere.

The patient's drawing of the cross improved and whether it has any pathological significance would be open to question. It might be noted that on both the square and the cross the patient had to return to the starting point in order to close the figure. The drawing of the key, however, contains a particular error that undoubtedly is a residual manifestation of right cerebral damage: note carefully the notches in the stem near the handle.

In summary, this woman continued to show significant generalized impairment of adaptive abilities as well as involvement of the middle part of the right cerebral hemisphere. Despite evidence of substantial improvement, the general pattern of test results was remarkably similar to the initial examination. One might predict that a degree of additional improvement will occur in the future, based particularly on the fact that lateralizing signs of right hemisphere dysfunction were still present. It is also likely that the patient will show some improvement on the general indicators as well, but how much of her deficit is due to the head injury and how much may be a result of chronic alcoholism would be a difficult question to answer.

CASE #27

Name: F.C.

Age: 51

Education: 16

Sex: Male

Handedness: Right

Occupation: Realtor

Background Information

Except for a long history of essential hypertension and excessive alcohol consumption, F.C. had no history of significant illnesses or medical disorders. During the prior three years he had been hospitalized four times because of problems stemming from these conditions. Medical examinations during these hospitalizations had indicated that his liver was enlarged and liver function was impaired. Each hospitalization resulted in a diagnosis of acute brain syndrome due to excessive alcohol consumption and fatty liver. The patient, who was obese and had occasional attacks of asthma as well as acute gastroenteritis, had been treated with antihypertensive drugs and vitamin and dietary supplements. He had sustained a number of head injuries from falls which occurred during episodes of intoxication but no brain injuries had been documented or diagnosed.

Eight days prior to the present hospitalization the patient had a tooth extracted and began drinking heavily. The following night he had bleeding from his left ear and a considerable amount of blood was found in his bed. He was seen by a physician the next day and was noted to be confused and dizzy and staggered when he attempted to walk. He showed no improvement over the next several days; he had great difficulty dressing himself, was disoriented for time and place, had severe generalized headaches, and walked with a wide-based gait. At that time (one month before neuropsychological testing) he was admitted to the hospital.

Neurological Examination

Medical examination showed the patient to be confused, somewhat stuporous, and unable to give reliable information when questioned about incidence of head trauma. Neurologic examination revealed sluggish but symmetrical reflexes, a stiff neck, a wide-based gait and difficulty with balance, confusion and disorientation, slowness in responses, and slurred speech. A plain skull film showed a linear skull fracture extending from the left temporal to the left parietal area. Bilateral cerebral angiograms and a radioisotopic brain scan demonstrated a lesion in the left temporal-parietal area.

Two days after being hospitalized the patient underwent surgery and had a subdural hematoma evacuated from the left cerebral convexity and an epidural hematoma removed from the left temporal tip. The neurosurgeon also noted contusion of the brain tissue in the left anterior temporal area.

Initially the patient was somnolent after surgery; he moved all extremities in response to painful stimuli but did not respond to verbal commands or show any recognition of speech. On the third post-operative day he began to regain alertness and started talking. On the fourth post-operative day F.C. had a clonic seizure that first involved his head, neck and right arm and then spread to the trunk and left leg. The patient was alert after this seizure but during the next several days he had episodes of confusion, incoherent verbalizations, and disorientation for time and place. Nevertheless, he was making gradual progress and neurological examination (done just after the neuropsychological testing) revealed no evidence of abnormalities.

Neuropsychological examination was done approximately four weeks after surgery. In a case of this kind one would expect to see evidence of generalized cerebral dysfunction, possibly due to longstanding essential hypertension as well as chronic alcoholism. The consequences of epidural and subdural hematomas are variable from one patient to another but it would be likely that F.C. would show some effects of the contusion of the left anterior temporal area.

The patient earned Verbal (96), Performance (92), and Full Scale (93) IQ values in the lower part of the Average range, exceeding 30%–39% of his age peers. The distribution of Verbal subtest scores suggests that F.C. has experienced some brain-related impairment, especially on the Similarities (3) subtest and possibly the Digit Span (3) subtest. It is unusual to see such a low Vocabulary score (7) in the presence of a considerably better performance on Information (13). The overall distribution of the Verbal subtests suggests that the patient was not performing as well as might be expected, especially considering the fact that he had completed college. How much of this impairment was due to generalized confusion and lack of alertness (contrasted with specific organic language deficit) would be difficult to postulate. The Performance subtests were consistently low, suggesting that F.C. has experienced deficit on these measures. Therefore, it seems likely that both the verbal and performance intelligence levels of this man have been adversely affected.

Although there may be some question of the extent to which his IQ values were impaired, F.C. showed unequivocal signs of significant deficit on the four most sensitive tests in the HRNTB. The generality of his deficits was shown by the Impairment Index of 1.0. The poor score (83) on the

Category Test indicates his difficulty in areas of logical analysis and reasoning and his general lack of alertness and inability to keep more than one idea in mind at a time (flexibility in thought processes) was shown by the impaired performance on Part B of the Trail Making Test (167 sec).

Finally, F.C. performed very poorly on the Memory (3) and Localization (1) components of the Tactual Performance Test. His difficulty adapting to this task demonstrated that he was generally impaired in his ability to deal with complex problem-solving tasks under unique conditions (blindfolded). Thus, the deficits that were shown on these tests indicate quite clearly that F.C. is much more significantly impaired in his general adaptive capability and efficiency of performance than would be presumed from his IQ values.

The patient did show that he had fair ability to pay attention and maintain concentration when required to deal with simple and well-defined stimulus material; this was demonstrated by his score on the Speech-sounds Perception Test (9). It is possible, though, that his score on this measure may also have been mildly impaired.

At this point in the analysis of the data it is clear that F.C. (1) is much more impaired on tasks that require immediate adaptive capabilities than on measures that reflect stored background information; and (2) performs worse on complex and difficult tasks than on tasks that are more simple in nature and well-defined.

Lateralizing indicators implicating each cerebral hemisphere were present. Signs of left cerebral damage included a somewhat slower finger tapping speed with the right hand (47) than the left hand (49) and considerably more difficulty in tactile finger recognition with the right hand (6 errors) than the left (0 errors).

The patient had slightly more difficulty in finger-tip number writing perception with his right hand (11 errors) than his left (8 errors), but the mistakes on the left hand are sufficiently frequent to require explanation. It is likely that the

THE HALSTEAD-REITAN
NEUROPSYCHOLOGICAL TEST BATTERY

Patient ___**F.C.**___ Age __**51**__ Sex __**M**__ Education __**16**__ Handedness __**R**__

WECHSLER-BELLEVUE SCALE

VIQ	96
PIQ	92
FS IQ	93

Information	13
Comprehension	9
Digit Span	3
Arithmetic	10
Similarities	3
Vocabulary	7

Picture Arrangement	6
Picture Completion	5
Block Design	5
Object Assembly	6
Digit Symbol	5

TRAIL MAKING TEST

Part A: __**59**__ seconds
Part B: __**167**__ seconds

STRENGTH OF GRIP

Dominant hand: __**27.5**__ kilograms
Non-dominant hand: __**23.5**__ kilograms

REITAN-KLØVE TACTILE FORM RECOGNITION TEST

Dominant hand: __**0**__ errors
Non-dominant hand: __**0**__ errors

REITAN-KLØVE SENSORY-PERCEPTUAL EXAM

Error Totals

RH___LH___	Both H:	RH___LH___	RH___LH___			
RH___LF___	Both H/F:	RH___LF___	RH___LF___			
LH___RF___	Both H/F:	LH___RF___	RF___LH___			
RE___LE **1**	Both E:	RE___LE **2**	RE___LE **2**			
RV___LV___	Both:	RV___LV___	RV **1** LV___			

___ ___
___ ___ **1**

TACTILE FINGER RECOGNITION

R 1___ 2___ 3 **2** 4 **4** 5___ R **6** / **20**

L 1___ 2___ 3___ 4___ 5___ L **0** / **20**

FINGER-TIP NUMBER WRITING

R 1 **4** 2 **1** 3 **2** 4 **2** 5 **2** R **11** / **20**

L 1 **3** 2 **1** 3 **2** 4 **1** 5 **1** L **8** / **20**

HALSTEAD'S NEUROPSYCHOLOGICAL TEST BATTERY

Category Test   83

Tactual Performance Test

Dominant hand:	**15.0 (4 blocks in)**
Non-dominant hand:	**15.0 (3 blocks in)**
Both hands:	**14.5**

Total Time	**44.5 (17 blocks in)**
Memory	3
Localization	1

Seashore Rhythm Test

Number Correct   **21**   10

Speech-sounds Perception Test

Number of Errors   9

Finger Oscillation Test

Dominant hand:	47	47
Non-dominant hand:	49	

Impairment Index   **1.0**

MINNESOTA MULTIPHASIC PERSONALITY INVENTORY

		Hs	54
		D	56
?	50	Hy	53
L	66	Pd	69
F	73	Mf	69
K	57	Pa	62
		Pt	52
		Sc	65
		Ma	73

REITAN-KLØVE LATERAL-DOMINANCE EXAM

Show me how you:

throw a ball	R
hammer a nail	R
cut with a knife	R
turn a door knob	R
use scissors	R
use an eraser	R
write your name	R

Record time used for spontaneous name-writing:

Preferred hand	**8** seconds
Non-preferred hand	**25** seconds

Show me how you:

kick a football	R
step on a bug	L

REITAN-INDIANA APHASIA SCREENING TEST

Form for Adults and Older Children

Name: _____F. C._____ Age: __51__

Copy SQUARE	Repeat TRIANGLE
Name SQUARE "A window."	Repeat MASSACHUSETTS
Spell SQUARE	Repeat METHODIST EPISCOPAL
Copy CROSS	Write SQUARE
Name CROSS "Red Cross"	Read SEVEN
Spell CROSS	Repeat SEVEN
Copy TRIANGLE	Repeat/Explain HE SHOUTED THE WARNING.
Name TRIANGLE "Square – a – a – can't remember."	Write HE SHOUTED THE WARNING.
Spell TRIANGLE	Compute 85 – 27 =
Name BABY	Compute 17 X 3 =
Write CLOCK	Name KEY
Name FORK	Demonstrate use of KEY
Read 7 SIX 2	Draw KEY
Read MGW	Read PLACE LEFT HAND TO RIGHT EAR.
Reading I	Place LEFT HAND TO RIGHT EAR
Reading II	Place LEFT HAND TO LEFT ELBOW

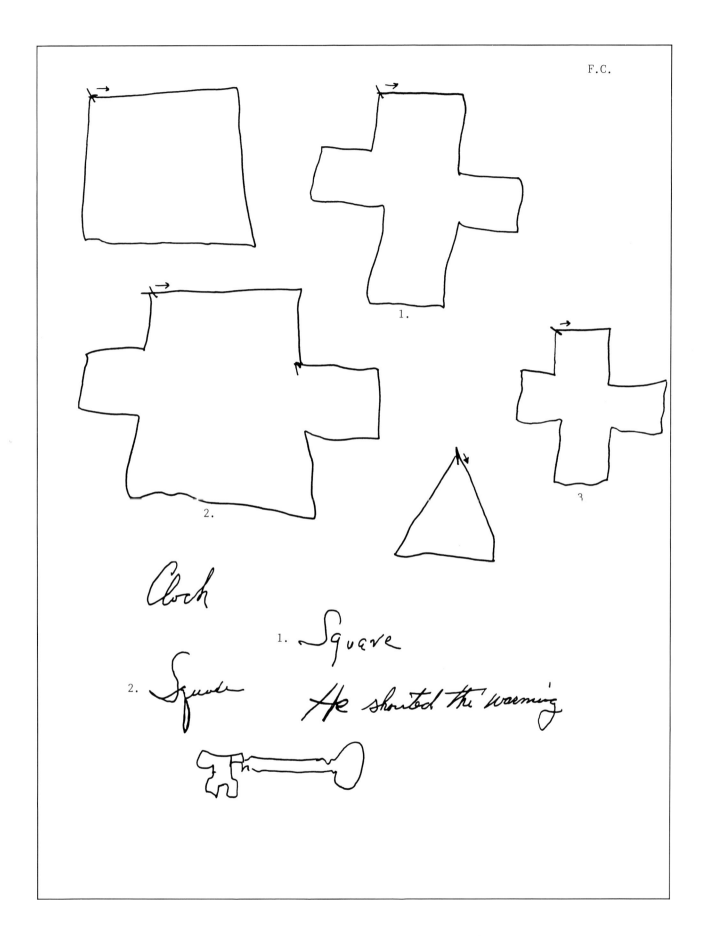

1.

2.

3

Clock

1. Square

2. Square

He shouted the warning

errors in finger-tip number writing perception on both hands were at least partly a reflection of the relatively complex nature of this task. This test requires careful and concentrated attention and the greater number of errors on this test than on tactile finger recognition probably reflects F.C.'s generalized impairment. Nevertheless, both primary motor and tactile-perceptual skills were more impaired on the right side of the body than the left.

On the Aphasia Screening Test the patient also showed mild deficits which are very probably indicative of left cerebral dysfunction. These difficulties were manifested in naming the SQUARE, CROSS, and TRIANGLE. The most significant deficit occurred when the patient named the TRIANGLE as a " square," followed by apparent recognition of the error but inability to give the correct name.

In summary, then, the specific deficits implicating the left cerebral hemisphere include motor, tactile, and language responses and suggest that the cerebral damage involves a fairly extensive area in the middle part of the hemisphere. In this case, however, considering the strong indications of generalized impairment, we would not be inclined to emphasize the left hemisphere findings as having localizing significance.

The patient also demonstrated right cerebral dysfunction. Although F.C. had a tendency to fail to perceive an auditory stimulus to his left ear when it was given simultaneously with a stimulus to the right ear, the examiner noted that the patient had a hearing deficit involving his left ear and this observation attenuates the significance of the results. F.C. had a mild deficit in grip strength with his left upper extremity (23.5 kg) compared with his right (27.5 kg) but this deviation was so minimal that it probably does not merit special attention.

On the Tactual Performance Test the patient did not perform quite as well with his left hand (second trial, three blocks placed in 15 min) as he did with his right (first trial, four blocks placed in 15 min), suggesting greater dysfunction of the right cerebral hemisphere than the left. However, it must be observed that these comparisons fall in the context of very serious generalized impairment and the poor overall performance attenuates the lateralizing significance.

Finally, F.C. showed definite constructional dyspraxia in his attempts to copy both the cross and the key. The indications of left cerebral dysfunction were probably stronger than the deficits suggesting right cerebral damage, but overall the lateralizing signs indicated significant and serious generalized impairment of brain functions.

Considering the patient's medical history and neurological findings, it appears that the neuropsychological test results are consistent with our expectations. The generalized impairment may be due to chronic alcoholism and essential hypertension, as well as undocumented instances of prior head trauma incurred during acute alcoholic states. Given these circumstances, it is not surprising that the patient showed some mild evidence of right as well as left cerebral dysfunction.

The more specific deficits relating to left cerebral damage were probably a result of the bleeding over the left cerebral hemisphere and contusion of the left anterior temporal area. We would expect F.C. to show some improvement in time as he recovers from the recent left cerebral damage; however, despite any improvement, it is likely that he will have permanent significant generalized impairment of neuropsychological functions that will compromise his occupational performance as well as his efficiency in more general aspects of everyday living.

CASE #28

Name: F.M.

Age: 44

Education: 12

Sex: Male

Handedness: Right

Occupation: Electrician

Background Information

F.M., a 42-year-old electrician, had been in good health until he awoke one morning unable to talk or move his right arm or leg. He was taken to the hospital and neurological examination indicated that he had suffered a thrombosis involving the left middle cerebral artery.

The patient was hospitalized for 10 weeks and participated in a vigorous rehabilitation program. He regained much of his speech and language functions as well as the use of his right extremities except for fine movements of the right hand. He was motivated to do well, returned to work, and was reported to have made an excellent recovery.

Fourteen months after suffering the stroke F.M. was involved in an automobile accident in which he sustained a severe head injury and multiple fractures. He was comatose for four months before gradually regaining consciousness. He had clear evidence of speech difficulty (although a detailed examination for aphasia was not conducted), a right hemiplegia, and inability to walk. He had developed contractures of the right upper and lower extremities and the limbs were essentially useless.

The patient's attitude was much different after the accident than after the stroke; now he was very depressed and discouraged, refused to try to help himself, and according to observers he essentially "gave up" any interest in trying to reach the level of his previous lifestyle. He became demanding, argumentative, and extremely difficult to get along with. His family members and others who knew F.M. said this was a complete change of personality and persisted in trying to help him recover.

Neurological Examination

Although F.M. had made relatively little progress, he was brought to a major medical center for complete neurological evaluation and intensive rehabilitation 21 months after the head injury (34 months after the stroke). In addition to the deficits noted above, neurological examination indicated that the patient had a pseudobulbar speech that was difficult to understand. Due to the severe contracture F.M. also required surgical lengthening of the right Achille's tendon.

During his three-month hospitalization the patient received physical therapy and speech therapy. He was a constant problem on the hospital ward because of his uncooperative and demanding behavior and he made minimal effort to participate in the rehabilitational program. The surgery for correcting the equinus deformity was not successful and it was finally decided that nothing more could be done to help the patient and he was discharged to the care of his family.

Neuropsychological Evaluation

Neuropsychological examination was done shortly after F.M. was admitted to the hospital for rehabilitation. Although results on the Minnesota Multiphasic Personality Inventory were essentially within normal limits, the patient's responses on the Cornell Medical Index Health Questionnaire indicated that he had a great number of somatic, psychophysiologic, and emotional complaints.

We originally did a "blind" interpretation of the neuropsychological test results and noted left cerebral damage to be present in a context of generalized impairment of brain functions. We inferred that the patient had diffuse and fairly severe cerebral vascular disease, possibly with a thrombosis involving the middle part of the left cerebral hemisphere. However, as will be explained below, we noted that the test results were not perfectly typical for such a condition and raised the possibility that some other complication (such as severe head trauma) might also have been contributory.

It is often difficult to dissociate two etiological conditions when both may cause severe impairment of brain functions and may result in serious lateralizing findings. Nevertheless, there are certain neuropsychological differences in persons with cerebral strokes and craniocerebral trauma, and the results for F.M. will be considered in light of these differential findings.

A brief review of F.M.'s test scores indicates that he was seriously and generally impaired. Considering his Verbal subtest scores on the Wechsler Scale (especially the score of 10 on Vocabulary), it would be reasonable to assume that F.M. had previously had average intelligence levels. At this time the patient earned a Verbal IQ (80) in the lower limit of the Low Average range (exceeding about 9% of his age peers) and a Performance IQ (87) in the upper part of the Low Average range (exceeding 19%). These values yielded a Full Scale IQ of 82, exceeding about 11% of his age peers.

A more detailed inspection of the Verbal subtest scores indicated that F.M. was able to make no progress whatsoever on Digit Span and seemed to be definitely impaired on the Similarities (4) subtest. Scores of 7, 8, and 10 for the other Verbal subtests suggest that the patient did have some residual stored verbal ability.

The Performance subtest scores were consistently at least one standard deviation below the mean, with particularly poor scores occurring on Block Design (5) and Digit Symbol (3). In summary, the overall results of the Wechsler Scale strongly suggest that impairment has occurred, but the findings would not implicate a strictly focal or lateralized lesion.

The patient performed very poorly on the four most sensitive measures in the Halstead-Reitan Battery. He earned an Impairment Index of 1.0, made 115 errors on the Category Test, required 426 seconds to complete Part B of the Trail Making Test and was not able to correctly localize any of the shapes in his drawing of the Tactual Performance Test board. In fact, none of the scores based upon scaled ability measurements even approached the average level.

F.M. demonstrated evidence of definite impairment even on tasks that basically required only close attention to specific and well-defined stimulus material (the first level of central processing). For example, note that on the Seashore Rhythm Test he made errors on 12 of the 30 items, a score almost worse than chance. He made 27 mistakes on the Speech-sounds Perception Test, almost twice the number of mistakes made by a group of heterogeneous brain-damaged subjects (Reitan, 1955d).

F.M.'s scores on the Tactual Performance Test illustrate his severe impairment on tasks that require adaptability and comprehension of the nature of the problem. In a total of 45 minutes the patient was able to place only seven blocks correctly (an average of more than six minutes per block).

After documenting the severity of this man's impairment on the Halstead-Reitan Battery, it is interesting to note that one of the principal complaints of the professional hospital staff working with him was that he took little interest in helping

THE HALSTEAD-REITAN
NEUROPSYCHOLOGICAL TEST BATTERY

Patient **F.M.** Age **44** Sex **M** Education **12** Handedness **R**

WECHSLER-BELLEVUE SCALE

VIQ	80
PIQ	87
FS IQ	82

Information	8
Comprehension	8
Digit Span	0
Arithmetic	7
Similarities	4
Vocabulary	10

Picture Arrangement	7
Picture Completion	7
Block Design	5
Object Assembly	7
Digit Symbol	3

TRAIL MAKING TEST

Part A: **88** seconds
Part B: **426** seconds

STRENGTH OF GRIP

Dominant hand: **—** kilograms

Non-dominant hand: **32.0** kilograms

REITAN-KLØVE TACTILE FORM RECOGNITION TEST

Dominant hand: **—** seconds; **—** errors

Non-dominant hand: **16** seconds; **0** errors

REITAN-KLØVE SENSORY-PERCEPTUAL EXAM

				Error Totals	
RH ___ LH ___	Both H: RH ___ LH ___	RH ___ LH ___
RH ___ LF ___	Both H/F: RH ___ LF ___	RH ___ LF ___
LH ___ RF ___	Both H/F: LH ___ RF ___	RF ___ LH ___
RE ___ LE ___	Both E: RE **3** LE ___	RE **3** LE ___
RV ___ LV ___	Both: RV ___ LV ___	RV **1** LV ___
___ ___	**1**	___
___ ___	___ ___	___ ___

TACTILE FINGER RECOGNITION

R 1___ 2___ 3___ 4___ 5___ COULD NOT DO

L 1___ 2___ 3 **1** 4 **2** 5 **1** L **4** / 20

FINGER-TIP NUMBER WRITING

R 1___ 2___ 3___ 4___ 5___ COULD NOT DO

L 1 **4** 2 **1** 3 **1** 4 **1** 5 **2** L **9** / 20

HALSTEAD'S NEUROPSYCHOLOGICAL TEST BATTERY

Category Test   **115**

Tactual Performance Test

Left hand:	**15.0 (2 blocks)**
Left hand:	**15.0 (2 blocks)**
Left hand:	**15.0 (3 blocks)**

Total Time	**45.0 (7 blocks)**
Memory	**2**
Localization	**0**

Seashore Rhythm Test

Number Correct **12**   **10**

Speech-sounds Perception Test

Number of Errors   **27**

Finger Oscillation Test

Dominant hand: **—**   **—**
Non-dominant hand: **21**

Impairment Index   **1.0**

MINNESOTA MULTIPHASIC PERSONALITY INVENTORY

		Hs	62
		D	53
?	50	Hy	53
L	53	Pd	41
J	50	Mf	43
K	57	Pa	38
		Pt	50
		Sc	50
		Ma	55

REITAN-KLØVE LATERAL-DOMINANCE EXAM

Show me how you:
throw a ball   _____
hammer a nail   _____
cut with a knife   _____
turn a door knob   _____ } PREVIOUSLY WAS STRONGLY RIGHT-HANDED.
use scissors   _____
use an eraser   _____
write your name   _____

Record time used for spontaneous name-writing:
Preferred hand   **—** seconds
Non-preferred hand   **53** seconds

Show me how you:
kick a football
step on a bug   **—** } NOT DONE

REITAN-INDIANA APHASIA SCREENING TEST

Form for Adults and Older Children

Name: _____ F. M. _____ Age: __44__

Copy SQUARE	Repeat TRIANGLE "Tianle"
Name SQUARE "Square D"	Repeat MASSACHUSETTS "Massthechewess"
Spell SQUARE	Repeat METHODIST EPISCOPAL "Besodis Episopal"
Copy CROSS	Write SQUARE
Name CROSS	Read SEVEN
Spell CROSS	Repeat SEVEN
Copy TRIANGLE	Repeat/Explain HE SHOUTED THE WARNING. "Help"
Name TRIANGLE	Write HE SHOUTED THE WARNING.
Spell TRIANGLE	Compute 85 – 27 =
Name BABY	Compute 17 X 3 =
Write CLOCK	Name KEY
Name FORK	Demonstrate use of KEY
Read 7 SIX 2	Draw KEY
Read MGW	Read PLACE LEFT HAND TO RIGHT EAR.
Reading I	Place LEFT HAND TO RIGHT EAR
Reading II	Place LEFT HAND TO LEFT ELBOW Right hand to left ear - self-corrected.

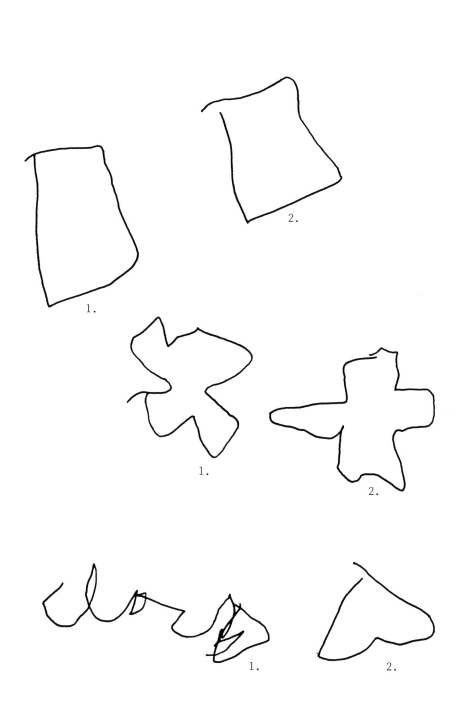

1.

2.

1.

2.

1.

2.

F.M.

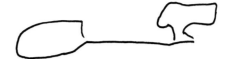

the month of wARTINB
89 - 27 = 23

1. SQUARE 51 (17 x 3)

2. Square

to develop and carry out his rehabilitational program. We can see that he was significantly impaired in his ability to pay attention to what was going on, grossly deficient in his capability to organize and understand circumstances and their relationships, and had few abilities except the ones related to skills acquired long in the past. Thus, a more realistic understanding of this man and his severe deficits would have lead to developing a program in which stimulation was offered without expecting much understanding from the patient. It is a mistake to expect a normal degree of cooperation, based on intellectual insight and understanding, from a patient with severe neuropsychological impairment.

We also see that F.M. had a number of lateralizing signs involving the left cerebral hemisphere to a much greater extent than the right. He had a right hemiplegia and contractures so severe that it was nearly impossible to open his right hand. He was unable to use his right hand on the Tactual Performance Test, the Finger Oscillation Test, or the measurement of grip strength. It was also impossible for him to do the Tactile Form Recognition Test, the Tactile Finger Recognition Test or the Finger-tip Number Writing Perception Test on the right hand. These problems involved the right upper extremity to a much greater extent than the left and have clear lateralizing significance.

We see, though, that the patient had relatively normal scores on certain aspects of the Sensory-perceptual Examination. For example, he made no errors in perception of bilateral simultaneous tactile stimulation and only one error (on the right side) with visual stimulation. Lateralization of sensory-perceptual functions was clearly manifested in the test for bilateral simultaneous auditory stimulation; the patient failed to perceive the stimulus to the right ear in three of the four trials. Therefore, we find that both sensory-perceptual and motor impairment (involving the right side of the body) implicated the biological status of the left cerebral hemisphere.

Seeing such lateralized deficits together with the indications of very severe generalized impairment one might predict that the patient had experienced a serious structural lesion of the left cerebral hemisphere which would produce serious aphasic losses. F.M. did, in fact, demonstrate some deficits suggesting mild difficulty in dealing with language symbols for communicational purposes, but his losses were much less severe than would be expected from a typical recent stroke patient with profound hemiplegia.

When asked to name the SQUARE he responded "square D," a term that probably had some significance with respect to his prior occupation as an electrician. He also had difficulty repeating words, omitting the "R" and "G" sounds in TRIANGLE, inserting a "th" and omitting an "a" and an "s" in MASSACHUSETTS, and there may have been some slurring of the sounds in METHODIST EPISCOPAL. These deficits probably involve peripheral enunciatory mechanisms primarily but they also represent at least a mild element of central dysarthria.

F.M. did not attempt to explain HE SHOUTED THE WARNING in any detail, but his single-word response ("Help") was appropriate. He initially showed some evidence of right-left confusion on PLACE LEFT HAND TO LEFT ELBOW but quickly corrected himself.

Because of the paresis and contractures of his right hand the patient had to use his left (non-preferred) hand to respond to the items on the Aphasia Screening Test. His difficulty drawing simple spatial configurations indicates at least mild constructional dyspraxia (e.g., the key was drawn backwards and upside down, representing an unusual manifestation of confusion in spatial relationships). In his attempts to write CLOCK and HE SHOUTED THE WARNING the patient also manifested dysphasic difficulty involving either dysgraphia or spelling dyspraxia or a combination of both deficits. Although it is somewhat difficult to read the numbers that he wrote, it appears that the patient also made a definite mistake in attempting to solve $85 - 27 =$. Note, however, that he was able to mentally compute 17×3 without error.

In summary, the results of the Aphasia Screening Test yielded information suggesting that F.M. has many brain-related difficulties, including dysnomia, central dysarthria, right-left confusion, spelling dyspraxia, dysgraphia, and constructional dyspraxia. His constructional dyspraxia was at least as pronounced as his difficulties in dealing with verbal symbols, suggesting that the patient has significant impairment of abilities related to *each* cerebral hemisphere. Obviously, this finding goes well beyond the inference of left cerebral damage that would be drawn from the evidence of right hemiplegia.

Even though the test results were generally indicative of more serious left cerebral damage, some of the findings were quite definite in implicating the right cerebral hemisphere as well: the poor drawings (constructional dyspraxia) and the fairly specific deficits on the left side of the body (four mistakes in twenty trials in tactile finger localization and nine mistakes in twenty trials in finger-tip number writing perception). Even the score on Block Design (5) might be a reflection of right cerebral damage.

As stated previously, we initially did a "blind" interpretation on this set of test results and noted the following: (1) indications of generalized impairment, including very slow finger tapping speed with the left hand; (2) profound motor impairment on the right side; and (3) the relative absence of aphasia. We concluded that the test results would be compatible with diffuse and relatively severe cerebral vascular disease with a probable thrombosis in the distribution of the left middle cerebral artery. The absence of significant dysphasia suggested that the lesion had probably occurred some time ago and the patient had had an opportunity for a significant degree of recovery of language functions.

We were puzzled, however, about how this recovery could have occurred in a brain so generally compromised. On this basis we postulated the possibility of another insult in addition to the stroke that could account for much of the severe generalized impairment. In this type of differential interpretation it is also necessary to consider the patient's age; while it is not unusual to see severe generalized impairment (as well as focal deficits) in an older person who has sustained a stroke, it is less common to see such severe generalized impairment in a younger person.

The reader will realize that differentiating between effects of cerebral vascular disease and head trauma may be very difficult when they occur in the same person. In this case both the test results and the history suggest that the patient had made significant recovery from the stroke (even returning to satisfactory performance of his work as an electrician) and then sustained significant additional neuropsychological deficits from the head injury.

CASE #29

Name: D.H.

Age: 25

Education: 11

Sex: Male

Handedness: Right

Occupation: Janitor

Background Information

D.H. was in involved in an automobile accident shortly after his 21st birthday. He suffered multiple injuries, including a basilar skull fracture, a depressed left frontal skull fracture, and a ruptured spleen with acute intra-abdominal hemorrhage. It was also noted that he had blood and cerebrospinal fluid draining from the right external auditory canal.

Neurosurgical evaluation done shortly after the accident indicated that D.H. had a left frontal cerebral contusion but it was not felt that surgery was necessary. The patient was almost entirely comatose for three weeks after the injury.

About four weeks post-injury an attempt was made to perform a neurological examination. D.H. was obtunded and verbal communication was very difficult to establish; he occasionally offered brief answers to verbal stimuli with weak, one-word responses that were rarely appropriate. It was difficult to examine the patient but the neurologist could determine that D.H. showed a right facial weakness and ptosis and external deviation of the left eye. He withdrew all four extremities in response to painful stimuli and his movements appeared to be spastic. The physician could not evaluate voluntary movement capabilities or complete any additional tests that required the patient's cooperation.

About one week later D.H. showed a considerable degree of improvement; he was alert, oriented, ambulatory and independent concerning self-care. However, he answered questions very briefly, usually in a whisper, and was sometimes confused.

The patient was transferred to a rehabilitation hospital and enrolled in a program of physical, occupational, and recreational therapy. The day after admission it was apparent that he still became very confused at times. For example, one day at lunch he placed his bacon in the empty milk carton on his tray; when the nurse told him what he was doing he took the bacon out of the carton and ate it.

During the first week of his hospitalization his speech improved spontaneously and speech therapy was discontinued. After participating in this rehabilitation program for about two weeks he was discharged to the care of two of his siblings.

D.H.'s brother and sister provided information about his pre-injury history. All nine of the siblings in this family had been abused and each left home as a teenager. D.H. was "kicked out" of the house at 17 and went to live with one of his older brothers. He quit high school in the 11th grade and worked at various jobs, including stock boy, clerk, and janitor. He was never able to hold a job for very long, principally because of his drug and alcohol abuse. He enlisted in the Army but received a dishonorable discharge eight months later because of his substance abuse problems. The siblings said that D.H. had many episodes of depression, frequently talked about suicide and led a very erratic lifestyle.

Between the date of discharge from the rehabilitation hospital and neuropsychological testing (approximately three years) D.H. continued to live very erratically and was hospitalized several times for drug abuse. Although it was difficult to establish which drugs D.H. had taken or the amounts involved, it was known that he had used marijuana, PCP, alcohol, amphetamines, and cocaine.

About 26 months after the head injury the patient had a major motor seizure and was hospitalized for evaluation. The neurological examination was entirely within normal limits but the electroencephalogram showed a left frontal intermittent slow-wave focus suggesting a focal, structural lesion that was probably serving as an epileptogenic focus. There also was diffuse slow-wave activity bilaterally. Computed tomography showed an area of structural damage centered in the left frontal lobe that was almost certainly a result of the previous injury.

Many persons who sustain head injuries have deviant lifestyles and a history of many complicating medical and psychiatric conditions. In many instances it is quite difficult to differentiate between the effects of head trauma and other brain-impairing influences. In the case of this patient there was a long history of being abused when he was a child. While this experience may have caused emotional problems of adjustment, it is less likely to have caused more brain damage than the drug and alcohol abuse.

Litigation was pending concerning the effects of D.H.'s head injury and it was necessary to attempt to separate the effects of the cerebrocranial trauma from possible adverse effects of drug and alcohol ingestion. To achieve any degree of success in such a differentiation it obviously would be necessary to be knowledgeable in the neuropsychological consequences of both traumatic brain injury as well as drug and alcohol abuse. (The reader who encounters problems of this type may be interested in reviewing the neuropsychological correlates of chronic alcoholism [Reitan & Wolfson, 1985b] and

the neuropsychological manifestations of drug and alcohol abuse [Reitan & Wolfson, 1985a]).

At the time of his neuropsychological examination (approximately three years post-injury) D.H. told us that he had been getting along relatively well at first and had been improving, but he felt that he had been progressively getting worse during the past six to twelve months. (Obviously, the patient was not a very accurate informant in assessing his own situation).

On the Cornell Medical Index Health Questionnaire D.H. gave positive answers to most of the questions. The results indicated that he had many somatic complaints, including severe nervous exhaustion. He also answered positively to most of the items concerned with emotional problems. Thus, in the patient's own judgement, he had numerous difficulties of various kinds.

Neuropsychological Examination

In general, the test results suggest that D.H. (1) has relatively low verbal intelligence; (2) shows impairment of adaptive abilities dependent upon brain functions of a type quite characteristic of craniocerebral trauma; and (3) demonstrates serious difficulties in the area of emotional and affective adjustment.

The patient earned a Verbal IQ (85) in the middle part of the Low Average range, exceeding about 16% of his age peers. He showed a significant degree of variability on the individual subtests, doing relatively well on some and poorly on others. He scored low on the Information (5) and Vocabulary (6) subtests, a finding frequently seen in persons who have not profited much from their educational experiences.

D.H. did better on the Performance subtests, earning a Performance IQ (106) in the upper part of the Average range (exceeding 66% of his age peers). These values yielded a Full Scale IQ in the lower part of the Average range (exceeding 34%).

THE HALSTEAD-REITAN
NEUROPSYCHOLOGICAL TEST BATTERY

Patient **D.H.** Age **25** Sex **M** Education **11** Handedness **R**

WECHSLER-BELLEVUE SCALE

VIQ	85
PIQ	106
FS IQ	94

Information	5
Comprehension	10
Digit Span	7
Arithmetic	7
Similarities	11
Vocabulary	6

Picture Arrangement	11
Picture Completion	11
Block Design	14
Object Assembly	10
Digit Symbol	8

TRAIL MAKING TEST

Part A: **38** seconds
Part B: **81** seconds

STRENGTH OF GRIP

Dominant hand: **54.0** kilograms
Non-dominant hand: **51.5** kilograms

REITAN-KLØVE TACTILE FORM RECOGNITION TEST

Dominant hand: **17** seconds; **0** errors
Non-dominant hand: **11** seconds; **0** errors

REITAN-KLØVE SENSORY-PERCEPTUAL EXAM

			Error Totals	
RH ___ LH ___	Both H:	RH **1** LH ___	RH **1** LH ___	
RH ___ LF ___	Both H/F:	RH **1** LF ___	RH **1** LF ___	
LH ___ RF ___	Both H/F:	LH ___ RF ___	RF ___ LH ___	
RE ___ LE ___	Both E:	RE **2** LE ___	RE **2** LE ___	
RV ___ LV ___	Both:	RV ___ LV ___	RV ___ LV ___	
___ ___		___ ___	___ ___	
___ ___		___ ___	___ ___	

TACTILE FINGER RECOGNITION

R 1 ___ 2 ___ 3 **1** 4 ___ 5 ___   R **1** / **20**

L 1 ___ 2 ___ 3 ___ 4 ___ 5 ___   L **0** / **20**

FINGER-TIP NUMBER WRITING

R 1 ___ 2 ___ 3 **1** 4 ___ 5 ___   R **1** / **20***

L 1 ___ 2 ___ 3 ___ 4 ___ 5 ___   L **0** / **20**

*SLOWER ON RIGHT HAND TRIALS

HALSTEAD'S NEUROPSYCHOLOGICAL TEST BATTERY

Category Test — Subtest V — 59 Errors; ___
Became more and more upset and finally refused to go on.

Tactual Performance Test

Dominant hand: **2.7**
Non-dominant hand: **6.8**
Both hands: **3.8**

Total Time	13.3
Memory	9
Localization	3

Seashore Rhythm Test

Number Correct **22**   **10**

Speech-sounds Perception Test

Number of Errors   **14**

Finger Oscillation Test

Dominant hand: **51**   **51**
Non-dominant hand: **40**

Impairment Index   0.6

MINNESOTA MULTIPHASIC PERSONALITY INVENTORY

		Hs	93
		D	94
?	50	Hy	84
L	53	Pd	83
F	90 +	Mf	80
K	48	Pa	94
		Pt	99
		Sc	113
		Ma	65

REITAN-KLØVE LATERAL-DOMINANCE EXAM

Show me how you:
throw a ball	R
hammer a nail	R
cut with a knife	R
turn a door knob	R
use scissors	R
use an eraser	R
write your name	R

Record time used for spontaneous name-writing:
Preferred hand	13 seconds
Non-preferred hand	49 seconds

Show me how you:
kick a football	R
step on a bug	R

REITAN-INDIANA APHASIA SCREENING TEST

Form for Adults and Older Children

Name: _____ D. H. _____ Age: __25__

Copy SQUARE	Repeat TRIANGLE
Name SQUARE	Repeat MASSACHUSETTS "Massasschusess"
Spell SQUARE	Repeat METHODIST EPISCOPAL
Copy CROSS	Write SQUARE
Name CROSS	Read SEVEN
Spell CROSS	Repeat SEVEN
Copy TRIANGLE	Repeat/Explain HE SHOUTED THE WARNING.
Name TRIANGLE	Write HE SHOUTED THE WARNING.
Spell TRIANGLE "T-R-I-N-G-L-E." Examiner asked him to try again. "T-R-Y-N-G-L-E."	Compute 85 – 27 =
Name BABY	Compute 17 X 3 = "41." Given 5 x 8 and answered correctly.
Write CLOCK	Name KEY
Name FORK	Demonstrate use of KEY
Read 7 SIX 2	Draw KEY
Read MGW	Read PLACE LEFT HAND TO RIGHT EAR.
Reading I	Place LEFT HAND TO RIGHT EAR
Reading II "He is a friendly animal, a famous winner of the dog show."	Place LEFT HAND TO LEFT ELBOW

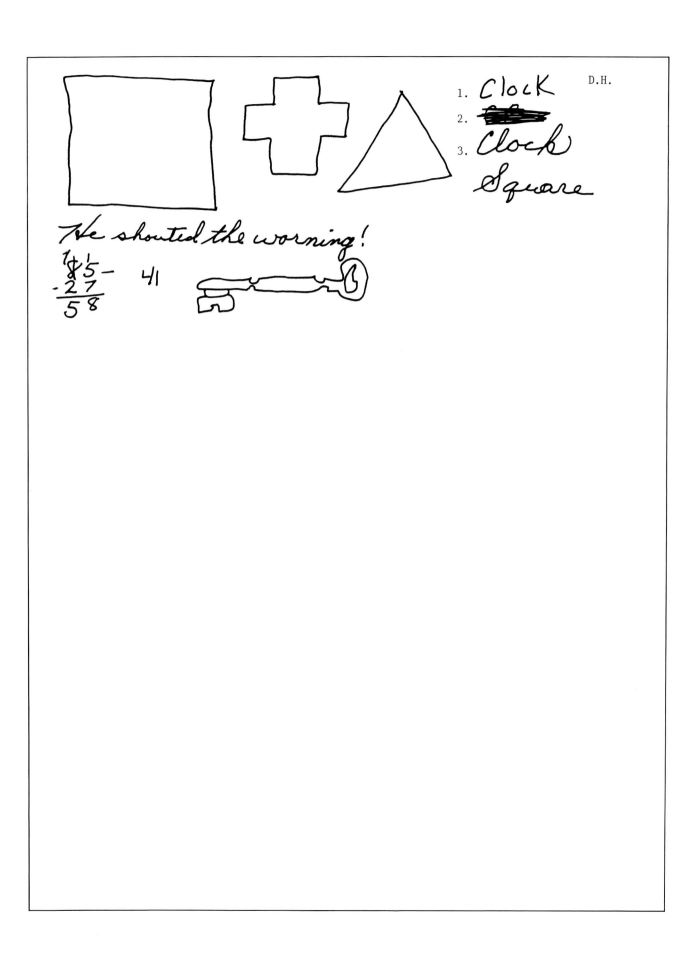

D.H.

1. Clock
2. ~~████~~
3. Clock
   Square

He shouted the worning!

1 ∂̸5̸¹ —   41
- 2 7
─────
  5 8

The neuropsychological examination revealed definite impairment of a number of abilities dependent upon the biological condition of the brain. D.H. earned a Halstead Impairment Index of 0.6 (approximately 60% of the tests had results in the brain-damaged range), a score distinctly beyond the normal range. He performed very poorly on the Category Test, scoring 59 errors by the time he reached subtest V. By that point he had become very upset and refused to continue taking the test. He scored in the impaired range on the Localization component of the Tactual Performance Test (3) and possibly was mildly impaired on Part B of the Trail Making Test, even though his score (81 sec) did not exceed the cut-off point.

The patient also had some difficulties in sensory-perceptual functions (especially on the right side of the body), some problems with motor functions on the left side, very mild impairment copying simple spatial configurations (constructional dyspraxia), mild deficits with memory and alertness, and very serious difficulties in the areas of abstraction, reasoning, and logical analysis.

This latter deficit undoubtedly is of major clinical significance: from his score on the Category Test we can predict that D.H. is seriously impaired in his ability to make observations, identify critical elements in analysis of the overall problem, and make progress in solving the problem. Therefore, he is likely to be very inefficient and ineffectual when a situation requires analyzing complex material, weighing alternatives, deciding upon the critical aspects of the problem, and being able to use sound judgement. This is one of the most common deficits and difficulties seen in head-injured persons and in this instance the patient shows even more impairment than we customarily see.

Lateralizing findings were of major significance in indentifying the presence of traumatic cerebral damage. Drug and alcohol abuse might have contributed to impaired level of performance (Grant, Mohns, Miller, & Reitan, 1976) but these factors generally cause diffuse impairment rather than dysfunction in each of the cerebral hemispheres.

Left cerebral indicators included (1) mild impairment in the ability to perceive a tactile stimulus to the right hand when simultaneously given with a stimulus to the left hand or left face; (2) more pronounced right auditory imperception; (3) slowness in tactile form perception with the right hand compared with the left; (4) possible mild impairment of the right hand (slower responses) in finger-tip number perception; and (5) a possible mild reduction of grip strength in the right upper extremity compared with the left.

On the Aphasia Screening Test the patient also manifested mild deficits in the ability to deal with simple verbal material (spelling, reading, and enunciating) but these mistakes may have stemmed from inadequate educational training. In summary, D.H.'s results definitely deviated from normal expectancy in terms of left cerebral functioning.

When persons with significant head injuries demonstrate lateralizing findings implicating one cerebral hemisphere, there is usually evidence to indicate dysfunction of the other hemisphere as well. In this case the patient performed adequately using his right hand on the first trial of the Tactual Performance Test (2.7 min) but was much less efficient on the second trial using his left hand (6.8 min). Since he clearly improved his performance on the third trial (3.8 min) using both hands, there would not be much support for attributing his poor performance to a lack of motivation.

It is difficult to discern the basis for the poor performance with the left hand on the TPT (since his tactile skills seemed to be more impaired in the right hand) and the inexperienced clinician may be tempted to relate such a finding to the mild impairment of finger tapping speed on the left side (fine motor skills). However, since there is generally minimal or no association between these variables with respect to lateralization (especially in head-injured subjects), this explanation is probably based only on the coincidental occurrence of reduced finger tapping speed and a poorer performance with the left hand on the TPT rather than on a consistent causal relationship. Of course, this lack of necessary (causal) association does not diminish the significance of the findings as indicators of right cerebral dysfunction (the TPT time with the left hand being more striking and definite than the finger tapping relationship). Although not unequivocally indicative of right cerebral damage, D.H.'s drawings (especially the key) do contribute to the total impression of cognitive impairment.

We used two instruments to assess the patient's emotional status — one that requires a relatively straightforward self-evaluation (Cornell Medical Index Health Questionnaire) and another technique that is somewhat more subtle in nature (Minnesota Multiphasic Personality Inventory).

In his own evaluation D.H. had many complaints of various types, including somatic symptoms, psychophysiological difficulties, and emotional problems of adjustment. It is apparent from his responses that he feels that his own physical and emotional status is filled with serious difficulties.

Similar results were obtained from the MMPI. Because of the elevated F scale on this instrument a question could be raised about the profile's validity; however, the score is probably part of the total picture of psychopathology. The overall profile suggests that this man is quite distressed, disturbed, and inconsistent in his behavior, has great difficulty controlling his behavior, and does not have a realistic understanding of his situation.

These emotional difficulties may very possibly interact with the indications of brain damage described above, but as the reader is undoubtedly aware, many people have serious emotional problems without evidence of any significant neuropsychological deficit related to brain damage. Considering D.H.'s severe impairment in the areas of logical analysis, reasoning, and abstraction, it is possible that the MMPI results reflect pre-existing emotional difficulties even though the patient's emotional stability has also been impaired by brain damage. Conversely, it is not probable that the neuropsychological deficits were present before the patient sustained a brain injury.

In terms of clinical implication and rehabilitation, the serious impairment shown by this man in the areas of abstraction, reasoning and logical analysis, coupled with his emotional and affective problems, may be the most important aspect of his test results. It is likely that his cognitive disorders are due to brain damage as well as environmental factors.

D.H.'s impairment undoubtedly has serious implications regarding his behavior in everyday living. Persons with serious deficits in abstraction and reasoning skills are frequently confused, do not get things organized properly, often complain of poor memory, are inconsistent in their behavior, do not analyze problems or understand the importance of doing things systematically, and generally are less competent than their apparent intelligence suggests. Comparisons of brain-damaged and affectively disturbed groups (Reitan, 1955d) suggest that impairment of abstraction abilities is due to brain damage; therefore, the combination of severe brain-related impairment and a significant affective disorder does not suggest a very favorable prognosis for this man.

Finally, we must emphasize that the key to identifying the comparative influence of various etiological factors on the neuropsychological test results is the conjoint use of the several methods of inference built into the Halstead-Reitan Battery. In the case of this man the methods based on intra-individual data comparisons were the most important sources of information. This is generally true in most cases because such comparisons are based on the very powerful procedure of assessing the patient's brain functions compared with him/herself (using the patient as his own control).

Comparisons of performances on the two sides of the D.H.'s body contributed the most definitive information, although comparisons of various performances within the overall protocol of test results were of definite clinical significance in (1) identifying his brain dysfunction as being relatively chronic and static in nature and (2) leading to an understanding of his brain-related cognitive deficits with relation to his affective problems.

Of the two intra-individual inferential methods, right-left comparisons are frequently more powerful than evaluation of patterns of higher-level scores, principally because identical performances are performed and direct intra-individual comparisons are possible, with only adjustments for hand preference being required in some instances.

CASE #30

Name: T.T.

Age: 25

Education: 12

Sex: Male

Handedness: Right

Occupation: Roofer

Background Information

T.T. was involved in an automobile accident at the age of 24 and suffered multiple injuries, including a linear right parietal skull fracture and fractures involving the right ankle, tibia, fibula, and clavicle. He also sustained a severe closed head injury and was unconscious for approximately 10 days.

Neurological Examination

A neurological examination done three months post-injury demonstrated that T.T.'s use of his right forearm and hand was impaired since the time of the injury; he could not make a fist or close his fingers. The patient also complained of an area of numbness along the lateral border of the right arm extending from the tip of the fifth finger to just above the elbow and involving the lateral half of the fourth finger.

Neurological examination was essentially normal except for this impairment of the right arm. Muscle strength was reduced in the triceps and biceps. Shoulder protraction was impaired and there was marked weakness of forearm extension and flexion and weakness of the digital muscles. There was a noticeable atrophy of the forearm as well as the supraspinatus muscle but no fasciculations were observed. Perception of touch and pain were diminished in the lateral part of the arm and hand from just above the elbow to the tip of

the fifth finger (including the lateral half of the fourth finger), approximately in the distribution of the eighth cervical and first thoracic nerve roots. Vibration sense was normal but proprioception and temperature sense were impaired in the fifth finger. Reflexes of the right upper extremity were generally hyperactive except in the right triceps, which was markedly hypoactive. The right forearm and hand had a mottled and somewhat cyanotic appearance.

The neurologist believed that the patient had sustained a brachial plexus injury and recommended that an electromyelogram be done prior to determining the advisability of surgical exploration. However, T.T. elected to defer any further treatment until entering the medical center for a complete evaluation.

The second neurological examination (done approximately seven months post-injury) continued to show findings involving the right upper extremity and generally concurred with the previous reports. The electromyelogram (EMG) was compatible with a right brachial plexus injury. The electroencephalogram was normal.

Neuropsychological Evaluation

Neuropsychological testing was done at this time (7 months post-injury) to evaluate higher-level cognitive functions. On direct questioning, the patient had no complaints except those relating to use of his right arm and hand. His responses on the Cornell Medical Index Health Questionnaire, however, indicated that he suffers from severe pains in his eyes, often has severe soaking sweats at night, has badly swollen ankles and frequent cramps in his legs, feels constant stiffness in his muscles and joints, has frequent severe headaches and spells of severe dizziness, and has burning pains while urinating and sometimes loses control of his bladder. He had absolutely no positive responses related to emotional or affective problems.

The reader is undoubtedly aware that the effective neuropsychological examination is dependent upon input to the brain, evaluation of central processing by the brain, and output from the brain. The medical history information and neurological examination of this man identified a serious output (expressive) problem involving the right upper extremity, probably due to peripheral nerve damage involving the right brachial plexus. Considering the fact that T.T. had been unconscious for 10 days following a severe head blow, it was possible that higher-level neuropsychological deficits were also present. As we frequently see among patients who have sustained head injuries, the clinical interpretation of the data required differentiation between peripheral nervous system dysfunction (in this case efferent or expressive) and deficits resulting from brain damage.

T.T. earned a Verbal IQ (129) in the Superior range (exceeding about 97% of his age peers) and a Performance IQ (116) in the High Average range (exceeding about 86%). These values yielded a Full Scale IQ (125) in the Superior range (exceeding about 95%).

It is apparent from these values that this man's general intelligence was well above average. The scores for the individual subtests indicated that only two measures were below the average level: Digit Span (9) and Picture Completion (9). His Arithmetic score (17) was exceptionally good, and of the Verbal subtests this measure is probably the most sensitive to brain damage. T.T. performed equivalently well on Similarities (17), the subtest in the Wechsler Scale that is probably most sensitive to left cerebral damage.

There was no significant impairment on Picture Arrangement (13) or Block Design (12) and the overall pattern of Performance subtest scores was probably within normal limits. With the exception of Digit Symbol, the subtests of the Wechsler Scale are either not particularly sensitive to cerebral damage or are selectively sensitive (Picture Arrangement and Block Design). Thus, even though in most cases it is clinically hazardous to depend upon the Wechsler Scale for a complete clinical neuropsychological assessment, in this instance the results would not suggest the presence of cerebral damage.

The four most sensitive indicators in the Halstead-Reitan Battery were also within the normal range. It is always important to consider the Impairment Index in terms of the tests that have contributed to it. In this case the scores contributing to the Impairment Index of 0.3 were the Total Time on the Tactual Performance Test (18.9 min) and finger tapping speed with the right hand (3). Both of these performances obviously depended heavily on adequacy of motor function (output) with the right upper extremity and poor scores can be due to peripheral involvement. It is possible that the slight slowness on Part B of the Trail Making Test may also have been limited by impaired motor proficiency with the right upper extremity, even though the score (75 sec) was still in the normal range. The Localization score of the TPT (6) was adequate. In summary, the results on the general indicators are well within the range of normal brain functioning.

Lateralizing results involved the right hand and arm in particular and showed definite deviations from normality. We have already noted the extremely poor performance with the right upper extremity on the Tactual Performance Test. The examiner observed that T.T. had trouble holding the blocks, manipulating the block so that it would

THE HALSTEAD-REITAN
NEUROPSYCHOLOGICAL TEST BATTERY

Patient _____ **T.T.** _____ Age __**25**__ Sex __**M**__ Education __**12**__ Handedness __**R**__

WECHSLER-BELLEVUE SCALE

VIQ	129
PIQ	116
FS IQ	125

Information	13
Comprehension	15
Digit Span	9
Arithmetic	17
Similarities	17
Vocabulary	15

Picture Arrangement	13
Picture Completion	9
Block Design	12
Object Assembly	14
Digit Symbol	12

TRAIL MAKING TEST

Part A: __57__ seconds
Part B: __75__ seconds

STRENGTH OF GRIP

Dominant hand: __0__ kilograms
Non-dominant hand: __31.0__ kilograms

REITAN-KLØVE TACTILE FORM RECOGNITION TEST

Dominant hand: __34__ seconds; __2__ errors
Non-dominant hand: __8__ seconds; __0__ errors

REITAN-KLØVE SENSORY-PERCEPTUAL EXAM — No errors

			Error Totals	
RH___ LH___	Both H:	RH___ LH___	RH___ LH___	
RH___ LF___	Both H/F:	RH___ LF___	RH___ LF___	
LH___ RF___	Both H/F:	LH___ RF___	RF___ LH___	
RE___ LE___	Both E:	RE___ LE___	RE___ LE___	
RV___ LV___	Both:	RV___ LV___	RV___ LV___	

TACTILE FINGER RECOGNITION

R 1___ 2___ 3___ 4___ 5___   R **0** / 20

L 1___ 2 **1** 3___ 4 **1** 5___   L **2** / 20

FINGER-TIP NUMBER WRITING

R 1___ 2___ 3___ 4___ 5 **2**   R **2** / 20

L 1 **1** 2___ 3___ 4___ 5___   L **1** / 20

HALSTEAD'S NEUROPSYCHOLOGICAL TEST BATTERY

Category Test		**32**

Tactual Performance Test

Dominant hand:	**15.9**		
Non-dominant hand:	**1.6**		
Both hands:	**1.4**		
		Total Time	**18.9**
		Memory	**9**
		Localization	**6**

Seashore Rhythm Test

Number Correct	**29**	**1**

Speech-sounds Perception Test

Number of Errors	**2**

Finger Oscillation Test

Dominant hand:	**3**	**3**
Non-dominant hand:	**51**	

Impairment Index __**0.3**__

MINNESOTA MULTIPHASIC PERSONALITY INVENTORY

		Hs	54
		D	63
?	50	Hy	58
L	46	Pd	74
F	60	Mf	63
K	66	Pa	56
		Pt	34
		Sc	44
		Ma	53

REITAN-KLØVE LATERAL-DOMINANCE EXAM

Show me how you:

throw a ball	_____
hammer a nail	_____
cut with a knife	_____
turn a door knob	_____
use scissors	_____
use an eraser	_____
write your name	_____

} WOULD HAVE USED RIGHT HAND EXCEPT FOR IMPAIRMENT

Record time used for spontaneous name-writing:

Preferred hand	**30**	seconds
Non-preferred hand	**28**	seconds

Show me how you:

kick a football	**R**
step on a bug	**L**

REITAN-INDIANA APHASIA SCREENING TEST

Form for Adults and Older Children

Name: _____T. T._____ Age: __25__

Patient used left hand because of impairment of right upper extremity.
Ordinarily prefers right hand, but says he has always been somewhat ambidextrous.

Copy SQUARE	Repeat TRIANGLE
Name SQUARE	Repeat MASSACHUSETTS 　　　　"Massachusess"
Spell SQUARE	Repeat METHODIST EPISCOPAL
Copy CROSS	Write SQUARE
Name CROSS	Read SEVEN
Spell CROSS	Repeat SEVEN
Copy TRIANGLE	Repeat/Explain HE SHOUTED THE WARNING.
Name TRIANGLE	Write HE SHOUTED THE WARNING.
Spell TRIANGLE	Compute 85 – 27 = Answered "58" before writing the problem on paper.
Name BABY	Compute 17 X 3 =
Write CLOCK	Name KEY
Name FORK	Demonstrate use of KEY
Read 7 SIX 2	Draw KEY
Read MGW	Read PLACE LEFT HAND TO RIGHT EAR.
Reading I 　　Added "period" at the end.	Place LEFT HAND TO RIGHT EAR
Reading II 　　Added "period" at the end.	Place LEFT HAND TO LEFT ELBOW

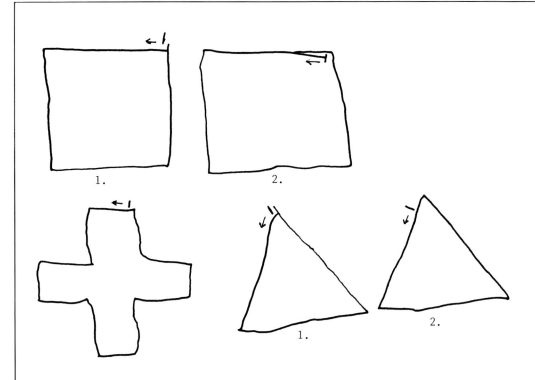

clock

square

He shouted the warning

85 - 27 = 58

51

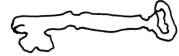

fit into the proper space, and was discouraged and mentioned several times that he was having so much trouble that he wanted to quit. He was extremely quick and proficient with his left hand and had no difficulties. It does not appear that the problem-solving element of the task was the limiting factor; T.T.'s difficulty related to the lack of manipulatory skills with his right hand. On the dynamometer he was not able to register any reading with his right hand.

The patient's finger tapping speed was also greatly reduced with his right hand, although it was well within normal limits for the left hand. For purposes of experimental collection of additional data, T.T. was also examined with the electronic tapper. With this apparatus he was able to register an average of 29 taps with his right hand and 48 taps with his left hand. The patient was able to do fairly well with his impaired right upper extremity by "jiggling" the key on the electronic tapper, but the manual tapper requires discrete movements of the index finger in order to register a score.

We should also note that T.T. had a great deal of difficulty on the Tactile Form Recognition Test with his right hand, requiring a total of 34 seconds and making two errors in the eight trials. His performance with his left hand was entirely within normal limits. The reader should be aware that some degree of motor function is required in this test because the patient must manipulate the stimulus figure with his fingers in order to provide input to the contralateral cerebral hemisphere. This man appeared to have difficulty handling the stimulus figures and therefore was impaired in the quickness and accuracy with which he could respond.

The patient had no difficulty with perception of bilateral simultaneous tactile, auditory, or visual stimuli and made no mistakes with his right hand on the Tactile Finger Recognition Test. The patient had a mild degree of deficit in finger-tip number writing perception (two errors on the right hand

and one error on the left hand). Thus, he showed striking evidence of impairment on tasks that could be limited by impaired motor function and, despite the numbness reported on the neurological examination, showed relatively little impairment on sensory-perceptual tests. Such a dissociation of motor and sensory-perceptual deficits is more commonly found in patients with peripheral damage rather than lateralized cerebral dysfunction.

The test results definitely deviate from normality and show a type of impairment of the right upper extremity that might be attributable exclusively to motor impairment. We must now evaluate the neuropsychological findings in relation to higher-level aspects of left cerebral function.

The patient had a Verbal IQ of 129, showed absolutely no signs of aphasia and (perhaps more impressively) made only two errors on the Speech-sounds Perception Test. The overall results demonstrate a pattern of peripheral rather than central damage: (1) the general indicators do not suggest brain damage; (2) the lateralizing results can be attributed principally (and perhaps exclusively) to motor impairment; and (3) tests of verbal and language functions are within the normal range.

The remainder of the lateralizing findings may possibly represent very mild right cerebral dysfunction. The patient had some difficulty in tactile finger recognition with his left hand and manifested some confusion dealing with the spatial characteristics of the key (particularly relating to the nose). He may have also had some problem achieving opposing symmetry of the notches of the key near the teeth. Although T.T. was using his left hand for the drawings, his proficiency with his left hand was well demonstrated when he wrote his name with his left hand (not shown to protect the patient's identity).

Obviously, with only this minimal evidence, it would be difficult to conclude definitively that T.T. had any significant degree of right cerebral damage, particularly considering his excellent scores with his left hand on other tasks and the good scores on the general indicators. The results suggest that any residual neuropsychological impairment from the head injury was minimal and the deficits involving the right upper extremity were reflections of peripheral (rather than central) involvement.

When reviewing neuropsychological findings of patients with head injuries, it must be remembered that regardless of the test battery used, the complete response cycle requires a satisfactory degree of input (receptive) functioning and responses may be limited by impaired output (expressive) capabilities. Differentiating between peripheral and central impairment requires a careful evaluation and categorization of the particular difficulties as well as observations of consistencies (or lack of

consistency) between the peripheral deficits and the corresponding deficits in central processing.

In the interpretation of this case, two points of information were critical: (1) there was a dissociation between the input and output measures; and (2) there were no higher-level deficits (either general or lateralized) to support the right-sided impairment as a central (left hemisphere) dysfunction. The history information obviously concurred with the interpretation; however, it is always advantageous to be able to interpret the neuropsychological data independently and confirm your expectation on the basis of the history rather than be dependent upon the history alone and thereby not in a position to make an independent contribution and prediction.

CASE #31

Name: A.E.

Age: 60

Education: 15

Sex: Female

Handedness: Right

Occupation: Registered Nurse

Background Information

A.E. was a 60-year-old woman who had completed high school and nurse's training. She had been in generally good health all of her life and had been employed as a registered nurse for many years. She took no medications, denied any allergies, and had been hospitalized only one time, for an appendectomy.

The patient was involved in a moving vehicle accident two weeks before this neuropsychological examination was done. She said that she had suffered a head blow in the accident, lost consciousness briefly, and was dazed for a few minutes afterwards. When asked about her problems she said that initially after the accident she was not able to focus her eyes properly, suffered some pain in her left ear, eye, and shoulder, and experienced numbness in her left arm. However, by the time of the neuropsychological examination two weeks later, she felt that she had shown definite improvement.

Since the accident A.E. had also been experiencing headaches that were most prominent in the frontal region but also involved the back of her head as well. She could recall events up to the time of the accident and starting again a few minutes after the accident. She was amnesic for events during her brief period of unconsciousness and the few minutes of confusion that followed.

Neurological Examination

The patient was able to move all four extremities well and showed no signs of localized weakness or atrophy. Muscle stretch reflexes were normal and equal on both sides. No other neurological signs were elicited and tests of cerebellar functions were normal. No dysphasic symptoms were discerned. A.E. did show evidence of hypalgesia over the left side of the face and the back of the head and hypalgesia as well as hypesthesia over the entire left side of the body. However, these indications of tactile deficits were variable on repeated examinations.

Testing of vibration sensitivity using a tuning fork also showed variable and inconsistent findings. In addition, A.E. seemed to show some loss in the temporal area of the left visual field. The inconsistency of findings on repeated neurological examinations raised the question of whether the indications of deficit might be a manifestation of hysteria.

Radioisotopic brain scans and the electroencephalogram done one day before neuropsychological testing were normal. Laboratory studies, including cerebral spinal fluid, revealed no abnormalities. Because of the possible visual field loss on the left side the patient was referred for ophthalmologic examination to rule out a retinal detachment. Although evidence of this condition was not found, the results did suggest a bilateral constriction of the temporal visual fields.

A.E. was also given additional examinations because of her complaints of occasional episodes of vertigo. Responses to caloric stimulation were normal bilaterally. Bone conduction (compared with air conduction) yielded somewhat inconsistent results; tests of auditory acuity suggested some impairment in the left ear.

In summary, the principal objective neurological finding was loss of touch and pain sensitivity, particularly on the left side of the body. Other findings were often variable from one examination to the next and the possibility of a conversion reaction was suggested; however, it was considered equally likely that the patient had sustained cerebral damage. A.E. was showing some improvement in her tactile deficits, was referred back to her local physician upon discharge from the hospital, and reportedly demonstrated continued improvement. The final diagnosis was recorded as encephalopathy secondary to brain trauma.

Neuropsychological Evaluation

Results from the Wechsler Scale indicated that this woman had previously developed intelligence levels that were within the normal range. The Verbal subtests showed perhaps slightly more variability than might normally be expected, but the distribution was clearly in the average range with some tests being slightly above average and others being somewhat below. The relatively low Information score (8) with relation to the Vocabulary score (11) suggests that A.E. may not have been very actively involved in reading and other intellectual pursuits.

Although the scores on the Performance subtests were consistently below the average level, this might be expected for a 60-year-old woman. In fact, the Wechsler-Bellevue Scale norms yielded a slightly higher Performance than Verbal IQ, although the norms for this particular version of the Wechsler Scales provides for a large increment in Performance IQ for older persons. Even though the Performance subtests scores generally might be considered to be within the range of normal variation for a person of this age, one must consider the low score (4) on the Picture Arrangement subtest to be a possible indicator of right anterior temporal lobe damage (Reitan, 1955c; Meier & French, 1966).

In summary, the general conclusion derived from evaluation of the Wechsler scores is that A.E., if she has not sustained any significant brain damage, should be expected to perform about as well as the average person of her age on brain-sensitive tests.

Next, evaluating A.E.'s performances on the four most sensitive measures in the HRNTB, we see that she showed at least mild impairment on each measure. The Impairment Index of 0.9 indicates that the patient consistently performed slightly worse than persons with normal brain functions, except on the Memory component (6) of the Tactual Performance Test. Research has shown that with normal aging, performances on the four most sensitive indicators in the HRNTB deteriorate more rapidly than the performances on the Verbal subtests of the Wechsler Scale (Reitan, 1956b). Therefore, it appears that these four measures are more sensitive to the accruing neuropathological changes that occur in the brains of older people. In this case, then, the question becomes one of whether the impairment shown by this woman is in line with expectation for a person of her age or whether it goes beyond that level.

Evaluating the test results independently, one sees that the Impairment Index (0.9) and the score on Part B of the Trail Making Test (142 sec) were particularly defective. The Category Test score (65) was slightly poor for a 60-year-old person; the Localization score (4) was probably within expected limits. From the scores on these four indicators one would conclude that there was a definite possibility that the patient had sustained some degree of cerebral damage over and beyond age-expected changes.

THE HALSTEAD-REITAN
NEUROPSYCHOLOGICAL TEST BATTERY

Patient __A.E.__ Age __60__ Sex __F__ Education __R.N.__ Handedness __R__

WECHSLER-BELLEVUE SCALE

VIQ	104
PIQ	108
FS IQ	104

Information	8
Comprehension	12
Digit Span	10
Arithmetic	7
Similarities	8
Vocabulary	11

Picture Arrangement	4
Picture Completion	8
Block Design	8
Object Assembly	8
Digit Symbol	7

TRAIL MAKING TEST

Part A: __81__ seconds
Part B: __142__ seconds

STRENGTH OF GRIP

Dominant hand: __28.0__ kilograms
Non-dominant hand: __15.5__ kilograms

REITAN-KLØVE TACTILE FORM RECOGNITION TEST

Dominant hand: __15__ seconds; __0__ errors
Non-dominant hand: __14__ seconds; __0__ errors

REITAN-KLØVE SENSORY-PERCEPTUAL EXAM

				Error Totals	
RH ___ LH ___	Both H:	RH ___ LH ___		RH ___ LH ___	
RH ___ LF ___	Both H/F:	RH _2_ LF ___		RH _2_ LF ___	
LH ___ RF ___	Both H/F:	LH ___ RF ___		RF ___ LH ___	
RE ___ LE ___	Both E:	RE ___ LE _1_		RE ___ LE _1_	
RV ___ LV ___	Both:	RV ___ LV _1_		RV ___ LV _2_	
___ ___		___ _1_			
___ ___		___ ___			

TACTILE FINGER RECOGNITION

R 1___ 2___ 3___ 4 _1_ 5___   R _1_ / 20
L 1___ 2___ 3 _1_ 4 _1_ 5___   L _2_ / 20

FINGER-TIP NUMBER WRITING

R 1 _3_ 2___ 3___ 4___ 5 _1_   R _4_ / 20
L 1 _2_ 2 _1_ 3 _1_ 4 _1_ 5___   L _5_ / 20

VISUAL FIELD EXAMINATION: MILD LEFT HOMONYMOUS CONSTRICTION.

HALSTEAD'S NEUROPSYCHOLOGICAL TEST BATTERY

Category Test	65

Tactual Performance Test

Dominant hand: __5.2__
Non-dominant hand: __12.8__
Both hands: __5.1__

Total Time	23.1
Memory	6
Localization	4

Seashore Rhythm Test

Number Correct __20__   10

Speech-sounds Perception Test

Number of Errors   8

Finger Oscillation Test

Dominant hand: __42__   42
Non-dominant hand: __31__

Impairment Index __0.9__

MINNESOTA MULTIPHASIC PERSONALITY INVENTORY

		Hs	68
		D	69
?	50	Hy	64
L	50	Pd	76
F	50	Mf	45
K	70	Pa	47
		Pt	58
		Sc	63
		Ma	43

REITAN-KLØVE LATERAL-DOMINANCE EXAM

Show me how you:
throw a ball	R
hammer a nail	R
cut with a knife	R
turn a door knob	R
use scissors	R
use an eraser	R
write your name	R

Record time used for spontaneous name-writing:
Preferred hand	15 seconds
Non-preferred hand	30 seconds

Show me how you:
kick a football	R
step on a bug	R

REITAN-INDIANA APHASIA SCREENING TEST

Form for Adults and Older Children

Name: _____ A. E. _____ Age: __60__

Copy SQUARE	Repeat TRIANGLE
Name SQUARE	Repeat MASSACHUSETTS "Massatusetts"
Spell SQUARE	Repeat METHODIST EPISCOPAL "Methodist Etistical"
Copy CROSS I. Broke pencil lead.	Write SQUARE
Name CROSS	Read SEVEN
Spell CROSS	Repeat SEVEN
Copy TRIANGLE II. Ran off edge of paper.	Repeat/Explain HE SHOUTED THE WARNING.
Name TRIANGLE	Write HE SHOUTED THE WARNING.
Spell TRIANGLE	Compute 85 – 27 =
Name BABY	Compute 17 X 3 =
Write CLOCK	Name KEY
Name FORK	Demonstrate use of KEY
Read 7 SIX 2	Draw KEY
Read MGW	Read PLACE LEFT HAND TO RIGHT EAR.
Reading I	Place LEFT HAND TO RIGHT EAR
Reading II	Place LEFT HAND TO LEFT ELBOW

A.E.

He shouted the warning!

clock

square

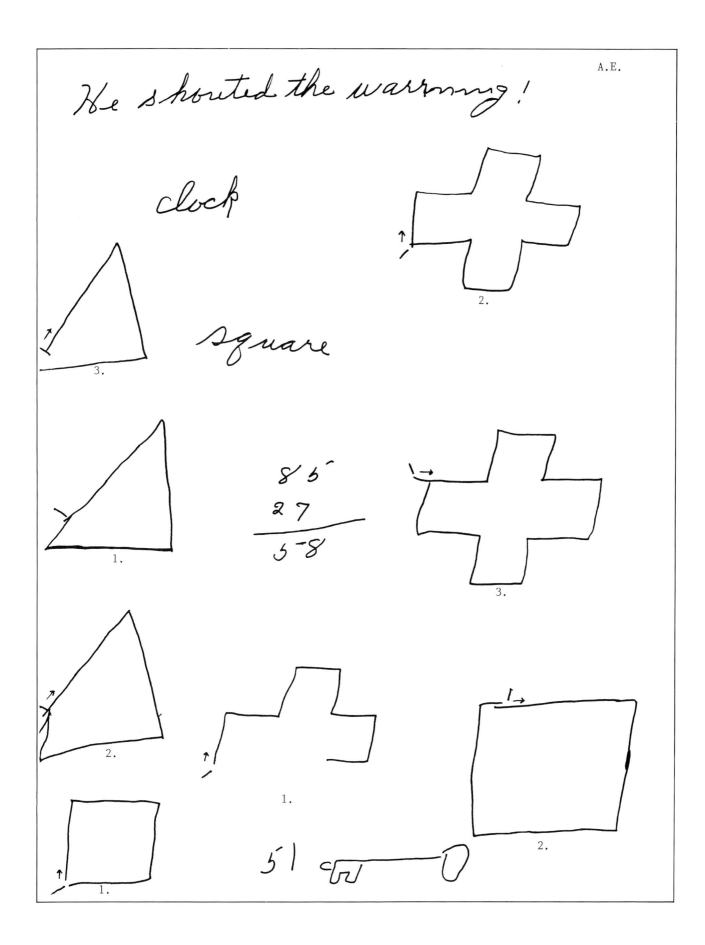

$$8\,5^-$$
$$2\,7$$
$$\overline{5^-8}$$

51

The lateralizing indicators add additional credence to the hypothesis that A.E.'s deficits are due to cerebral damage. Taking into account that the measures of lateral dominance indicated that A.E. was strongly right-handed, she performed quite poorly with her left hand (compared with her right) on measurements of motor speed (Finger Oscillation), motor strength, (Strength of Grip), and complex psychomotor performances (Tactual Performance Test). From these results there is no doubt that the patient has motor difficulties involving her left upper extremity.

Conversely, many of her performances with her right upper extremity could be considered to be within the normal range for a woman of her age, although her finger tapping speed (RH-42; LH-31) was not up to the expected level for non-brain-damaged persons. (Women usually tap somewhat slower than men and an additional decrement in speed appears to begin at about 55 years of age.) Grip strength is difficult to evaluate in absolute terms because of the great variability in musculoskeletal structure, but, in general, men are somewhat stronger than women. The performance with the right hand on the Tactual Performance Test (5.2 min) must certainly be considered to be within normal limits. The relative impairment on Total Time (23.1 min) is essentially a function of the poor performance with the left hand (12.8 min).

If these indications of dysfunction of the left upper extremity were restricted to motor tests one would have difficulty establishing that they were results of right cerebral damage rather than signs of peripheral impairment. There are two points of information in the test results that help the interpreter to resolve this question. First, the patient showed a degree of generalized impairment of brain functions that probably goes beyond age-expectancy. Therefore, if A.E.'s brain is involved in producing the deficits, the likelihood of her right cerebral hemisphere being more seriously involved than the left is increased.

Second, and more importantly, is the fact that certain sensory (receptive) deficits were also present, even though they were not as pronounced as the motor impairment. Except for the evidence of a mild left homonymous constriction of both visual fields, these deficits did not have lateralizing significance. The temporal portion of the visual field for the left eye and the nasal portion for the right eye were constricted. We are not in a position to relate these findings to the somewhat variable results obtained from the visual fields examination by the referring neurological surgeon or by the ophthalmology consultants. However, on the basis of our examination, it seemed that this woman did have a mild but definite left homonymous visual field constriction.

The other sensory-perceptual deficits were not strongly lateralizing. The patient had difficulty in tactile finger recognition and approximately equivalent difficulty on both hands in finger-tip number writing perception. Even though these findings were not lateralizing, the fact that A.E. made as many mistakes as she did on finger-tip number writing (9 errors in 40 trials) adds to the general impression of cerebral damage. The errors in tests of bilateral simultaneous tactile, auditory, and visual stimulation have essentially the same significance.

Next, we see that the patient showed signs of mild but definite difficulty in dealing with simple spatial configurations. She tended to press very hard when drawing and broke the lead of her pencil on her first attempt to draw the cross. She asked if she could start over again and was allowed to do so. Both the second and third drawings of the cross show a mild deviation from correspondence of the opposing extremities.

More pronounced deficits were shown in A.E.'s attempts to draw the triangle. She had some difficulty with the symmetry of the figure, and in her initial attempt the second line was too long. In order to draw a horizontal line as the base, it was necessary for her to come back across and then finally close the figure. In her second attempt to draw the triangle she had not evaluated the available space with relation to her drawing and had even more difficulty. Note that this same kind of problem occurred on her third attempt; it was obviously difficult for this patient to deal with the left margin of the paper with relation to her drawing of figures and such an inability to deal effectively with spatial configurations is frequently observed in persons with right cerebral damage. Even A.E.'s second attempt to draw the square was highly suspicious; she proceeded too far with the third (lower horizontal) line and, upon completing the fourth line, found it necessary to close the figure.

Although it was only a skeletal figure, A.E.'s drawing of the key was equally revealing. Failure to originally include the nose of the key and having to add it on later may be considered a pathognomonic sign for right cerebral damage.

One could question whether A. E.'s consistent difficulty in drawing the left side of the figures is related to the evidence of a left homonymous visual field constriction. In the individual case it is difficult to predict when a visual field defect will produce problems in dealing with spatial relationships; however, we have observed many patients *without* visual field constrictions or losses demonstrate the same type of difficulty with spatial relationships when they also have a lesion of the right cerebral hemisphere. *Thus, we can say with certainty that a patient does not have to have a homonymous visual field loss in order to demonstrate impaired drawings or difficulty with the left side of space.* Because both of these findings correlate with damage of the right cerebral hemisphere it would therefore seem that the basic deficit relates to right cerebral damage rather than a left homonymous visual field loss.

In summary, these lateralizing findings, together with the indications of mild impairment on brain-sensitive tests (taking the patient's age into account), reinforce the impression that the motor

deficits on the left side are part of the total picture of cerebral damage that involves the right hemisphere to a greater extent than the left.

A review of other test results suggests that there is mild generalized impairment in addition to the right cerebral damage. For example, the patient had difficulty perceiving a tactile stimulus to her right hand when it was given simultaneously with a stimulus to the left face. She also made an error typical of brain-damaged persons in her enunciation of METHODIST EPISCOPAL. The difficulty, an obvious confusion of consonant sounds, occurred with EPISCOPAL. Together with the general results pointing toward diffuse cerebral damage, these mild left cerebral indicators and the results on finger-tip number writing perception all suggest that A.E.'s brain impairment is not strictly lateralized to the right cerebral hemisphere.

In addition, we find that the patient did relatively well on several measures, including the Speech-sounds Perception Test (8) and the first trial on the Tactual Performance Test (5.2 min). Good performances such as these generally rule out an acutely destructive focal lesion (e.g., an intrinsic tumor or a stroke). The small disparity between Verbal and Performance IQ scores (4 points) and the lack of gross impairment in copying simple spatial configurations also support the hypothesis that A.E. did not have a devastating right cerebral lesion.

At this point the test findings clearly indicate that this woman (1) had developed brain-behavior relationships relatively normally; (2) shows some degree of impairment associated with her age; (3) demonstrates additional evidence of a pathological nature that involves her right cerebral hemisphere much more than her left and has some diffuse components as well; and (4) has cerebral damage that is not acutely devastating and appears to be relatively stabilized.

Considering these various findings, it would not be likely that either a stroke or an intrinsic tumor were responsible and an extrinsic tumor would not explain the generalized impairment. Results of this kind could conceivably be associated with early generalized cerebral vascular deterioration together with thrombosis of a small branch of the right middle cerebral artery, but in such a case we would have expected at least somewhat poorer scores on the Speech-sounds Perception Test and the first trial on the Tactual Performance Test.

The test performances demonstrated by this woman are compatible with a closed head injury that damaged the right cerebral hemisphere to a greater extent than the left. Retrospectively, it would appear that head trauma is the most likely cause of A.E. performances but in the "blind" interpretation done initially we were reluctant to specify the likely causative factors and recommended that the etiology of the brain damage be considered with relation to the patient's history.

As noted previously, the better scores on the HRNTB suggest that A.E.'s brain damage is in a relatively stabilized rather than progressive state. Although we would not have been able to predict that the left-sided hypesthesia was gradually resolving at this time, this finding is entirely consistent with the test results. In fact, considering the overall circumstances, it was likely that the patient would gradually show improvement and this was later reported to us by her physician.

Although we are not able to explain the inconsistent findings on the clinical neurological examination, problems of this type are not a factor in neuropsychological interpretation. Two circumstances seem to be particularly responsible for this. First, the Halstead-Reitan Battery is organized as a *battery* of tests. If certain tests from the Battery were selected for repetition, it is entirely possible that the results would not be exactly the same. In other words, a degree of inconsistency in specific test results might occur if individual tests from the neuropsychological examination were repeated. However, the Halstead-Reitan Battery has been developed to reflect brain-behavior relationships for

the individual subject rather than merely report results obtained on individual tests. If the focus were upon individual tests and variability in results were found, one might wonder about the possibility of hysterical manifestations.

It appears that brain-damaged persons are not able to show the degree of consistency in stimulus-response situations that characterizes the performances of persons with normal brain functions; therefore, it was necessary to develop an examination that reflected the status of the individual *brain* rather than an individual test. We feel that the Halstead-Reitan Battery accomplishes this purpose. It has not been achieved as effectively with the clinical neurological examination or the examinations of neuropsychologists who select different tests to evaluate each patient based upon the complaints of the patient or the clinical history.

Considering the test results that were obtained with A.E., it is not surprising to learn that she was gradually and progressively showing some resolution of her left-sided hypesthesia. In all probability this was actual improvement. Over time we would expect additional improvement on the neuropsychological tests as well, since only two weeks had elapsed since the injury when this evaluation was done.

As often occurs in instances of relatively mild brain injuries, this woman was not referred for any type of specific rehabilitation. It seems that physical therapy might have been indicated, especially in light of A.E.'s prominent motor difficulties involving her left upper extremity. Physical therapy might also have improved her performances on the left side on measures of finger tapping speed, grip strength, and complex psychomotor performances. It is likely that the patient will show some spontaneous improvement in these areas but facilitation of such a recovery trend would certainly have been advantageous.

We also saw that A.E. had difficulties in dealing with spatial relationships and some problems with tasks that required abstraction, reasoning, and keeping various elements of a situation in mind at the same time (e.g., Category Test and Part B of the Trail Making Test). In a case of this kind we would certainly recommend use of REHABIT. In this particular situation we would start with Track C and gradually work through various parts of Tracks D and E.

Finally, results on the Minnesota Multiphasic Personality Inventory suggest that this woman may have certain personality and emotional problems that are relevant to her overall adjustment. It does not seem likely that the deviant results on the MMPI are a direct effect of brain damage; in all probability these personality traits existed before the brain injury was sustained. Nevertheless, her personality characteristics may be a factor that need attention and psychological counseling, and in the context of the overall recovery process, should be carefully considered.

REFERENCES

Adams, G.F. (1963). Prospects for patients with strokes. *British Medical Journal, 2,* 253–259.

Adams, J.H. (1975). The neuropathology of head injuries. In P.J. Vinken & G.S. Bruyn (Eds.), *Handbook of clinical neurology.* Vol. 23. Amsterdam: North Holland Publishing Co.

Adams, J.H., & Graham, D.I. (1976). The relationship between ventricular fluid pressure and the neuropathology of raised intracranial pressure. *Neuropathology and Applied Neurobiology, 2,* 323–332.

Adams, J.H., Graham, D.I., Murray, L.S., & Scott, G. (1982). Diffuse axonal injury due to nonmissile injury in humans: An analysis of forty-five cases. *Annals of Neurology, 12,* 557–563.

Adams, J.H., Mitchell, D.E., Graham, D.I., et al. (1977). Diffuse brain damage types. *Brain, 100,* 482–502.

Adams, J.H., Mitchell, D.E., Graham, D.I., & Doyle, D. (1977). Diffuse brain damage of immediate impact type. Its relationship to "primary brain stem damage" in head injury. *Brain, 100,* 489–502.

Adams, J.H., Scott, Grace, et al. (1980). The contusion index. A quantitative approach to cerebral contusions in head injury. *Neuropathology and Applied Neurobiology, 6,* 319–324.

Aita, J.A., Armitage, S.G., Reitan, R.M., & Rabinovitz, A. (1947). The use of certain psychological tests in the evaluation of brain injury. *Journal of General Psychology, 37,* 25–44.

Aita, J.A., & Reitan, R.M. (1948). Psychotic reactions in late recovery period following brain injury. *American Journal of Psychiatry, 105,* 161–169.

Aita, J.A., Reitan, R.M., & Ruth, J.M. (1947). Rorschach's Test as a diagnostic aid in brain injury. *American Journal of Psychiatry, 103,* 770–779.

Anderson, D.W., Kalsbeek, W.D., & Hartwell, T.D. (1980). The National Head and Spinal Cord Injury Survey: Design and methodology. *Journal of Neurosurgery* (Suppl.), *53,* 11–18.

Annegers, J.F., Grabow, J.D., Kurland, L.T., & Laws, E.R. (1980). The incidence, causes, and secular trends of head trauma in Olmsted County, Minnesota. *Neurology, 30,* 912–919.

Armitage, S.G. (1946). An analysis of certain psychological tests used for evaluation of brain injury. *Psychology Monographs,* No. 1 (Whole No. 277), *60.*

Babcock, H. (1930). An experiment in the measurement of mental deterioration. *Archives of Psychology, 18,* 5–105.

Bakay, L. & Glasauer, F.E. (1980). *Head injury.* Boston: Little, Brown and Company.

Baker, H.L., Campbell, J.K., Houser, O.W., et al. (1974). Computer-assisted tomography of the head. *Mayo Clinic Proceedings, 49,* 17–27.

Becker, D.F., Miller, J.D., & Greenberg, R.P. (1982). Prognosis after head injury. In J.R. Youmans (Ed.), *Neurological surgery.* Philadelphia: W.B. Saunders & Company.

Becker, D.P., Miller, J.D., Young, H.F., Selhorst, J.B., Kishore, P.R.S., Greenberg, R.P., Rosner, M.J., & Ward, J.D. (1982). Diagnosis and treatment of head injury in adults. In J.R. Youmans (Ed.), *Neurological surgery.* Philadelphia: W.B. Saunders & Company.

Bond, M.R., (1975). Assessment of the psychosocial outcome after severe head injury. *CIBA Foundation Symposium, 34,* 141–57.

Bond, M.R., & Brooks, D.N. (1976). Understanding the process of recovery as a basis for the investigation of rehabilitation for the brain injured. *Scandinavian Journal of Rehabilitational Medicine, 8,* 127–133.

Brenner, C., Friedman, A.P., Merritt, H.H., & Denny-Brown, D.E. (1944). Post-traumatic headache. *Journal of Neurosurgery, 1,* 379–391.

Brooks, D.N. (1972). Memory and head injury. *Journal of Nervous and Mental Disease, 155,* 350–355.

Brooks, D.N. (1974). Recognition memory and head injury. *Journal of Neurology, Neurosurgery, and Psychiatry, 37,* 794–801.

Brooks, D.N. (1976). Wechsler memory scale performance and its relationship to brain damage after severe closed head injury. *Journal of Neurology, Neurosurgery, and Psychiatry, 39,* 593–601.

Brooks, D.N., Aughton, M.E., Bond, M.R., Jones, P., & Rizvi, S. (1980). Cognitive sequelae in relationship to early indices of severity of brain damage after severe blunt head injury. *Journal of Neurology, Neurosurgery, and Psychiatry, 43,* 529–534.

Bruce, D.A., Shute, L., Bruno, L.A., Wood, J.H., & Sutton, L.N. (1978). Outcome following severe head injuries in children. *Journal of Neurosurgery, 48,* 679–688.

Cartlidge, N.E.F. (1978). Post-concussional syndrome. *Scottish Medical Journal, 23,* 103.

Caveness, W.F. (1976). Epilepsy, a product of trauma of our time. *Epilepsia, 17,* 207–215.

Caveness, W.F. (1977). Incidence of craniocerebral trauma in the United States, 1970–1975. *Annals of Neurology, 1,* 507.

Cockrill, H.H., Jiminez, J.P., & Gorse, J.A. (1977). Traumatic false aneurysm of the superior cerebellar artery simulating posterior fossa tumor. Case report. *Journal of Neurosurgery, 46,* 377–380.

Corkin, S. (1968). Acquisition of motor skill after bilateral medial temporal-lobe excision. *Neuropsychologia, 6,* 225–265.

Corkin, S. (1979). Hidden figures test performance: Lasting effects of unilateral penetrating injury and transient effect of bilateral cingulotomy. *Neuropsychologia, 17,* 585–605.

Corsellis, J.A.N., Bruton, C.J., & Freeman-Browne, D. (1973). The aftermath of boxing. *Psychological Medicine, 3,* 270–303.

Courville, C.D. (1962). Traumatic intracerebral hemorrhages with special reference to the mechanics of their production. *Bulletin of the Los Angeles Neurological Society, 27,* 22.

Cronholm, B., & Jonsson, I. (1957). Memory functions after cerebral concussion. *Acta Chirurgica Scandanavica, 113,* 263–271.

DeMyer, W. (1980). *Technique of the neurologic examination.* Third edition. New York: McGraw-Hill.

Dikmen, S., & Reitan, R.M. (1974). MMPI correlates of localized structural cerebral lesions. *Perceptual and Motor Skills, 39,* 831–840.

Dikmen, S., & Reitan, R.M. (1976). Psychological deficits and recovery of functions after head injury. *Transactions of the American Neurological Association, 101,* 72–77.

Dikmen, S., & Reitan, R.M. (1977a). Emotional sequelae of head injury. *Annals of Neurology, 2,* 492–494.

Dikmen, S., & Reitan, R.M. (1977b). MMPI correlates of adaptive ability deficits in patients with brain lesions. *Journal of Nervous and Mental Disease, 165,* 247–254.

Dikmen, S., Reitan, R.M., & Temkin, N.R. (1983). Neuropsychological recovery in head injury. *Archives of Neurology, 40,* 333–338.

Doehring, D.G., & Reitan, R.M. (1962). Concept attainment of human adults with lateralized cerebral lesions. *Perceptual and Motor Skills, 14,* 27–33.

Doehring, D.G., Reitan, R.M., & Kløve, H. (1961). Changes in patterns of intelligence test performances associated with homonymous visual field defects. *Journal of Nervous and Mental Disease, 132,* 227–233.

Ducker, T.B., Kempe, L.G., & Hayes, G.J. (1969). The metabolic background for peripheral nerve surgery. *Journal of Neurosurgery, 30,* 270–280.

Dye, O.A., Milby, J.B., & Saxon, S.A. (1979). Effects of early neurological problems following head trauma on subsequent neuropsychological performance. *Acta Neurologica Scandinavica, 59,* 10–14.

Ewing, R., McCarthy, D., Gronwall, D., & Wrightson, P. (1980). Persisting effects of minor head injury observable during hypoxic stress. *Journal of Clinical Neuropsychology, 2,* 147–155.

Feuchtwanger, E. (1923). Die Funktionen des Stirnhirn, ihre Pathologie und Psychologie. *Monog. a.d. Ges. d. Neurol. u. Psychiat., No. 38.*

Fishbone, H. (1976). Irreversible injury of the last four cranial nerves (Collet-Sicard syndrome). In P.J. Vinken & G.W. Bruyn (Eds.), *Handbook of clinical neurology.* Amsterdam: Elsevier-North Holland Publishing Co.

Fitzhugh, K.B., Fitzhugh, L.C., & Reitan, R.M. (1961). Psychological deficits in relation to acuteness of brain dysfunction. *Journal of Consulting Psychology, 25,* 61–66.

Fitzhugh, K.B., Fitzhugh, L.C., & Reitan, R.M. (1962a). The relationship of acuteness of organic brain dysfunction to Trail Making Test performances. *Perceptual and Motor Skills, 15,* 399–403.

Fitzhugh, K.B., Fitzhugh, L.C., & Reitan, R.M. (1962b). Wechsler-Bellevue comparisons in groups with "chronic" and "current" lateralized diffuse brain lesions. *Journal of Consulting Psychology, 26,* 306–310.

Fitzhugh, K.B., Fitzhugh, L.C., & Reitan, R.M. (1963). Effects of "chronic" and "current" lateralized and non-lateralized cerebral lesions upon Trail Making Test performances. *Journal of Nervous and Mental Disease, 137,* 82–87.

Fitzhugh, L.C., Fitzhugh, K.B., & Reitan, R.M. (1962). Sensorimotor deficits of brain-damaged subjects in relation to intellectual level. *Perceptual and Motor Skills, 15,* 603–608.

Fodor, I.E. (1972). Impairment of memory functions after acute head injury. *Journal of Neurology, Neurosurgery, and Psychiatry, 35,* 818–824.

Foster, Jaine M. (1982). Processing of verbal and non-verbal auditory information in brain-injured vs. control subjects. Unpublished master's thesis. University of Arizona.

French, B.N., & Dublin, A.B. (1977). The value of computerized tomography on one thousand consecutive head injuries. *Surgical Neurology, 7,* 171–183.

Fuld, P.A., & Fisher, P. (1977). Recovery of intellectual ability after closed head injury. *Developmental Medicine and Child Neurology, 19,* 495–502.

Gabor, A.J. (1982). Post-traumatic epilepsy. In J.R. Youmans (Ed.), *Neurological surgery.* Philadelphia: W.B. Saunders and Company.

Gilroy, J., & Meyer, R. (1979). *Medical neurology.* New York: MacMillan Publishing Company.

Gissane, W. (1963). The nature and causation of road injuries. *Lancet, 2,* 695–698.

Golden, C.J. (1981). A standardized version of Luria's neuropsychological tests. In S. Filskov & T. J. Boll (Eds.), *Handbook of clinical neuropsychology.* New York: Wiley-Interscience.

Goldstein, K. (1936). The significance of the frontal lobe for mental performances. *Journal of Neurology and Psychopathology, 17,* 27–40.

Goldstein, K. (1939). Clinical and theoretical aspects of lesions of the frontal lobes. *Archives of Neurology and Psychiatry, 41,* 865–867.

Goldstein, K. (1940). *Human nature.* Cambridge, MA: Harvard University Press.

Goldstein, K. (1942). *After-effects of brain injuries in war, their evaluation and treatment.* New York: Grune and Stratton.

Goldstein, K., & Scheerer, M. (1941). Abstract and concrete behavior: An experimental study with special mental tests. *Psychological Monographs,* 239.

Goodglass, H., & Kaplan, E. (1972). *The assessment of aphasia and related disorders.* Philadelphia: Lea & Febiger.

Graham, D.I., & Adams, J.H. (1971). Ischemic brain damage in fatal head injuries. *Lancet, 1,* 265–266.

Graham, D.E., Adams, J.H., & Doyle, D. (1978). Ischemic brain damage in fatal non-missile head injuries. *Journal of Neurological Sciences, 39,* 213–234.

Grant, I., Mohns, L., Miller, M., & Reitan, R.M. (1976). A neuropsychological study of polydrug users. *Archives of General Psychiatry, 33,* 973–978.

Greenberg, R.P., Becker, D.P., Miller, J.D., & Mayer, D.J. (1977). Evaluation of brain function in severe head trauma with multimodality evoked potentials. Part II. Localization of brain dysfunction and correlation with post-traumatic neurological condition. *Journal of Neurosurgery, 47,* 163–177.

Groher, M. (1977). Language and memory disorders following closed head trauma. *Journal of Speech and Hearing Research, 20,* 212–223.

Gronwall, D. (1977). Paced auditory serial-addition task: A measure of recovery from concussion. *Perceptual and Motor Skills, 44,* 367–373.

Gronwall, D., & Sampson, H. (1974). *The psychological effects of concussion.* Aukland, New Zealand: Aukland University Press.

Gronwall, D., & Wrightson, P. (1974). Delayed recovery of intellectual function after minor head injury. *Lancet, 2,* 605–609.

Gronwall, D., & Wrightson, P. (1975). Cumulative effect of concussion. *Lancet, 2,* 995–997.

Grossman, R.G. (1972). Alterations in the microphysiology of glial cells and neurones and the environment in the injured brain. *Clinical Neurosurgery, 19,* 69–83.

Grossman, R.G., & Seregin, A.I. (1976). Effects of traumatically induced edema on membrane potentials of cortical glial cells and neurones. In R.L. McLaurin (Ed.), *Head injuries: Second Chicago symposium on neural trauma.* New York: Grune & Stratton.

Guilford, J.P. (1936). *Psychometric methods.* New York: McGraw-Hill.

Gurdgian, E.S. (1975). *Impact head injury: Mechanistic, clinical and preventive correlations.* Springfield, IL: Charles C Thomas.

Guttman, E. (1946). Late effects of closed head injuries: Psychiatric observations. *Journal of Mental Science, 92,* 1–18.

Halstead, W.C. (1947). *Brain and intelligence: A quantitative study of the frontal lobes.* Chicago: University of Chicago Press.

Hammon, W.M. (1971). Analysis of 2,187 consecutive penetrating wounds of the brain from Vietnam. *Journal of Neurosurgery, 34,* 127–131.

Hannay, H.J., Levin, H.S., & Grossman, R.G. (1979). Impaired recognition memory after head injury. *Cortex, 15,* 269–283.

Hannay, H.J., Levin, H.S., & Kay, M. (1981). Tachistoscopic visual perception after closed head injury. *Journal of Clinical Neuropsychology.*

Harwood-Hash, D.C., Hendrick, E.D., & Hudson, A.R. (1971). The significance of skull fracture in children: A study of 1,187 patients. *Radiology, 101,* 155.

Hawthorne, V.M. (1978). Epidimiology of head injuries. *Scottish Medical Journal, 23,* 92.

Head, H. (1926). *Aphasia and kindred disorders of speech.* Volume I. Cambridge, England: The University Press.

Hendrick, E.B., Harwood-Hash, D.C.F., & Hudson, A.R. (1964). Head injuries in children: A survey of 4,465 consecutive cases at the Hospital for Sick Children, Toronto Canada. *Clinical Neurosurgery, 11,* 46–59.

Hirsh, C.A., & Kaufman, B. (1975). Contrecoup skull fractures. *Journal of Neurosurgery, 42,* 530–534.

Holbourne, A.H.S. (1943). Mechanics of head injuries. *Lancet, 2,* 438–441.

Holbourne, A.H.S. (1945). The mechanics of brain injuries. *The Medical Bulletin, 3,* 147–149.

Hom, J., & Reitan, R.M. (1982). Effects of lateralized cerebral damage upon contralateral and ipsilateral sensorimotor performances. *Journal of Clinical Neuropsychology, 4,* 249–268.

Hom, J., & Reitan, R.M. (1984). Neuropsychological correlates of rapidly vs. slowly growing intrinsic neoplasms. *Journal of Clinical Neuropsychology, 6,* 309–324.

Illingworth, G., & Jennett, B. (1965). The shocked head injury. *Lancet, 2,* 511–514.

Jacobsen, S.A. (1963). *The posttraumatic syndrome following head injury.* Springfield, IL: Charles C Thomas.

Jamieson, K.G., & Yelland, J.D.N. (1968). Extradural haematoma. Report of 167 cases. *Journal of Neurosurgery, 29,* 13–23.

Jamieson, K.G., & Yelland, J.D.N. (1972). Surgically treated traumatic subdural hematomas. *Journal of Neurosurgery, 37,* 137–149.

Jasper, H.H. (1970). Physiopathological mechanisms of post-traumatic epilepsy. *Epilepsia, 11,* 73–80.

Jennett, B. (1965). Predicting epilepsy after blunt head injury. *British Medical Journal, 1,* 1215–1216.

Jennett, B. (1975). *Epilepsy after non-missile head injury.* Second Edition. London: William Heinemann Ltd.

Jennett, B. (1977). *An introduction to neurosurgery.* Third Edition. Chicago: Year Book Medical Publishers.

Jennett, B., Snoek, J., Bond, M.R., & Brooks, N. (1981). Disability after severe head injury: Observation on the use of the Glasgow Outcome Scale. *Journal of Neurology, Neurosurgery, and Psychiatry, 44,* 285–293.

Jennett, B., & Teasdale, G. (1977). Aspects of coma after severe head injury. *Lancet, 1,* 878–881.

Jennett, B., & Teasdale, G. (1981). *Management of head injuries.* Philadelphia: F.A. Davis Company.

Johnson, G.W., & Sinkler, W.H. (1961). Subdural hematoma: A complex and insidious neurosurgical disease. A review of 100 cases. *Journal of the National Medical Association, 53,* 238.

Kalsbeek, W.D., McLaurin, R.L., Harris, B.S.H., III, & Miller, J.D. (1980). The National Head and Spinal Cord Injury Survey: Major findings. *Journal of Neurosurgery, Supplement, 53,* 19–31.

Kay, D.W.K., Kerr, T.A., & Lassman, L.P. (1971). Brain trauma and post-concussional syndrome. *Lancet, 2,* 1052–1055.

Kimura, D. (1963). Right temporal-lobe damage. *Archives of Neurology, 8,* 264–271.

Klatzo, I. (1967). Neuropathological aspects of brain edema. *Journal of Neuropathology and Experimental Neurology, 24,* 1.

Klonoff, H. (1971). Head injuries in children: Predisposing factors, accident conditions, accident proneness and sequelae. *American Journal of Public Health, 61,* 2405–2417.

Kløve, H., & Cleeland, C.S. (1972). The relationship of neuropsychological impairment to other indices of severity of head injury. *Scandanavian Journal of Rehabilitational Medicine, 4,* 55–60.

Kløve, H. & Matthews, C.G. (1969). Neuropsychological evaluation of the epileptic patient. *Wisconsin Medical Journal, 68,* 269–301.

Kløve, H., & Reitan, R.M. (1958). The effect of dysphasia and spatial distortion on Wechsler-Bellevue results. *Archives of Neurology and Psychiatry, 80,* 708–713.

Kraus, J.F. (1980). Injury to the head and spinal cord: The epidemiological relevance of the medical literature published from 1960 to 1978. *Journal of Neurosurgery, Supplement, 53,* 3–10.

Lee, J.C., & Bakay, L. (1966). Ultrastructural change in the edematous central nervous system. II. Cold induced edema. *Archives of Neurology, 14,* 36.

Levin, H.S., Benton, A.L., & Grossman, R.G. (1982). *Neurobehavioral consequences of closed head injury.* New York: Oxford University Press.

Levin, H.S., & Grossman, R.G. (1978). Behavioral sequelae of closed head injury: A quantitative study. *Archives of Neurology, 35,* 720–727.

Levin, H.S., Grossman, R.G., Kelly, P.J. (1976). Aphasic disorder in patients with closed head injury. *Journal of Neurology, Neurosurgery, and Psychiatry, 39,* 1062–1070.

Levin, H.S., Grossman, R.G., & Kelly, P.J. (1977). Impairment of facial recognition after closed head injuries of varying severity. *Cortex, 13,* 119–130.

Levin, H.S., O'Donnell, V.M., & Grossman, R.G. (1979). The Galveston Orientation and Amnesia Test: A practical scale to assess cognition after head injury. *Journal of Nervous and Mental Disease, 167,* 675–684.

Lezak, M.D. (1979). Recovery of memory and learning functions following traumatic brain injury. *Cortex, 15,* 63–72.

Lindgren, S.O. (1966). Experimental studies of mechanical effects in head injury. *Acta Chirurgica Scandinavica, Supplement, 132,* 1.

Lindenberg, R., & Freytag, E. (1957). Morphology of cortical contusions. *Archives of Pathology, 63,* 23.

Lishman, W.A. (1973). The psychiatric sequelae of head injury: A review. *Psychological Medicine, 3,* 304–318.

Lundberg, N. (1960). Continuous recording and control of ventricular fluid pressure in neurosurgical practice. *Acta Neurologica et Psychiatrica Scandanavica, 36,* 149, 1–193.

McKissock, W., Taylor, J.E., Bloom, W.H., & Till, K. (1960). Extradural haematoma. *Lancet, 2,* 167.

McLaurin, R.L., & King, L.R. (1975). Metabolic effects of head injury. In P.J. Vinken & G.W. Bruyn (Eds.), *Handbook of Clinical Neurology.* Volume 23, Injuries of the brain and skull. Part I. Amsterdam: Elsevier-North Holland Publishing Company.

McLaurin, R.L., & Titchener, J.L. (1982). Post-traumatic syndrome. In J.R. Youmans (Ed.), *Neurological surgery.* Philadelphia: W.B. Saunders and Company.

Mandleberg, I.A. (1975). Cognitive recovery after severe head injury. 2. Wechsler Adult Intelligence Scale during post-traumatic amnesia. *Journal of Neurology, Neurosurgery and Psychiatry, 38,* 1127–1132.

Mandleberg, I.A. (1976). Cognitive recovery after severe head injury. 3. WAIS verbal and performance IQs as a function of post-traumatic amnesia duration and time from injury. *Journal of Neurology, Neurosurgery, and Psychiatry, 39,* 1001–1007.

Mandleberg, I.A., & Brooks, D.N. (1975). Cognitive recovery after severe head injury. 1. Serial testing on the Wechsler Adult Intelligence Scale. *Journal of Neurology, Neurosurgery, and Psychiatry, 38,* 1121–1126.

Meier, M.J., & French, L.A. (1966). Longitudinal assessment of intellectual functioning following unilateral temporal lobectomy. *Journal of Clinical Psychology, 22,* 22–27.

Merino, J., deVillasante, J., & Tavares, J.M. (1976). Computerized tomography (CT) in acute head trauma. *American Journal of Roentgenology, 126,* 765–778.

Merskey, H., & Woodforde, J.M. (1972). Psychiatric sequelae of minor head injury. *Brain, 95,* 521–528.

Miller, J.D., & Becker, D.P. (1982). General principles and pathophysiology of head injury. In J.R. Youmans (Ed.), *Neurological surgery.* Philadelphia: W.B. Saunders Co.

Miller, J.D., Becker, D.P., Ward, J.D., Sullivan, H.G., Adams, W.E., & Rosner, M.J. (1977). Significance of intracranial hypertension in severe head injury. *Journal of Neurosurgery, 47,* 503–516.

Miller, J.D., & Jennett, W.B. (1968). Complications of depressed skull fractures. *Lancet, 2,* 991–995.

Mitchell, D.E., & Adams, J.H. (1973). Primary focal impact damage to the brainstem in blunt head injuries: Does it exist? *Lancet, 2,* 215–218.

Moruzzi, G., & Magoun, H.W. (1949). Brainstem reticular function and activation of the EEG. *Electroencephalography and Clinical Neurophysiology, 1,* 455–473.

Newcombe, F. (1969). *Missile wounds of the brain.* London: Oxford University Press.

Ommaya, A.K. (1982). Mechanisms of cerebral concussion, contusion, and other effects of head injury. In J.R. Youmans (Ed.), *Neurological surgery.* Philadelphia: W.B. Saunders Company.

Ommaya, A.K., & Gennarelli, T. (1974). Cerebral concussion and traumatic unconsciousness. Correlation of experimental and clinical observations on blunt head injuries. *Brain, 97,* 633–654.

Ommaya, A.K., & Gennarelli, R.A. (1976). A physiopathologic basis for noninvasive diagnosis and prognosis of head injury severity. In R.L. McLaurin (Ed.), *Head injuries.* New York; Grune & Stratton Inc.

Ommaya, A.K., Grubb, R.L., & Naumann, R.A. (1970). Coup and contrecoup cerebral contusions: An experimental analysis. *Neurology, 20,* 388–389.

Ommaya, A.K., & Yarnall, P., (1969). *Subdural haematoma after whiplash injury.* Lancet ii, 237–239.

Oppenheimer, D.R. (1968). Microscopic lesions in the brain following head injury. *Journal of Neurology, Neurosurgery, and Psychiatry, 31,* 299.

Paxton, R., & Ambrose, J. (1974). The EMI scanner. A brief review of the first 650 patients. *British Journal of Radiology, 47,* 530–565.

Penfield, W. & Roberts, L. (1959). *Speech and brain mechanisms.* Princeton, NJ: Princeton University Press.

Piotrowski, Z. (1937). On the Rorschach method and its application in organic disturbances of the central nervous system. *Rorschach Research Exchange, 1,* 23.

Piotrowski, Z. (1938). The Rorschach ink-blot method in organic disturbances of the central nervous system. *Journal of Nervous and Mental Disease, 86,* 525.

Plum, F., & Posner, J.B. (1980). *Diagnosis of stupor and coma.* Third Edition. Philadelphia: F.A. Davis.

Porter, R.J., & Miller, R.A. (1948). Diabetes insipidus following closed head injury. *Journal of Neurology, Neurosurgery, and Psychiatry, 11,* 258–262.

Potter, J.M., & Braakman, R. (1976). Injury to the facial nerve. In P.J. Vinken & G.W. Bruyn (Eds.), *Handbook of clinical neurology.* Amsterdam: Elsevier-North Holland Publishing Co.

Pudenz, R.H., & Shelden, R.H. (1946). The Lucite calvarium — A method for direct observation of the brain. II. Cranial trauma and brain movement. *Journal of Neurosurgery, 3,* 487–505.

Raimondi, A.I., & Samuelson, G.H. (1970). Cranio-cerebral gunshot wounds in civilian practice. *Journal of Neurosurgery, 17,* 483–485.

Reed, H.B.C. (May, 1963). Effects of head trauma, intrinsic tumor, and cerebrovascular lesions on verbal and performance IQ differences. Paper presented at the Midwestern Psychology Association, Chicago, IL.

Reitan, R.M. (1955a). Affective disturbances in brain-damaged patients: Measurements with the Minnesota Multiphasic Personality Inventory. *AMA Archives of Neurology and Psychiatry, 73,* 530–532.

Reitan, R.M. (1955b). Certain differential effects of left and right cerebral lesions in human adults. *Journal of Comparative and Physiological Psychology, 48,* 474–477.

Reitan, R.M. (1955c). Discussion: Symposium on the temporal lobe. *Archives of Neurology and Psychiatry, 74,* 569–570.

Reitan, R.M. (1955d). An investigation of the validity of Halstead's measures of biological intelligence. *Archives of Neurology and Psychiatry, 73,* 28–35.

Reitan, R.M. (1956a). Investigation of relationships between "psychometric" and "biological" intelligence. *Journal of Nervous and Mental Disease, 123,* 536–541.

Reitan, R.M. (1956b). The relationship of the Halstead Impairment Index and the Wechsler-Bellevue Weighted Score to chronological age. *Journal of Gerontology, 2,* 4.

Reitan, R.M. (1958). The validity of the Trail Making Test as an indicator of organic brain damage. *Perceptual and Motor Skills, 8,* 271–276.

Reitan, R.M. (1959a). The comparative effects of brain damage on the Halstead Impairment Index and the Wechsler-Bellevue Scale. *Journal of Clinical Psychology, 15,* 281–285.

Reitan, R.M. (1959b). Effects of brain damage on a psychomotor problem-solving task. *Perceptual and Motor Skills, 9,* 211–215.

Reitan, R.M. (1959c). Impairment of abstraction ability in brain damage: Quantitative versus qualitative changes. *Journal of Psychology, 48,* 97–102.

Reitan, R.M. (1960). The significance of dysphasia for intelligence and adaptive abilities. *Journal of Psychology, 50,* 355–376.

Reitan, R.M. (1962a). Psychological deficit. *Annual Review of Psychology, 13,* 415–444.

Reitan, R.M. (1962b). Problems in evaluating the psychological effects of brain lesions. Special supplement. *APA Division 22 Newsletter.*

Reitan, R.M. (1966). A research program on the psychological effects of brain lesions in human beings. In N.R. Ellis (Ed.), *International review of research in mental retardation.* Volume I. New York: Academic Press.

Reitan, R.M. (1967a). Problems and prospects in identifying the effects of brain lesions with psychological tests. *Sinai Hospital Journal, 14,* 37–55.

Reitan, R.M. (1967b). Psychological assessment of deficits associated with brain lesions in subjects with normal and subnormal intelligence. In J.L. Khanna (Ed.), *Brain damage and mental retardation: A psychological evaluation.* Springfield, IL: Charles C Thomas.

Reitan, R.M. (1984). *Aphasia and sensory-perceptual deficits in adults.* Tucson, AZ: Neuropsychology Press.

Reitan, R.M. (1985). Relationships between measures of brain functions and general intelligence. *Journal of Clinical Psychology, 41,* 245–253.

Reitan, R.M., & Sena, D.A. (1983, August). The efficacy of the REHABIT technique in remediation of brain-injured people. Paper presented at the meeting of the American Psychological Association, Anaheim, California.

Reitan, R.M., & Wolfson, D. (1984). The emergence of clinical neuropsychology: Practical applications for psychologists. *Texas Psychologist, 36,* 5–13.

Reitan, R.M., & Wolfson, D. (1985a). *The Halstead-Reitan Neuropsychological Test Battery: Theory and clinical interpretation.* Tucson, AZ: Neuropsychology Press.

Reitan, R.M., & Wolfson, D. (1985b). *Neuroanatomy and neuropathology: A clinical guide for neuropsychologists.* Tucson, AZ: Neuropsychology Press.

Reitan, R.M., & Wolfson, D. (In press). *Traumatic brain injury.* Volume II: Recovery and Rehabilitation. Tucson, AZ: Neuropsychology Press.

Richardson, J.T. (1979a). Mental imagery, human memory, and the effects of closed head injury. *British Journal of Social and Clinical Psychology, 18,* 319–327.

Richardson, J.T. (1979b). Signal detection theory and the effects of severe head injury upon recognition memory. *Cortex, 15,* 145–148.

Roberts, M. (1976). Lesions of the ocular motor nerves (III, IV, and VI). In P.J. Vinken & G.W. Bruyn (Eds.), *Handbook of clinical neurology.* Amsterdam: Elsevier-North Holland Publishing Co.

Ruesch, J. (1944). Intellectual impairment in head injuries. *American Journal of Psychiatry, 100,* 480–496.

Ruesch, J., Harris, R.E., & Bowman, K. (1945). Pre- and post-traumatic personality in head injuries. In *Trauma of the central nervous system.* Vol. 24. Proceedings of the Association for Research in Nervous & Mental Disease, Baltimore: Williams & Wilkins.

Russell, W.R. (1960). Injury to cranial nerves and optic chiasm. In S. Brock (Ed.), *Injuries of the brain and spinal cord and their coverings.* Fourth edition. New York: Springer-Verlag.

Rutherford, W.H., Merrett, J.D., & McDonald, J.R. (1977). Sequelae of concussion caused by minor head injuries. *Lancet, 1,* 1–4.

Ryan, G.A. (1967). Injuries in traffic accidents. *New England Journal of Medicine, 276,* 1066.

Salazar, A.M., Jabbari, B., Vance, S.C., Grafman, J., Amin, D. & Dillon, J.D. (1985). Epilepsy after penetrating head injury. I. Clinical correlates: a report of the Vietnam Head Injury Study. *Neurology, 35,* 1406–14.

Sarno, M.T. (Ed.). (1981). *Acquired aphasia.* New York: Academic Press.

Schacter, D.L., & Crovitz, H.F. (1977). Memory function after closed head injury: A review of the quantitative research. *Cortex, 13,* 150–176.

Schilder, P. (1934). Psychic disturbances after head injuries. *American Journal of Psychiatry, 91,* 155–188.

Schneider, R.C., Reifel, E., Crisler, H.O., & Oosterbaan, B.G. (1961). Serious and fatal football injuries involving head and spinal cord. *Journal of the American Medical Association, 177,* 362.

Semmes, J., Weinstein, S., Ghent, L., & Teuber, H.L. (1960). *Somatosensory changes after penetrating brain wounds in man.* Cambridge: Harvard University Press.

Simonsen, J. (1963). Traumatic subarachnoid hemorrhage in alcohol intoxication. *Journal of Forensic Sciences, 8,* 97.

Spearman, C. (1927). *Abilities of man.* New York: The MacMillan Co.

Sperry, R.W. (1961). Cerebral organization and behavior. *Science, 133,* 1749.

Strich, S.J. (1961). Shearing of nerve fibres as a cause of brain damage due to head injury. *Lancet, 2,* 443–448.

Summer, D. (1976). Disturbances of the senses of taste and smell after head injuries. In. P. J. Vinken & G.W. Bruyn (Eds.), *Handbook of clinical neurology.* Amsterdam: Elsevier-North Holland Publishing Co.

Sweet, R.C., Miller, J.D., Lipper, M., Kishore, P.R. & Becker, D.P. (1978). Significance of bilateral abnormalities on the CT scan in patients with severe head injury. *Neurosurgery, 3,* 16–21.

Symonds, C.P. (1928). The differential diagnosis and treatment of cerebral states consequent upon head injuries. *British Medical Journal, 4,* 829–832.

Talbert, O.R. (1982). General methods of clinical examination. In J.R. Youmans (Ed.), *Neurological surgery.* Philadelphia: W.B. Saunders Company.

Teasdale, G., & Galbraith, S. (1981). Acute traumatic intracranial haematomas. *Progress in Neurological Surgery, 10.*

Teasdale, G., & Jennett, B. (1974). Assessment of coma and impaired consciousness. *Lancet, 2,* 81–84.

Teasdale, G., & Jennett, B. (1976). Assessment and prognosis of coma after head injury. *Acta Neurochirurgica, 34,* 45–55.

Testa, C., Bollini, C., & Columella, F. (1970). Cerebral capillaries in the evolution of traumatic lacerations in man: An ultrastructural study. *Folia Angiol., 96,* 83.

Teuber, H.-L., & Weinstein, S. (1954). Performance on a formboard-task after penetrating brain injury. *Journal of Psychology, 38,* 177–190.

Teuber, H.-L. (1962). Effects of brain wounds implicating right or left hemisphere in man. In V.B. Mountcastle (Ed.), *Interhemispheric relations and cerebral dominance.* Baltimore: Johns Hopkins Press.

Teuber, H.-L. (1964). The riddle of frontal-lobe function in man. In J.M. Warren and K. Akert (Eds.), *The frontal granular cortex and behavior.* New York: McGraw-Hill.

Teuber, H.-L. (1966). Alterations of perception after brain injury. In J.C. Eccles (Ed.), *Brain and conscious experience.* New York: Springer.

Teuber, H.-L. (1968). Disorders of memory following penetrating missile wounds of the brain. *Neurology* (Minneapolis), *18,* 278.

Teuber. H.-L., Battersby, W.S., & Bender, M.B. (1949). Alterations in pattern vision following trauma of occipital lobes in man. *Journal of General Psychology, 40,* 37.

Teuber, H.-L., Battersby, W.B., & Bender, M.B. (1960). *Visual field defects after penetrating missile wounds of the brain.* Cambridge, MA: Harvard University Press.

Teuber, H.-L., Battersby, W.S., & Bender, M.B. (1951). Performance of complex visual tasks after cerebral lesions. *Journal of Nervous and Mental Disease, 114,* 413–429.

Teuber, H.-L., Milner, B., & Vaughn, H. (1968). Persistent anterograde amnesia after stab wound of the basal brain. *Neuropsychologia, 6,* 267.

Teuber, H.-L., & Mishkin, M. (1954). Judgment of visual and postural vertical after brain injury. *Journal of Psychology, 38,* 161.

Teuber, H.-L., & Weinstein, S. (1956). Ability to discover hidden figures after cerebral lesions. *Archives of Neurology and Psychiatry, Chicago, 76,* 369–379.

Teuber, H.-L., & Weinstein, S. (1958). Equipotentiality versus cortical localization. *Science, 127,* 240.

Thurstone, L.L. (1931). Multiple factor analysis. *Psychological Review, 88,* 406–427.

Toglia, J.U. (1969). Dizziness after whiplash injury of the neck and closed head injury. In A.E. Walker, W.F. Caveness & M. Critchley (Eds.), *Late effects of head injury.* Springfield, IL: Charles C Thomas.

Toglia, J.U., & Katinsky, S. (1976). Neuro-otological aspects of closed head injury. In P.J. Vinken and G.W. Bruyn (Eds.), *Handbook of clinical neurology.* Amsterdam: Elsevier-North Holland Publishing Co.

U.S. Department of Health, Education, & Welfare. (1974). Facts of life and death. Publication No. (HRS) 74–1222. Rockville, MD: National Center for Health Statistics.

Van Vliet, A.G.M. (1976). Post-traumatic ocular imbalance. In P.J. Vinken & G.W. Bruyn (Eds.), *Handbook of clinical neurology.* Amsterdam: Elsevier-North Holland Publishing Co.

Van Zomeren, A.H. & Deelman, B.G. (1978). Long-term recovery of visual reaction time after closed head injury. *Journal of Neurology, Neurosurgery, and Psychiatry, 41,* 452–457.

Walpole, L. (1966). Injuries to cranial nerves and visual pathways. In L. Walpole (Ed.), *The management of head injuries.* Baltimore: Williams & Wilkins.

Watts, C., & Pulliam, M. (1982). Problems associated with multiple trauma. In J.R. Youmans (Ed.), *Neurological surgery.* Philadelphia: W.B. Saunders Co.

Wechsler, D. (1955). *Manual for the Wechsler Adult Intelligence Scale.* New York: The Psychological Corporation.

Weinstein, S. (1954). Weight judgment in somesthesis after penetrating injury to the brain. *Journal of Comparative and Physiological Psychology, 48,* 203–207.

Weinstein, S., Ghent, L., & Teuber, H.-L., (1958). Roughness discrimination after penetrating brain injury in man: analysis according to locus of lesion. *Journal of Comparative Physiology and Psychology, 51,* 269–75.

Weinstein, S., Semmes, J., Ghent, L., & Teuber, H.-L. (1956). Spatial orientation in man after cerebral injury. II. Analysis according to concomitant defects. *Journal of Psychology, 42,* 249–263.

Weinstein, S., & Teuber, H.-L. (1957). The role of preinjury education and intelligence level in intellectual loss after brain injury. *Journal of Comparative and Physiological Psychology, 50,* 535.

Wepman, J.M. (1951). *Recovery from aphasia.* New York: The Ronald Press.

Westrum, L.E., White, L.E., & Ward, A.A. (1964). Morphology of the experimental epileptic focus. *Journal of Neurosurgery, 21,* 1033–1046.

Wheeler, L., & Reitan, R.M. (1962). The presence and laterality of brain damage predicted from responses to a short aphasia screening test. *Perceptual and Motor Skills, 15,* 783–799.

Zimmerman, R.A., Bilaniuk, L.T., & Gennarelli, T. (1978). Computed tomography of shearing injuries of the cerebral white matter. *Radiology, 127,* 393–396.

INDEX OF PLATES

Plate 1   Skull Fractures

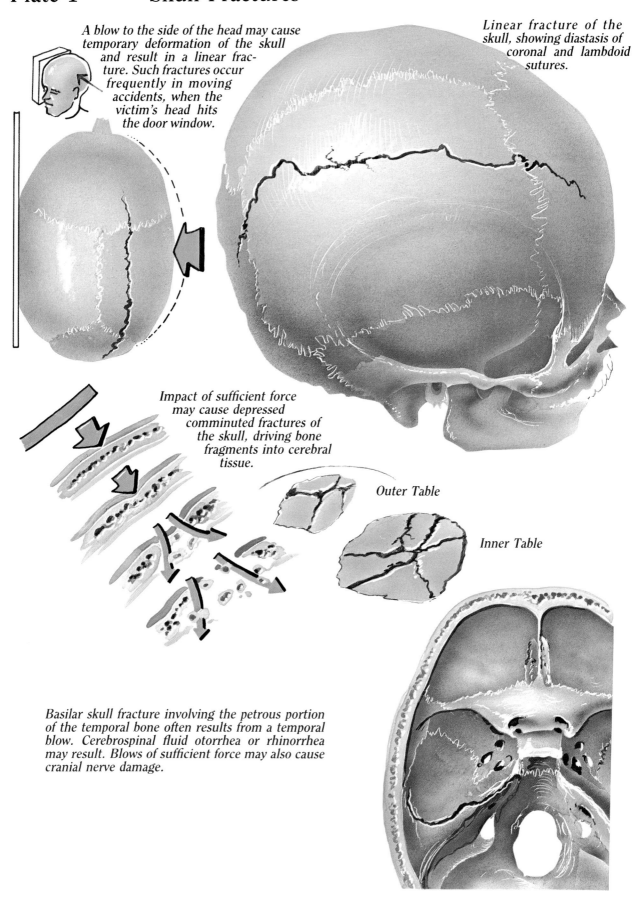

A blow to the side of the head may cause temporary deformation of the skull and result in a linear fracture. Such fractures occur frequently in moving accidents, when the victim's head hits the door window.

Linear fracture of the skull, showing diastasis of coronal and lambdoid sutures.

Impact of sufficient force may cause depressed comminuted fractures of the skull, driving bone fragments into cerebral tissue.

Outer Table

Inner Table

Basilar skull fracture involving the petrous portion of the temporal bone often results from a temporal blow. Cerebrospinal fluid otorrhea or rhinorrhea may result. Blows of sufficient force may also cause cranial nerve damage.

Plate 2   Compound Depressed Skull Fracture

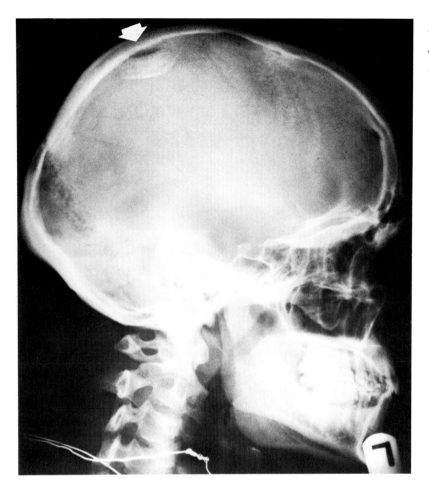

Right lateral skull film showing right parietal depressed skull fracture.

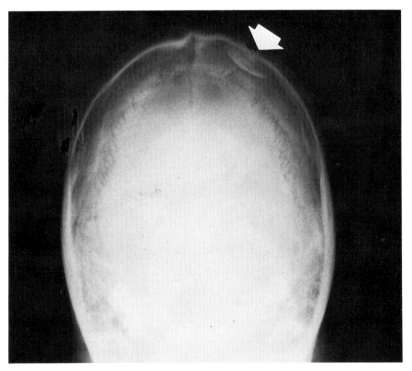

Posterior skull film, demonstrating right parietal depressed skull fracture.

Plate 3   Depressed Comminuted Skull Fracture

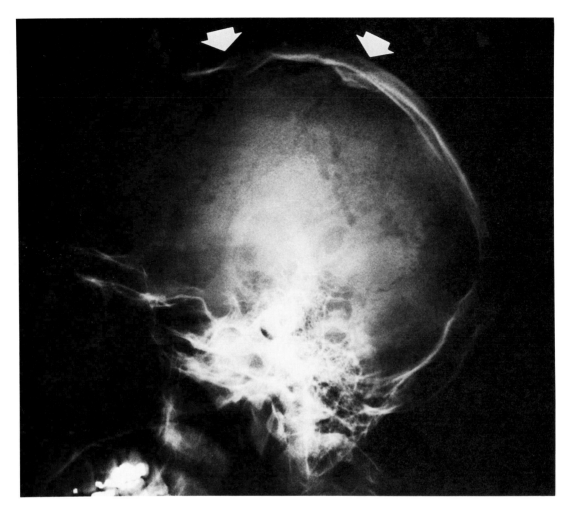

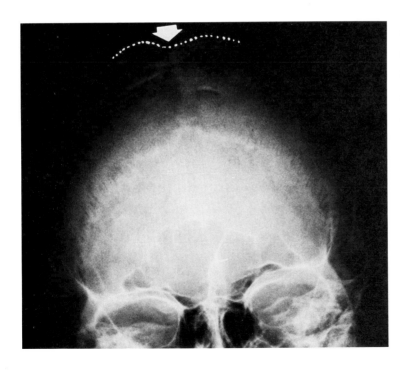

Lateral and anterior skull films showing depressed comminuted skull fractures.

Plate 4   Craniotomy for Compound Depressed Fracture

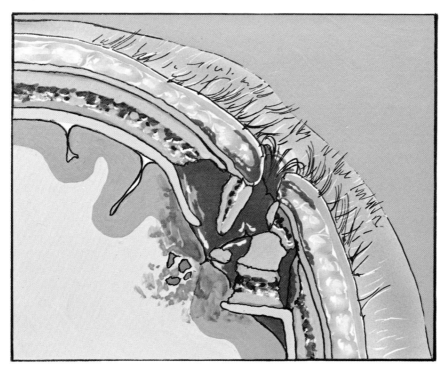

(Left) A compound depressed skull fracture may tear the dura and drive bone fragments, hair and foreign material directly into cerebral tissue.
(Below) If the area of injury is small, an incision is made around the wound.

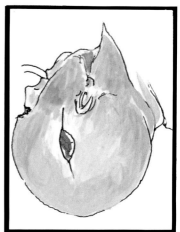

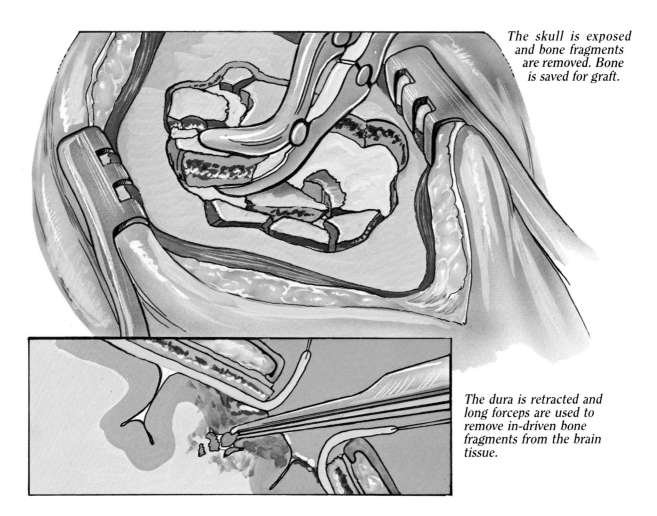

The skull is exposed and bone fragments are removed. Bone is saved for graft.

The dura is retracted and long forceps are used to remove in-driven bone fragments from the brain tissue.

Plate 5   Craniotomy for Compound Depressed Fracture (Con't)

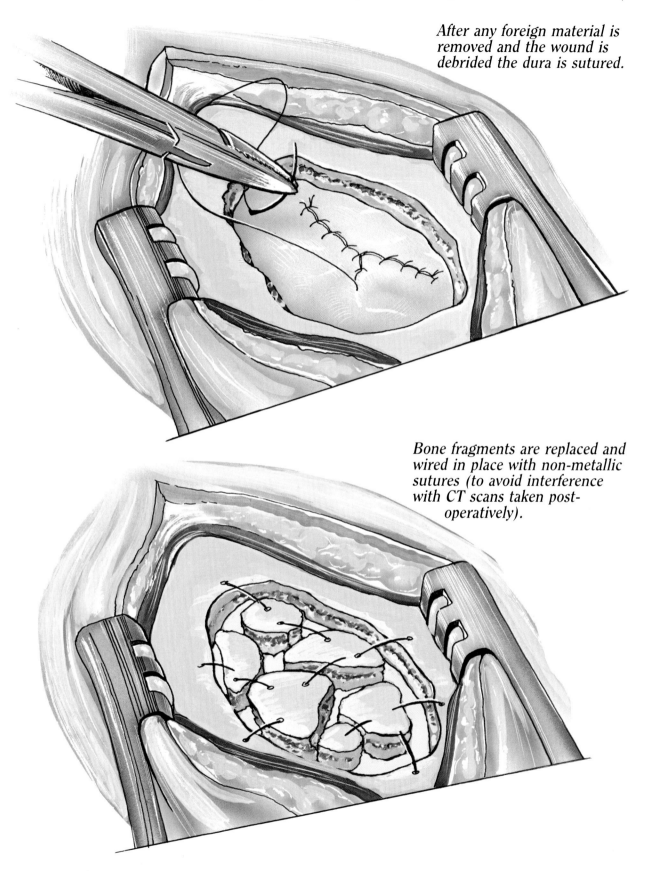

After any foreign material is removed and the wound is debrided the dura is sutured.

Bone fragments are replaced and wired in place with non-metallic sutures (to avoid interference with CT scans taken post-operatively).

Plate 6   Sagittal Sinus Injury

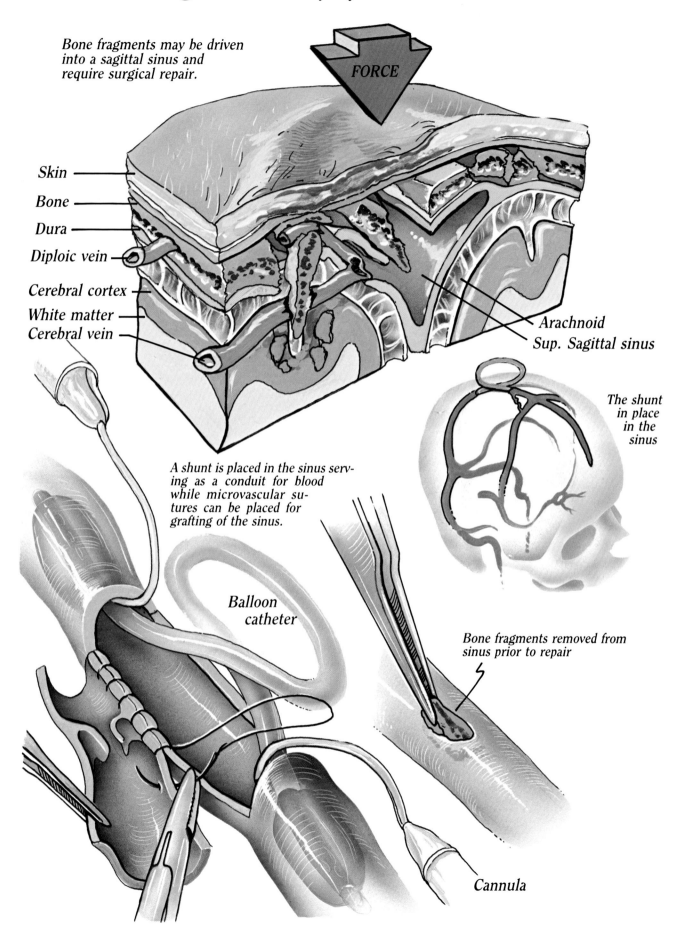

Bone fragments may be driven into a sagittal sinus and require surgical repair.

FORCE

Skin

Bone

Dura

Diploic vein

Cerebral cortex

White matter

Cerebral vein

Arachnoid

Sup. Sagittal sinus

The shunt in place in the sinus

A shunt is placed in the sinus serving as a conduit for blood while microvascular sutures can be placed for grafting of the sinus.

Balloon catheter

Bone fragments removed from sinus prior to repair

Cannula

Plate 7 Tangential and Penetrating Missile Wounds

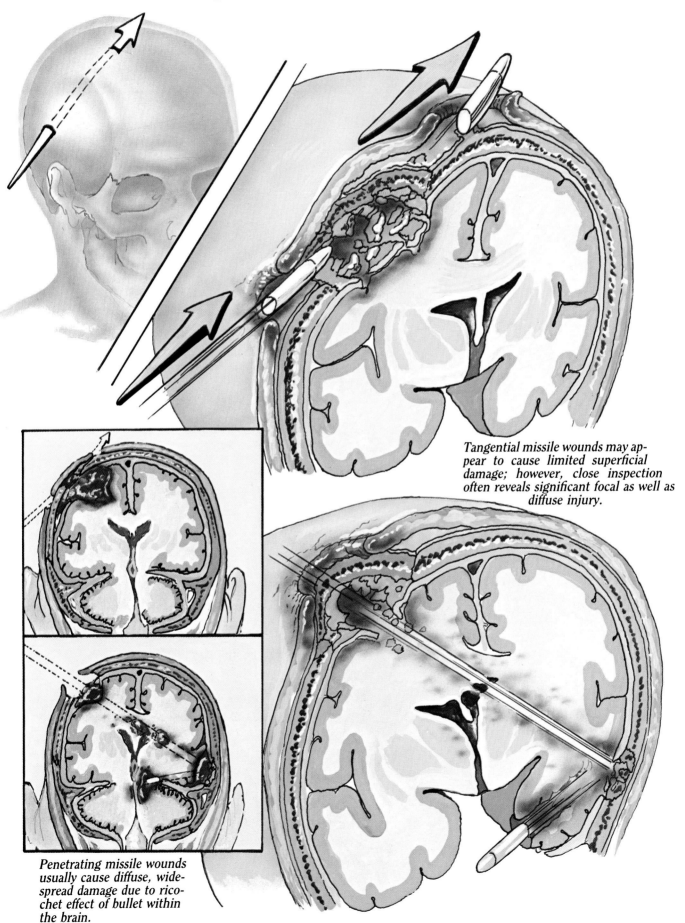

Tangential missile wounds may appear to cause limited superficial damage; however, close inspection often reveals significant focal as well as diffuse injury.

Penetrating missile wounds usually cause diffuse, widespread damage due to ricochet effect of bullet within the brain.

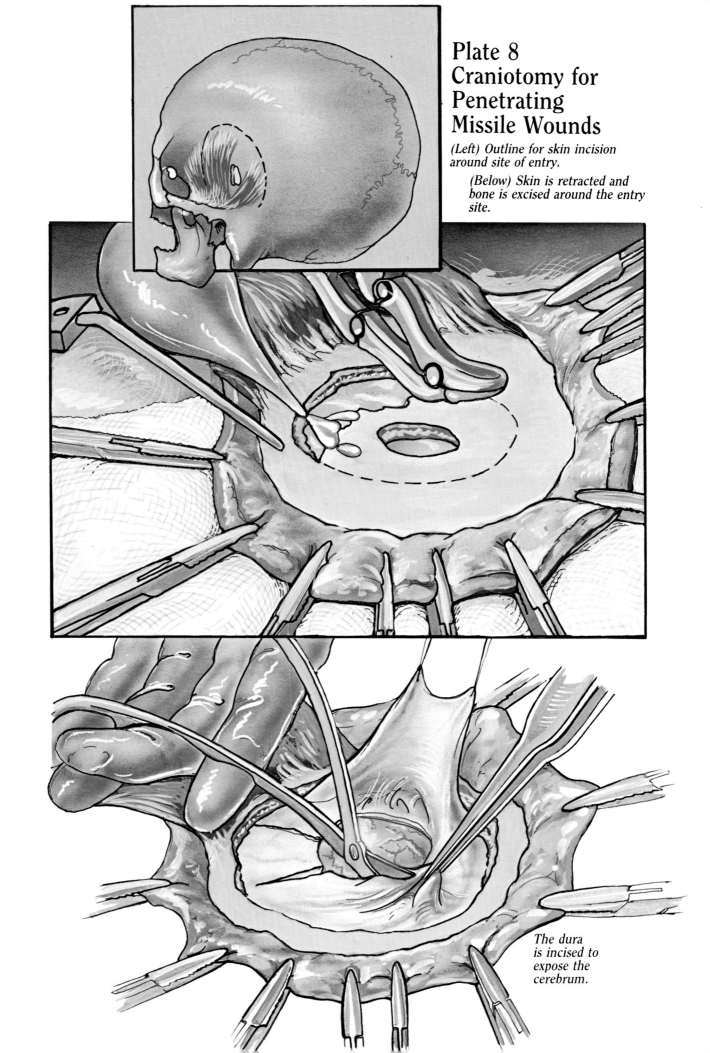

Plate 8
Craniotomy for Penetrating Missile Wounds

(Left) Outline for skin incision around site of entry.

(Below) Skin is retracted and bone is excised around the entry site.

The dura is incised to expose the cerebrum.

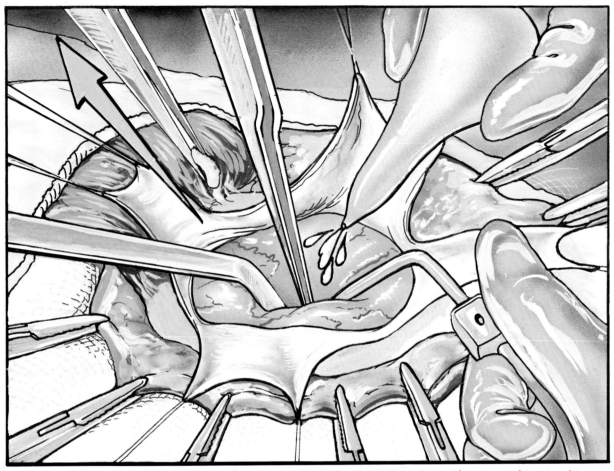

(Above) The cerebral tissue is inspected and debrided. Superficial hematomas and debris are removed by suction.

(Below) The brain tissue is gently separated to reveal indriven bone fragments.

The dura is closed with a watertight seal, using a graft if necessary, to prevent the brain from herniating through the craniotomy site.

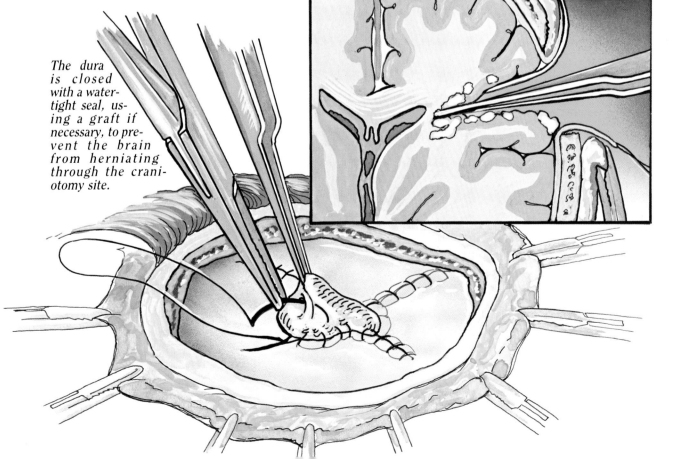

Plate 10   Traumatic Aneurysms

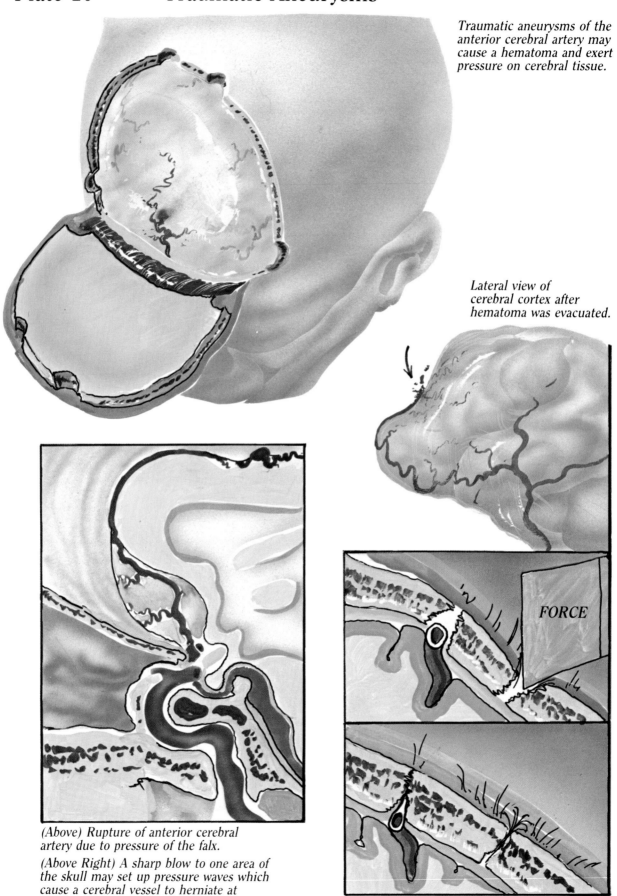

Traumatic aneurysms of the anterior cerebral artery may cause a hematoma and exert pressure on cerebral tissue.

Lateral view of cerebral cortex after hematoma was evacuated.

FORCE

(Above) Rupture of anterior cerebral artery due to pressure of the falx.

(Above Right) A sharp blow to one area of the skull may set up pressure waves which cause a cerebral vessel to herniate at another site.

(Right) Vessel becomes "trapped" as bone returns to normal position.

Plate 11 Traumatic Aneurysms of the Cavernous Sinus and Neurovascular Relationships

A). Circle of Willis

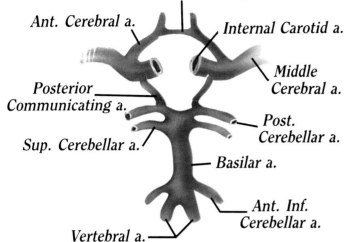

Ant. Communicating a.

Ant. Cerebral a.

Internal Carotid a.

Middle Cerebral a.

Posterior Communicating a.

Post. Cerebellar a.

Sup. Cerebellar a.

Basilar a.

Ant. Inf. Cerebellar a.

Vertebral a.

1. Stalk of pituitary
2. Optic tract
3. Internal carotid a.
4. Oculomotor n.
5. Abducens n.

6. Pituitary
7. Cochlear n.
8. Ophthalmic branch of Trigeminal

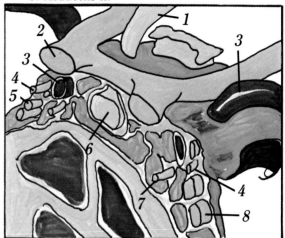

B). Normal neurovascular anatomy

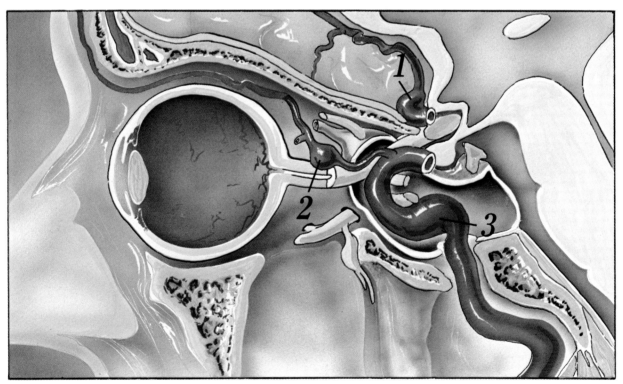

1. Aneurysm of anterior cerebral artery. 2. Aneurysm of ophthalmic artery.
3. Aneurysm of middle cerebral artery in the cavernous sinus.

Plate 12   Epidural Hematoma

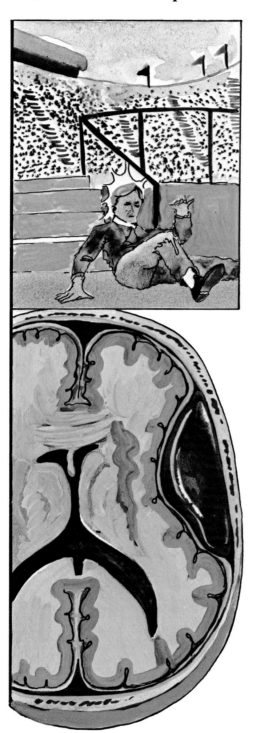

Epidural hematomas often result from minor accidents, such as a fall. They are usually the result of damage to the middle meningeal artery. As the hematoma enlarges it will impinge on cerebral tissue and displace midline structures to the opposite side. If not treated promptly, the temporal fossa epidural hematoma may cause herniation of the temporal lobe under the falx cerebelli.

Plate 13

Drainage of Epidural Hematoma

If the hematoma has not solidified, it may be drained via a catheter. A craniostomy is performed over the hematoma (A) and a catheter is threaded through the craniostomy hole into the hematoma (B).

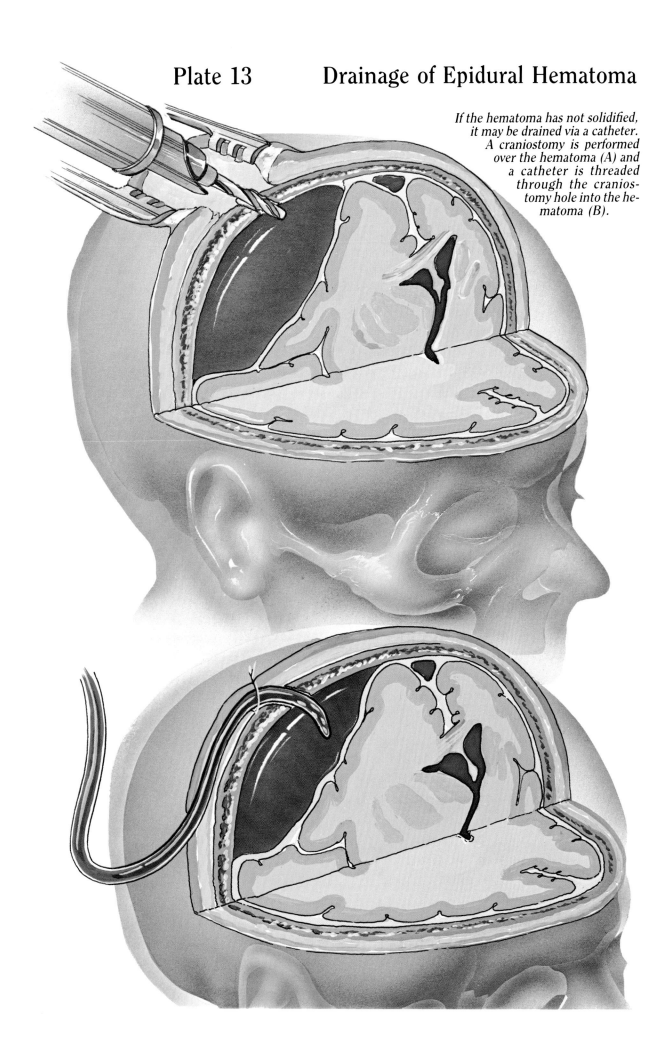

Plate 14   Craniotomy for Acute Hematomas

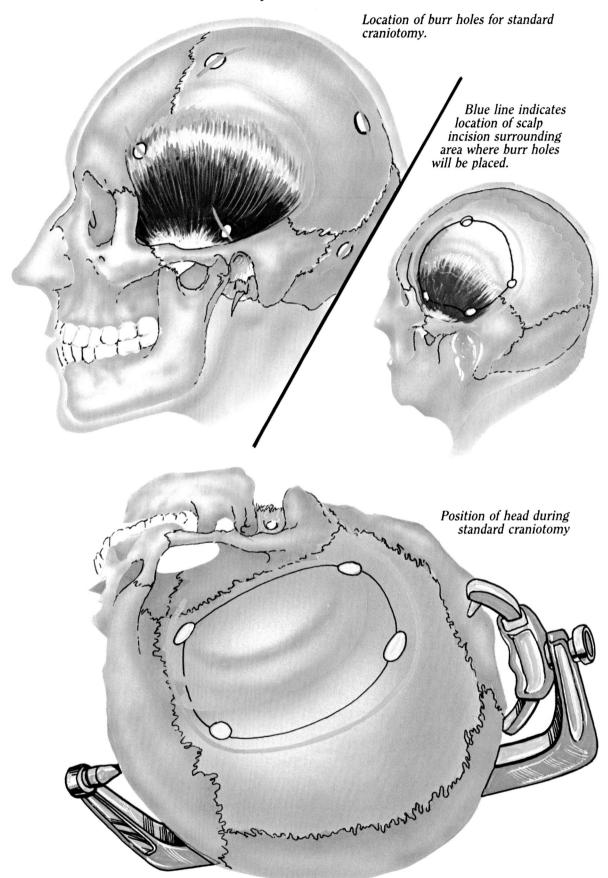

Location of burr holes for standard craniotomy.

Blue line indicates location of scalp incision surrounding area where burr holes will be placed.

Position of head during standard craniotomy

Plate 15   Craniotomy for Acute Hematomas (Con't)

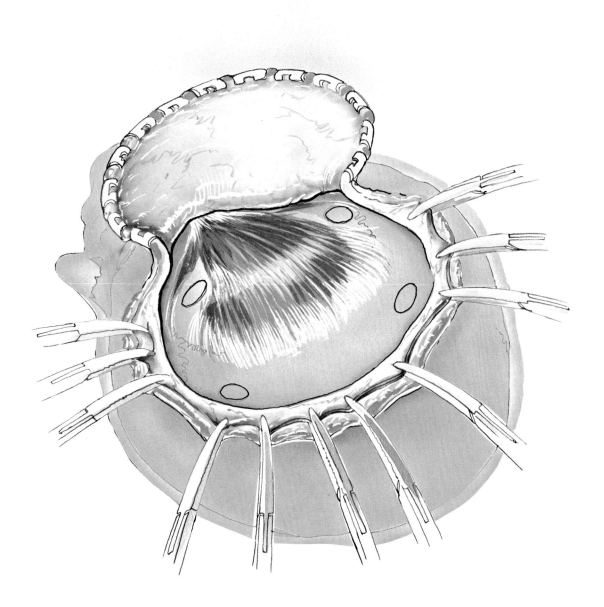

The skin is incised and a bone flap is turned back on the temporalis muscle. This type of craniotomy flap will provide exposure to the areas of the brain most commonly damaged in rotational injuries.

Plate 16   Craniotomy for Acute Hematomas (Con't)

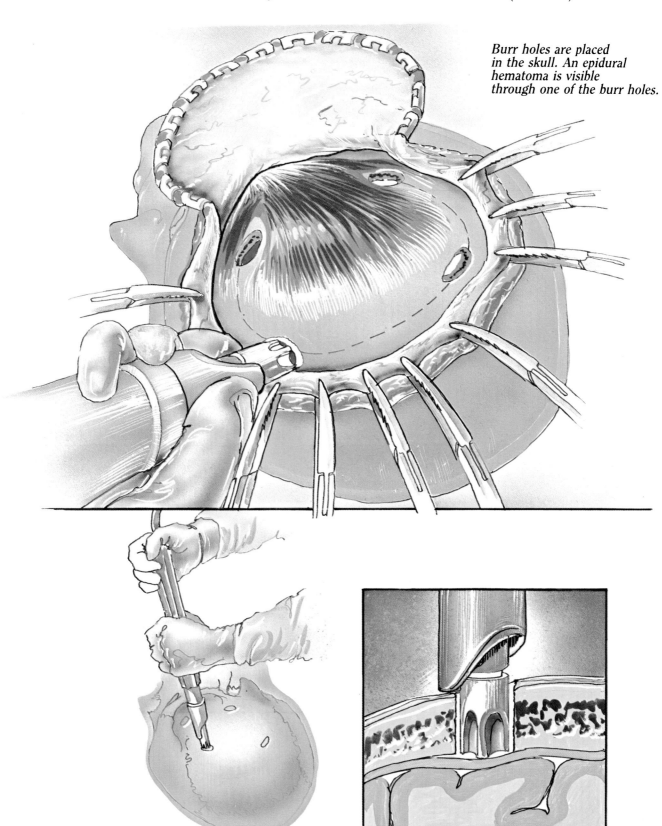

Burr holes are placed
in the skull. An epidural
hematoma is visible
through one of the burr holes.

Burr holes being drilled
with craniotome.

Safety mechanism on craniotome
protects soft tissues.

Plate 17   Craniotomy for Acute Hematomas (Con't)

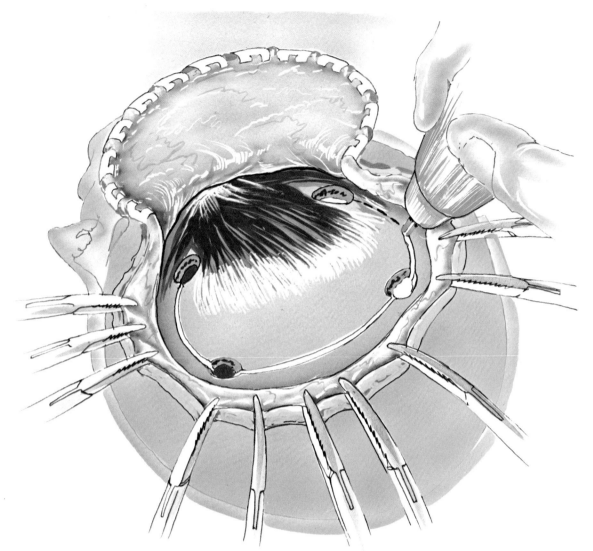

Craniotome is used to connect burr holes.

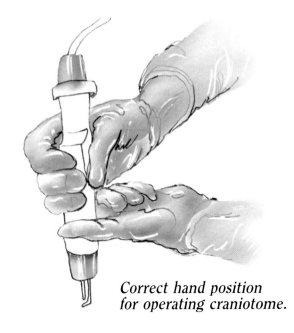

*Correct hand position
for operating craniotome.*

*Safety mechanism prevents
penetration of dura.*

Plate 18   Craniotomy For Acute Hematomas (Con't)

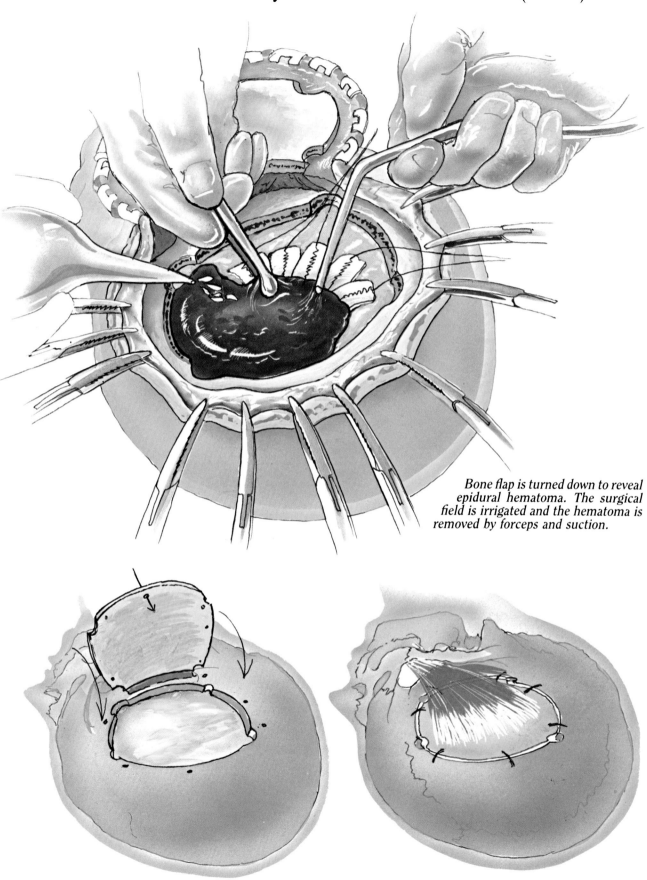

Bone flap is turned down to reveal epidural hematoma. The surgical field is irrigated and the hematoma is removed by forceps and suction.

Burr holes drilled for placement of sutures.

Sutures in place to secure bone flap.

Plate 19   Chronic Subdural Hematoma

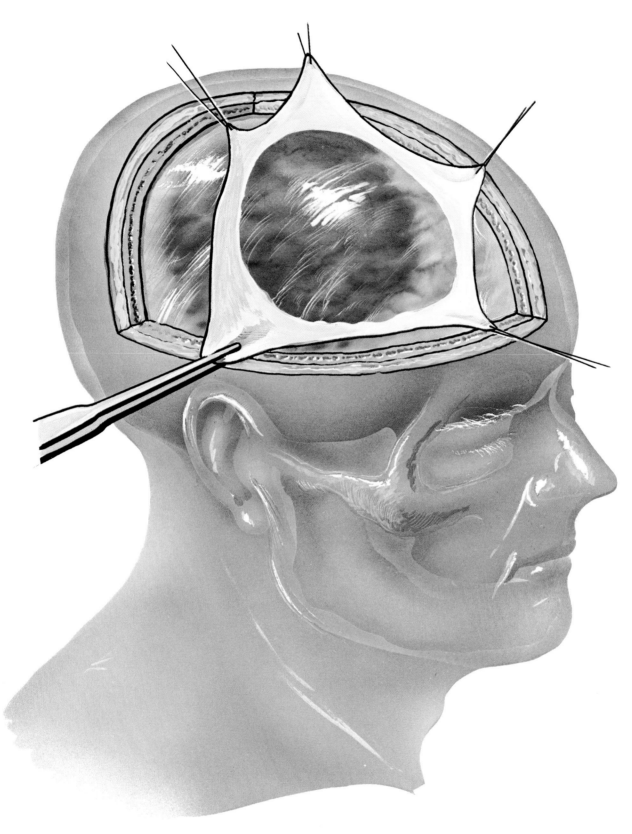

Chronic subdural hematomas are often caused by minor trauma. Persons with some degree of brain atrophy (e.g., alcoholics and the aged) are particularly at risk because of the increase in the size of the subdural space that usually accompanies these conditions. The hematoma may become quite large before producing symptoms.

Plate 20   Epidural Hematomas

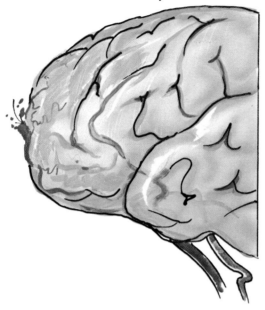

Linear fractures of the skull may cause damage to the anterior cerebral artery.

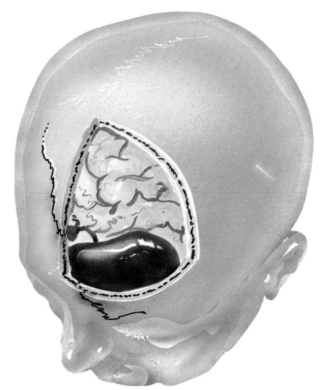

Hematoma forms as blood accumulates between the dura and the inner table of the skull.

Dura retracted to expose epidural hematoma on base of skull.

Frontal epidural hematoma displacing midline structures.

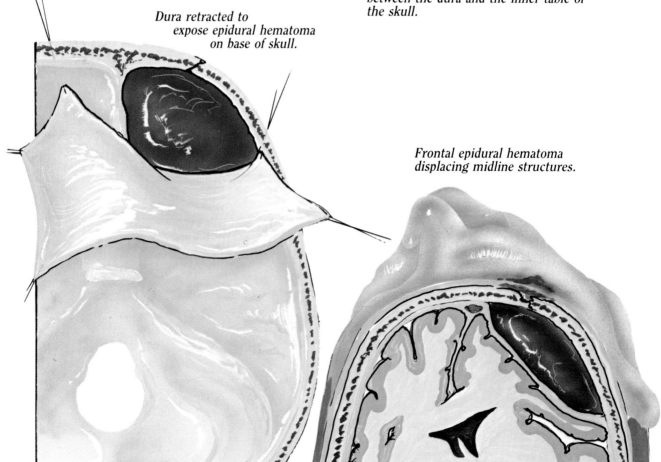

Plate 21

Craniotomy for Acute Subdural Hematoma

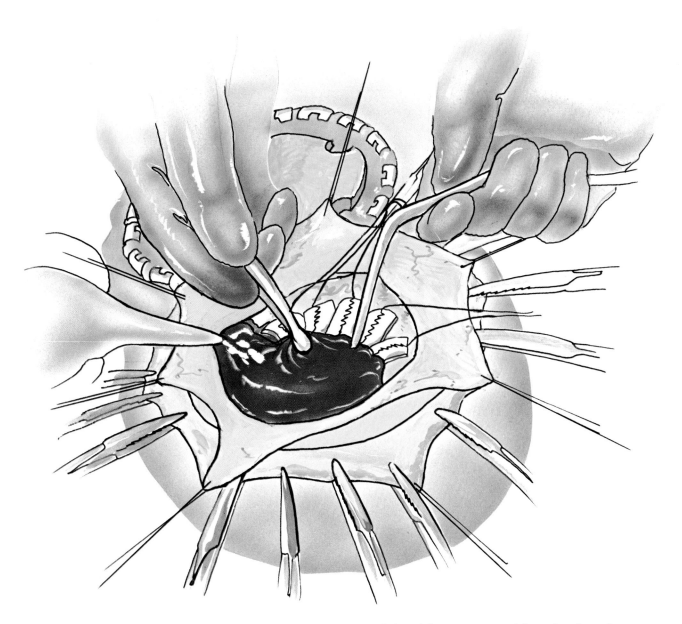

A standard craniotomy flap is used to evacuate subdural hematomas. After the dura is exposed it can be incised to reveal the subdural hematoma, which can then be removed by suction, irrigation and forceps extraction.

Plate 22   Cerebral Hematomas

A. Frontal epidural hematoma

B. Temporal fossa epidural hematoma resulting from injury to the middle meningeal artery

C. Posterior fossa epidural hematoma

D. Occipital subdural hematoma

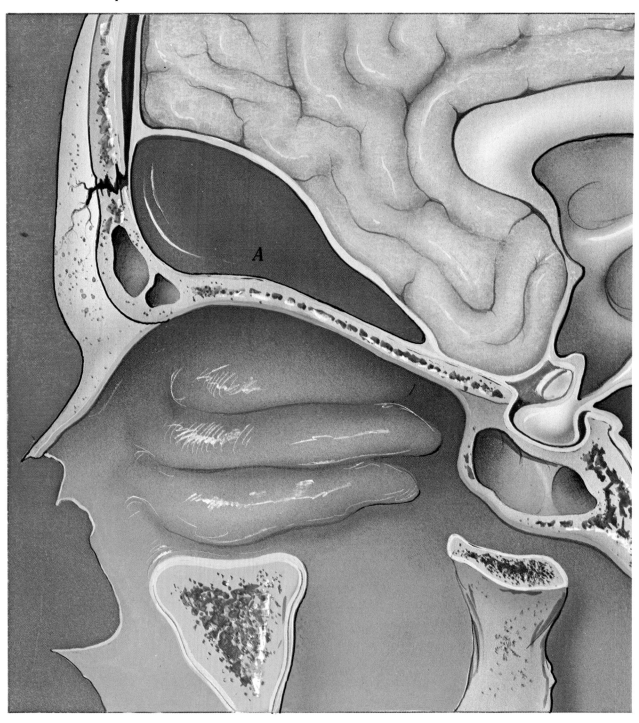

Plate 23   Cerebral Hematomas

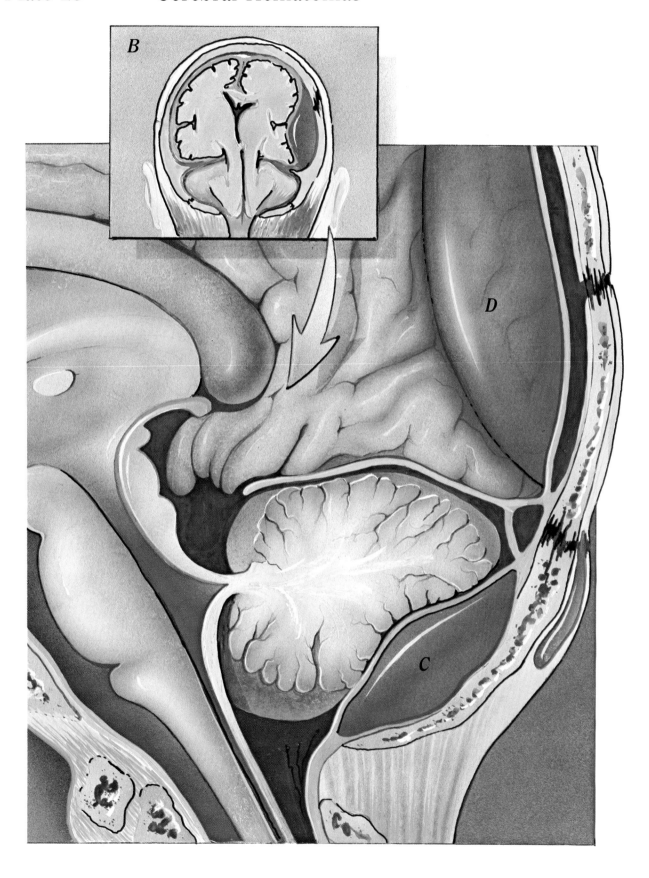

Plate 24   Intracerebral Hemorrhage

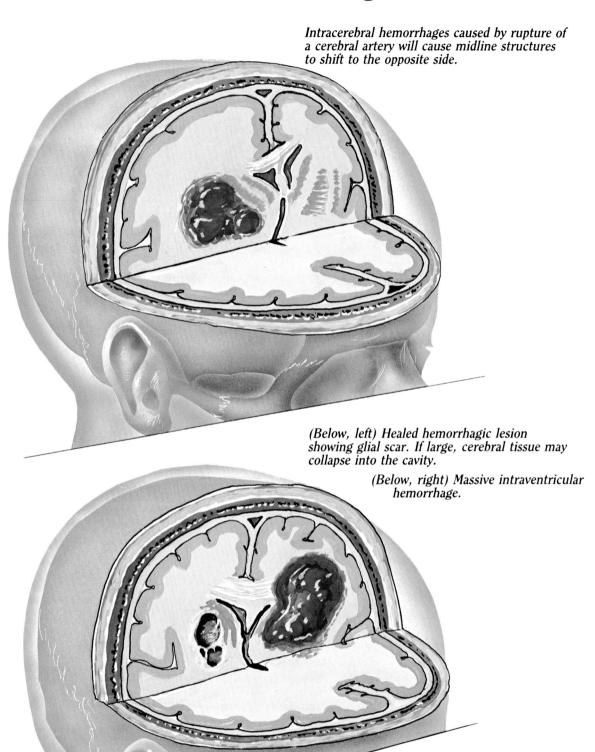

Intracerebral hemorrhages caused by rupture of a cerebral artery will cause midline structures to shift to the opposite side.

(Below, left) Healed hemorrhagic lesion showing glial scar. If large, cerebral tissue may collapse into the cavity.

(Below, right) Massive intraventricular hemorrhage.

Plate 25   Intracerebral Hematomas

Intracerebral hematomas may be caused by the rupture of an aneurysm. As the hematoma enlarges it will cause shift of midline structures.

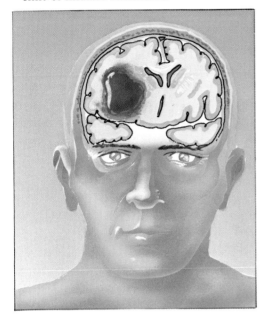

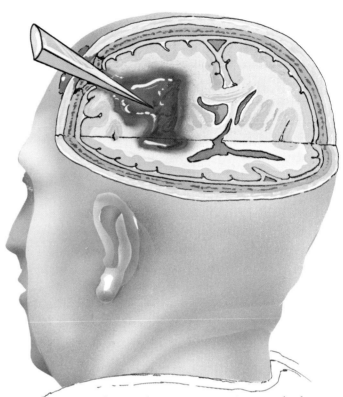

Penetrating stab wounds may cause an intracerebral hematoma along the path of penetration.

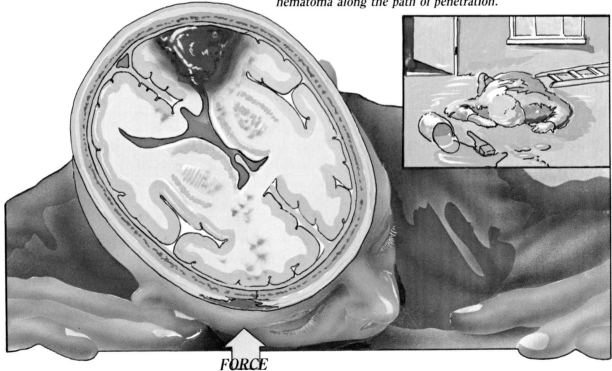

FORCE

A forceful blow to the frontal area may cause a contre-coup injury which may result in intraventricular hemorrhage.

Plate 26   Geniculostriate Visual Pathway

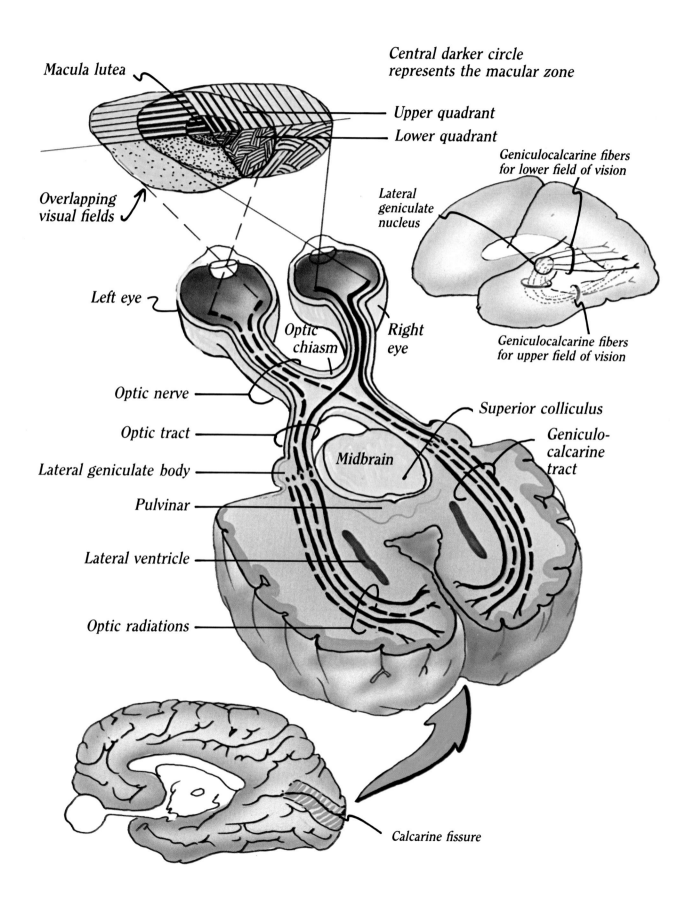

Macula lutea

Central darker circle
represents the macular zone

Upper quadrant

Lower quadrant

Geniculocalcarine fibers
for lower field of vision

Lateral
geniculate
nucleus

Overlapping
visual fields

Left eye

Optic
chiasm

Right
eye

Geniculocalcarine fibers
for upper field of vision

Optic nerve

Optic tract

Superior colliculus

Geniculo-
calcarine
tract

Midbrain

Lateral geniculate body

Pulvinar

Lateral ventricle

Optic radiations

Calcarine fissure

Plate 27   Visual Field Defects

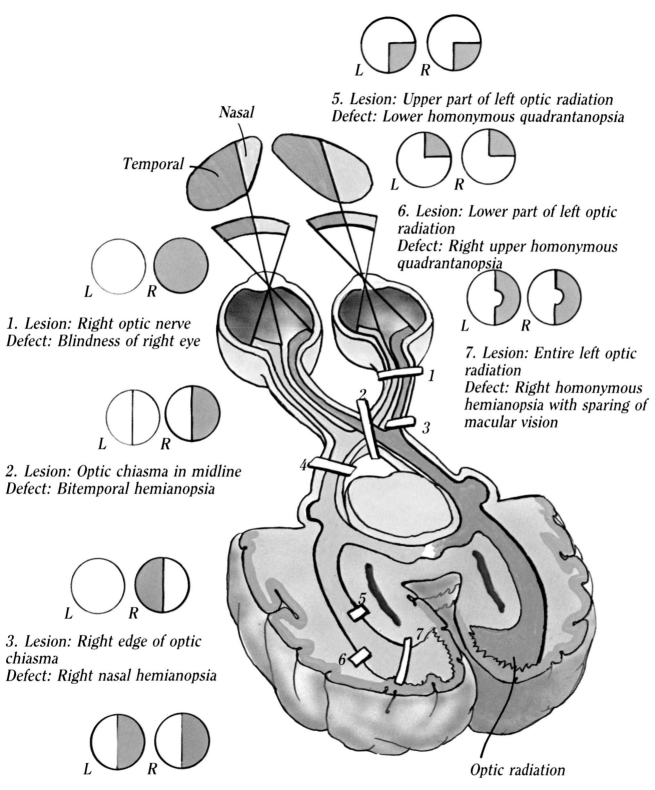

5. Lesion: Upper part of left optic radiation
Defect: Lower homonymous quadrantanopsia

Nasal

Temporal

1. Lesion: Right optic nerve
Defect: Blindness of right eye

6. Lesion: Lower part of left optic radiation
Defect: Right upper homonymous quadrantanopsia

2. Lesion: Optic chiasma in midline
Defect: Bitemporal hemianopsia

7. Lesion: Entire left optic radiation
Defect: Right homonymous hemianopsia with sparing of macular vision

3. Lesion: Right edge of optic chiasma
Defect: Right nasal hemianopsia

Optic radiation

4. Lesion: Left optic tract
Defect: Right homonymous hemianopsia

Plate 28

Neuromuscular Manifestations Associated With Cerebral Aneurysms

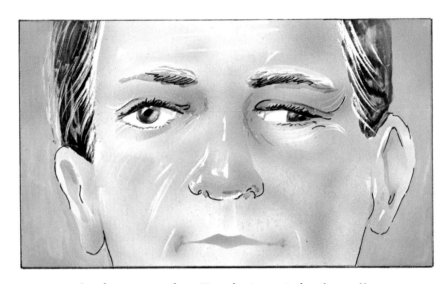

Oculomotor palsy. Eye deviates inferolaterally.

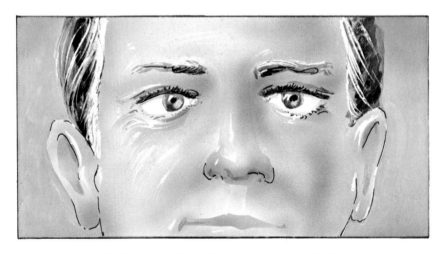

Abducens palsy. Eye deviates medially.

Plate 29   Retinal Changes Frequently Associated With Cerebral Aneurysms

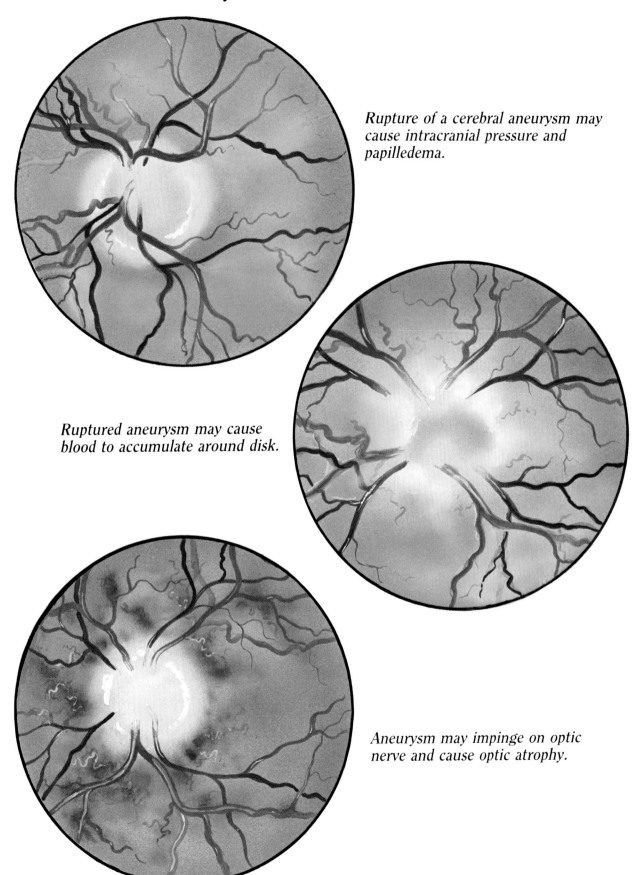

Rupture of a cerebral aneurysm may cause intracranial pressure and papilledema.

Ruptured aneurysm may cause blood to accumulate around disk.

Aneurysm may impinge on optic nerve and cause optic atrophy.

Plate 30   Computed Tomography (CT)

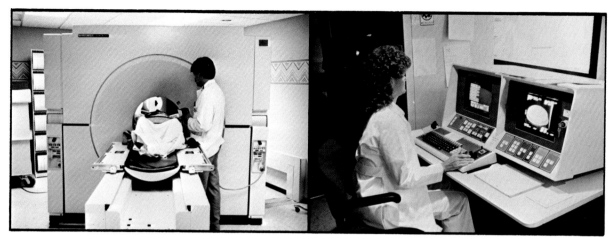

CT Scanner

Operator's Terminal

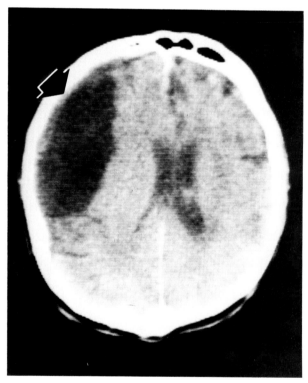

CT scan showing chronic right epidural hematoma (dark area).

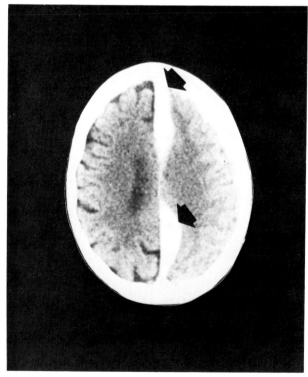

CT scan demonstrating acute left subdural hematomas (white areas) resulting from a fall.

Plate 31   Computed Tomography (CT)

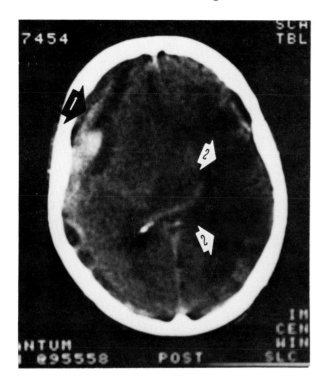

1. *Chronic subdural hematoma (diagonal lines) with acute hemorrhage.*

2. *Old infarction (dotted line). Note shift of midline structures to left.*

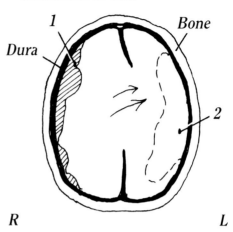

3. *Acute subdural hematoma in anterior and posterior portions of left cerebral hemisphere (stipled areas).*

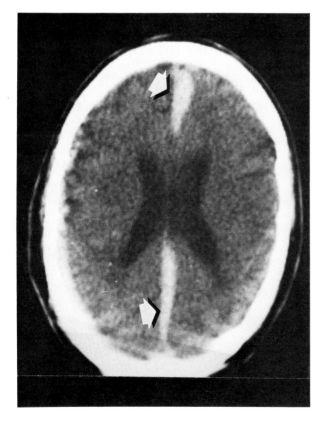

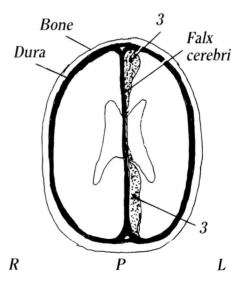

Plate 32   Computed Tomography (CT)

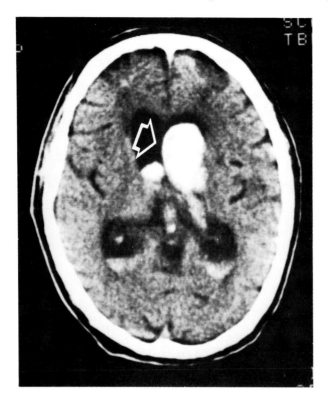

Intraventricular
hemorrhage

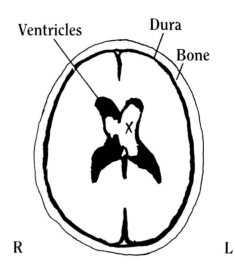

Ventricles   Dura
                         Bone

R   L

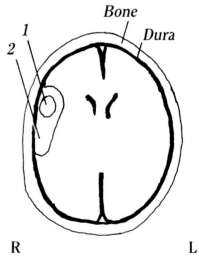

Hemorrhagic infarction
secondary to middle
cerebral artery aneurysm.
 1. Ischemic infarction
 2. Hemorrhagic infarction

Bone
      Dura
1
2

R   L

Plate 33   Magnetic Resonance Imaging (MRI)

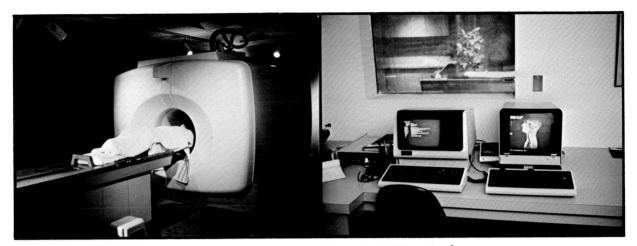

Operator's Terminal

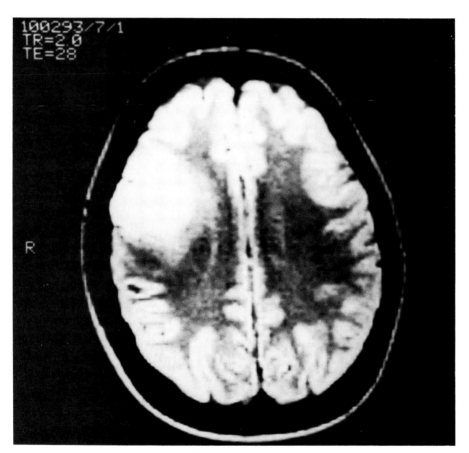

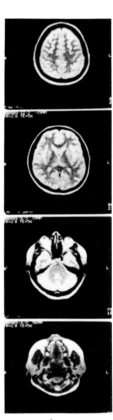

*Axial views
(normal)*

*MRI of a ruptured cerebral aneurysm in the
right fronto-temporal area.*

SUBJECT INDEX